Accountability

HASTINGS CENTER STUDIES IN ETHICS

A SERIES EDITED BY

Gregory Kaebnick and Daniel Callahan

This series of books, published by The Hastings Center and Georgetown University Press, examines ethical issues in medicine and the life sciences. Established in 1969, The Hastings Center, located in Garrison, New York, is an independent, nonprofit, and nonpartisan research organization. The work of the Center is mainly carried out through research projects, the publication of the *Hastings Center Report* and *IRB: A Review of Human Subjects Research,* and numerous workshops, conferences, lectures, and consultations. The *Hastings Center Studies in Ethics* series brings the ongoing research of The Hastings Center to a wider audience.

Accountability

Patient Safety and Policy Reform

Virginia A. Sharpe

Editor

Georgetown University Press
Washington, D.C.

Georgetown University Press, Washington, D.C.
©2004 by Georgetown University Press. All rights reserved.
Printed in the United States of America

10 9 8 7 6 5 4 3 2 1   2004

Library of Congress Cataloging-in-Publication Data
Accountability : patient safety and policy reform / Virginia A. Sharpe, editor.
    p. cm. — (Hastings Center studies in ethics)
  Includes bibliographical references and index.
  ISBN 1-58901-023-X (cloth : alk. paper)
  1. Medical errors—United States.   2. Health care reform—United States.   I. Sharpe, Virginia A. (Virginia Ashby), 1959–   II. Series.
  R729.8.A25   2004
    362.1'0425—dc22   2004005622

For all whose lives have been changed by medical error

CONTENTS

PREFACE

In October 2000, the Hastings Center initiated a two-year project to analyze the ethical issues and values at stake in policy proposals on patient safety and the reduction of medical error. The catalyst for the project was the publication of the Institute of Medicine (IOM) report *To Err Is Human: Building a Safer Health System* (Kohn, Corrigan, and Donaldson 2000) as well as reforms already underway within institutions charged with oversight or provision of health care.

To conduct this work, we assembled an interdisciplinary group of experts to help us make sense of the complex phenomenon of patient safety reform. Working group members brought their expertise as people who had suffered from devastating medical harms and as institutional leaders galvanized to reform by tragic events in their own health care institutions. They brought expertise as clinicians, chaplains, and risk managers working to deliver health care, to face its downsides, and to make it safer for current and future patients. They brought expertise in systems thinking from air traffic control and from the military. The project group also brought critical insight on the issue of patient safety from their work in medical history and sociology, economics, health care purchasing, health policy, law, philosophy, and religion. I am grateful for all of the time and intelligence that the group brought to the project and am pleased to bring their expertise together in this volume.

The introduction lays out the rationale for the project, the broad topics of the volume—disclosure, reporting, compensation, and error prevention—and notes in some detail the ways in which these topics are addressed by each author. After a brief overview of the IOM report, the introduction identifies the ethical values and issues at stake in proposed reforms, placing particular emphasis on the need for policymakers to grapple simultaneously with the demands of accountability, justice, and safety.

Chapters 1 through 3, by Sandra M. Gilbert, Carol Levine, and Roxanne Goeltz, respectively, are powerful narratives about the losses that they and their loved ones have suffered not simply as a result of medical error, but also as a result of the inhumanities of the health care system. Sandra Gilbert is a poet and literary critic whose husband died as a result of still-unexplained causes following a routine prostatectomy. She describes the multiple ways in which she and others who seek redress for catastrophic medical events are silenced in their attempts to right the wrong that has occurred. Carol Levine writes about a medical error that resulted in her husband's loss of his arm following a devastating brain-stem injury in an automobile accident. Levine, director of the Project on Families and Health Care at the United Hospital Fund of New York, places her experience in the broader context of health care financing and delivery, describing what it means for patients and their family-caregivers to live with the consequences of medical error in a system ill-prepared to support long-term care for the injured. Roxanne Goeltz provides a searing account of her brother's death as the result of omissions in his hospital care. This experience, as well as her own postsurgical pulmonary embolism in an understaffed hospital unit, has led Goeltz to become a pioneer in patient safety, bringing the insights of her field, air traffic control, to health care delivery. As a safety advocate, Goeltz recommends that during hospital care, patients have a friend or family member with them twenty-four hours a day, seven days a week.

Chapters 4 through 8, by Bryan A. Liang, Edmund D. Pellegrino, Carol Bayley, Nancy Berlinger, and Albert W. Wu, focus on the institutional, cultural, and moral contexts in which errors occur and are revealed or concealed. Bryan Liang describes how the traditional response of "shame and blame"—that emphasizes individual culpability for error—is counterproductive both in improving institutional safety and in delivering justice to harmed parties. Liang argues that shifting our focus from individual culpability to system failures will allow for all members of a health care team—including patients—to contribute to the safety enterprise. Edmund Pellegrino, by contrast, argues that a systems approach cannot and should not replace individual accountability for error and its aftermath. He calls for the creation of institutional cultures that foster rather than discourage individual virtue both in preventing and in responding to error. Carol Bayley, vice president for ethics and justice education at Catholic Healthcare West (CHW), describes the development and implementation at CHW of an approach to mistakes and patient disclosure that is informed by the institution's core values of dignity, collaboration, stewardship, justice, and excellence. Nancy Berlinger examines the meanings of error, confession, forgiveness, and reconciliation in religious traditions and cautions against expectations of forgiveness from God, one's superiors or peers, or one's patients after a harmful error. Rather, she says, forgiveness should be understood as a (possible) outcome of concrete efforts to ensure justice for injured parties. Taking a closer look at the obligation to disclose harmful errors to patients, Albert Wu examines whether there might be an obligation to disclose "near-misses," that is, errors that have not caused harm. He argues that disclosure of near-misses is not obligatory but may be desirable as an opportunity to enhance a therapeutic relationship.

Chapters 9 and 10, by Kenneth De Ville and William M. Sage, provide social histories of medical error and malpractice in America. Tracing different explanations of medical misfortune from the nineteenth century to the present, De Ville suggests that the apparent "rash" of errors today is in many respects an inevitable feature of technological innovation. The lesson, then, is that events currently identified as errors are likely to be replaced by new ones as innovative technologies bring new expectations, new demands, and new opportunities for error. De Ville points to the implications of increasingly sophisticated medical technologies for malpractice and the assignment of responsibility for medical error. In chapter 10, William Sage describes in detail the ways in which physicians' efforts to preserve their reputations and management science's emphasis on corporate responsibility and reputation bear on legal and extralegal means of policing medical quality and safety. Sage argues that although alternatives to malpractice litigation—such as no-fault liability—that require physicians to openly discuss error may be hobbled by the medical profession's defensiveness about error, the "corporatization" of health care delivery may bring greater clarity to reputation as a competitive and social benefit.

Chapters 11 through 13, by Edward A. Dauer, David M. Studdert, and E. Haavi Morreim, focus specifically on the ethical pros and cons of compensation schemes for adverse patient outcomes. These chapters look at tort liability (malpractice), enterprise liability, no-fault, and mediation as means of achieving justice for harmed parties and as background conditions for safety-improvement efforts. Dauer and Studdert each point to the failure of tort liability to justly compensate harmed parties and to act as a deterrent. For example, regarding compensation, malpractice's costs often make it an inaccessible remedy to groups who are already marginalized and vulnerable in society and the health care system. Both Dauer and Studdert also identify the ways in which malpractice drives error underground and inhibits safety improvement. Edward Dauer offers interest-based mediation as an alternative that can satisfy nonmonetary outcomes that harmed parties seek after a medical error, including apology and participation in the quality-improvement process. David Studdert offers no-fault as an instrument of social justice, advancing equity, efficiency, and predictability in the distribution of due compensation.

In chapter 13, E. Haavi Morreim argues that there are many ways that safety can be promoted and systems improved that do not require either replacing the tort system or depriving injured parties of information or compensation. According to Morreim, the tort system, properly understood as a way of assigning the burdens of injury, should be rehabilitated to reflect a process-oriented rather than an outcome-oriented standard of reasonable care in medicine and should seek to accommodate a more complex notion of causality than it currently does. Even within the currently flawed tort process, progress is already being made, Morreim argues, regarding collection and disclosure of information about error. The best-case scenario regarding justice and error prevention, Morreim argues, would include universal access to a reasonable level

of health care for all citizens and voluntary disclosures and offers of compensation by individual and institutional health care providers. Without universal
access to care, there are fundamental distortions in error management in the
United States, distortions that continue to hobble just compensation whether
through tort or no-fault.

I thank all of the individuals who made this project possible: the contribu-
tors to the volume and to project meetings, the Hastings Center staff who supported the work, the project codirector, Nancy Berlinger, and the Patrick and
Catherine Weldon Donaghue Medical Research Foundation for the generous
grant that supported this book and the project as a whole. Together, it is our
hope that this work will shed light on the most ethically promising patient
safety reforms.

Accountability and Justice in Patient Safety Reform

VIRGINIA A. SHARPE

Introduction and Background

The Institute of Medicine (IOM) report *To Err Is Human* presented the most comprehensive set of public policy recommendations on medical error and patient safety ever to have been proposed in the United States. Prompted by three large insurance industry–sponsored studies on the frequency and severity of preventable adverse events, as well as by a host of media reports on harmful medical errors, the report offered an array of proposals to address *at the policy level* what is being identified as a new "vital statistic": that as many as 98,000 Americans die each year as a result of medical errors—a figure higher than deaths due to motor vehicle accidents, breast cancer, or AIDS. And this figure does not include those medical harms that are serious but nonfatal.

The IOM recommendations resulted in a surge of media attention to the issue of medical error and in swift bipartisan action by President Clinton and the 106th and then the 107th Congress. Shortly after the report was issued in 2000, President Clinton lent his full support to efforts aimed at reducing medical error by 50 percent over five years. In Congress, the report prompted hearings and the introduction of a host of bills including the SAFE (Stop All Frequent Errors) Act of 2000 (S. 2378), the Medication Errors Reduction Act of 2001 (S. 824 and H.R. 3292), and recently the Patient Safety and Quality Improvement Act of 2002 (S. 2590) and the Patient Safety Improvement Act of 2002 (H.R. 4889). Although none of these bills has made it into law, each represents ongoing debate about the recommendations in the IOM report. Because the IOM recommendations have been either a catalyst or a touchstone for all subsequent patient safety reform proposals—whether by regulation or by institutions hoping to escape regulatory mandates—I introduce this volume with a brief description of the IOM report's point of departure, the problem it seeks to address, and the solutions it identifies. From there, this chapter maps out the ethical values and issues that subsequent chapters address as a basis for policy deliberation.

The Institute of Medicine Report

The Institute of Medicine report is a public policy document. That is, it proposes the need for government intervention to address a problem of serious concern to public health and health care financing. Although there was an immediate flurry of resistance to the report's statistics on the number of deaths associated with preventable medical error—a key premise in the argument establishing the scope and significance of the problem—these challenges have been effectively silenced by the preponderance of evidence that the rate of harmful medical error—with its enormous human and financial consequences in death, disability, lost income, lost household production, and health care costs—is unacceptable.

The report observes that health care has lagged behind other industries in safety and error prevention, in part because, unlike aviation or occupational safety, medicine has no designated agency to set and communicate priorities or to reward performance for safety. As a result, the IOM's keystone recommendation is the establishment of a center for patient safety to be housed at the Agency for Health Care Quality and Research under the auspices of the Department of Health and Human Services. The center's charge: to set and oversee national goals for patient safety. In order to track national and institutional performance, and to hold institutions accountable for harm, the IOM also proposes mandatory, public, standardized reporting of serious adverse events. In addition to mandatory reporting, the IOM advocates efforts to encourage voluntary reporting. To motivate participation in a voluntary reporting system, the IOM recommends legislation to extend peer review protections, that is, confidentiality, to data collected in health care quality improvement and safety efforts.

To complement the national initiative, the IOM recommends that patient safety be included as a performance measure for individual and institutional health care providers and that institutions and professional societies commit themselves to sustained, formal attention to continuous improvement on patient safety. Finally, regarding medication safety, the IOM recommends increased attention by the Food and Drug Administration (FDA) and by health care organizations to identify and address latent errors in the production, distribution, and use of drugs and medical devices.

A unifying theme in the report is the role that systems play in the occurrence of medical mistakes. Over the last few decades, research conducted on error in medicine and other high-risk, high-variability industries has revealed that the majority of quality failures in these industries result not from poor, incompetent, or purposefully harmful individual performance but, rather, from the complexity of systems. In the hospital setting, systems of drug dissemination or infection control, for example, can be designed either to prevent or to facilitate error by individual providers. Recognizing the system dimensions of the problem, the IOM recommendations promote human factors research—which examines the interface between humans and machines in complex work environments—to get at the root causes of error and adverse events. The report encourages nonpunitive, voluntary reporting as an essential ingredient in understanding lesser injuries and "near-misses"—those errors that have the potential to cause harm but haven't yet.

Although the IOM acknowledges the role that professional ethics and norms play in motivating health care quality, it bases its recommendations on the premise that internal motivations are insufficient to assure quality and patient safety consistently throughout the health care system. Thus, the IOM's aim is to create external regulatory and economic structures that will create both a level playing field and "sufficient pressure to make errors so costly . . . that [health care] organizations must take action" (Kohn, Corrigan, and Donaldson 2000, 18).

Given its aims as a comprehensive policy document, it is understandable that the IOM report places only minimal emphasis on professional norms or the moral motivation of health care providers as the principal catalyst for change. Change of the scope being proposed requires a uniform set of incentives and accountabilities. Further, if it is systems rather than individuals that are the most appropriate targets for improvement, then appeals to individual virtue would seem to be the wrong focus. I will come back to the relationship between individuals and systems, but, for the moment, I will point out that the role of ethics in public policy goes well beyond the question of moral *motivation*. Ethics also plays an essential role in the *justification* of public policy and the critique of policies already in place.

Underlying all public policy deliberations are specific social values and assumptions about how these values should be weighed and balanced or prioritized. In order to understand and assess the legitimacy of proposed policies in a democratic society, therefore, those underlying values and assumptions can be made explicit and subject to critical appraisal. The analysis and arguments that follow are an attempt to provide the framework for such deliberation. I begin with a brief look at the ethical values central to the IOM recommendations.

Patient Safety

The Obligation to "Do No Harm"

The guiding value of the IOM report is patient safety. This value can be understood to derive from two long-standing principles of health care ethics: beneficence, the positive obligation to prevent and remove harm, and nonmaleficence, the negative obligation to refrain from inflicting harm. As far as medical error is concerned, the principle of beneficence grounds a moral argument against errors of omission such as a misdiagnosis or failure to provide required treatments. The principle of nonmaleficence grounds an argument against errors of commission, such as surgical slips, drug administration to the wrong patient, or the transmission of nosocomial infection. Together, these two principles constitute the obligation to "do no harm" (Sharpe and Faden 1998; Beauchamp and Childress 1994). It is important to point out here that not all errors are harmful and not all patient harms are the result of error. The focus of the IOM report is on that subset of errors that have caused harm or have the potential do so.

Traditionally, the relationship between the clinician and the patient has been regarded as a *fiduciary* relationship. That is, the power disparity between doctor and patient, the patient's vulnerability, and the doctor's offer to help are understood to place special obligations on health care providers, as professionals, to promote a patient's health interests, to respect the patient's autonomy, and to hold his or her good "in trust" (Pellegrino 1979; Pellegrino and Thomasma 1988).

Every medical error and injury happens to an identifiable individual. From the point of view of fiduciary ethics—that is, professionalism—the individual patient is the focus of the obligation to do no harm (Pellegrino, this volume). This patient-centered focus is acknowledged by the IOM in its definition of safety as "freedom from accidental injury." This definition, says the report, "recognizes that this is the primary safety goal from the patient's perspective" (Kohn, Corrigan, and Donaldson 2000, 4).

The Principle of Utility

The goal of patient safety is also justified by the principle of utility, understood in the simplest terms as the achievement of the greatest good for the greatest number or the net aggregate benefit across a population. Insofar as the IOM recommendations are aimed at patient safety as a public health problem requiring strategies to improve overall safety in the health care system, they are based on the principle of utility. From the point of view of public health ethics, the patient population *in the aggregate* is the normative focus, and safety improvements are measured in terms of population-based, or epidemiological, statistics such as the IOM's target goal of a "50 percent reduction in errors over five years" (Kohn, Corrigan, and Donaldson 2000, 4).

The value of patient safety is also understood to derive from its *economic* utility. As the IOM report states on page 2 of its executive summary, the total national cost of preventable medical error is between seventeen and twenty-nine billion dollars a year. The assumption behind the report's recommendations is that efforts to reduce error by the target of 50 percent over five years will be justified by the reduction of associated costs.

These different justifications, grounded in either utility or fiduciary responsibility, are largely implicit in the IOM report. By making them explicit, we see where they come into tension and where further justifications will be required to resolve those tensions. For example, although it is possible that the incentive to reduce the extra costs associated with preventable error will coincide with the imperative to protect patients from harmful outcomes, such a coincidence is by no means assured. One can easily imagine a cost-conscious hospital deciding against certain strategies to improve safety because the up-front costs are prohibitive. Likewise, without a clear prioritization of the fiduciary justification for safety—which gives priority to patient welfare as a policy objective—it is easy to imagine safety proposals being reduced to their economic value. Under such circumstances, policymakers might suppose certain safety trade-offs to be justified by economic considerations alone (Brennan 2000).

The IOM report has also left largely implicit the ways in which strategies to improve *overall* patient safety have the potential to compromise obligations to individual patients. For example, the IOM recommends mandatory reporting of serious adverse events and voluntary reporting of lesser harms and near-misses. To the extent that institutions direct their resources to meeting the standards for *mandatory* reporting, they may de-emphasize *voluntary* reporting and the follow-up necessitated by it. This could have the paradoxical effect of making safety improvement activities contingent on a patient having been seriously harmed. To fully appreciate what is at stake here, we need to understand the report's emphasis on accountability.

Accountability of Health Care Organizations

Accountability is another value guiding the IOM recommendations. It is expressed in the IOM's call for a nationwide mandatory system for reporting of serious adverse events and in its call for performance standards on patient safety and quality improvement for health care organizations (Kohn, Corrigan, and Donaldson 2000, 87–88, 133). In the report, accountability is grounded in the public's right to know about and be protected from hazards. It also derives from the principle of fairness.

From a regulatory perspective, hazards in the health care setting are matters of public safety. The IOM's recommendations regarding mandatory reporting are designed to generate standardized information that can be used to understand and track known hazards and to take preventive action. As the report states: "The public has the right to expect health care organizations to respond to evidence of safety hazards by taking whatever steps are necessary to make it difficult or impossible for a similar event to occur in the future. The public also has a right to be informed about unsafe conditions" (Kohn, Corrigan, and Donaldson 2000, 102).

The principle of fairness operates on two levels in the mandatory reporting proposal. First, mandatory reporting is intended to level the playing field for health care institutions so that none is exempt from data collection on safety or from exposure to penalties or civil liability in the case of serious patient harms. Second, mandatory reporting to oversight bodies is intended to provide an avenue for harmed patients to gain access to information regarding the circumstances surrounding an injury and use it to seek justice for negligent harm associated with care.[1]

Although a number of states currently mandate external reporting of serious adverse events—usually to the state health department—in most cases, the information collected is intended to be protected by law from potential claimants.[2] Many state programs fail to provide public access to the information and most require a subpoena or court order for release of information. By contrast, the IOM proposes meaningful public access to information about serious harms, stating that "requests by providers for confidentiality and protection from liability seem inappropriate in this context" (Kohn, Corrigan, and Donaldson 2000, 102).

It is useful to conceptually distinguish between reporting and disclosure. Reporting refers to the provision of information to oversight bodies such as state agencies, or the proposed Center for Patient Safety. Disclosure, by contrast, refers to the provision of information to patients and their families. It is important to point out that the IOM's emphasis on accountability and the public's right to know in the context of mandatory *reporting* has nothing to do with active *disclosure* of information by health care institutions to harmed parties. Although the mandatory reporting of serious or fatal adverse events would, in principle, trigger meaningful investigation and administrative action, it does not automatically direct that information to the patients who have been harmed (Gilbert, this volume). Thus, the "right to know" invoked by the IOM is *not* an endorsement of the *individual's* right to know or the obligation of respect for the autonomy of individuals. In this way, the IOM's understanding of accountability is extremely narrow and points up one of the ways in which a public health or safety approach overlooks obligations to specific individuals.

Although it is not a feature of the IOM's recommendations, the need for disclosure, understood as a prima facie obligation of professionalism, *is* being addressed on other fronts in the patient safety movement. For example, in 2002, the Joint Commission on Accreditation of Healthcare Organizations (JCAHO) put into effect a disclosure standard setting forth the expectation that hospitals and physicians will inform patients (and families) about "unanticipated outcomes" associated with their care.[3] This requirement is included in the JCAHO's Patient Rights and Organizational Ethics standards. Likewise, a number of forward-looking health care institutions, such as the Veterans Affairs (VA) Medical Center of Lexington, Kentucky, have embraced disclosure as an institutional obligation and one that has the added advantage, from a consequentialist point of view, of not resulting in a negative financial impact on the hospital (Kraman and Hamm 1999). As Steve Kraman of the Lexington VA hospital says, "We didn't start doing this to try to limit payments; we did it because we decided we weren't going to sit on or hide evidence that we had harmed a patient just because the patient didn't know it. . . . We started doing it because it was the right thing to do, and after a decade of doing it decided to look back to see what the experience had been. The indication that it's costing us less money was really unexpected" (Osterweil 1999). Implicit in Kraman's remark is an endorsement of disclosure as an obligation of professionalism, that is, "the right thing to do."

The IOM report also calls for accountability of health care institutions to performance standards regarding continuous improvement in safety and quality. The emphasis here is on pressure that will be applied by regulators, accreditors, and purchasers to evaluate and compare hospitals according to their demonstrated commitment to safety. Because of its public policy focus, the IOM report focuses on accountability of *organizations*, not of *individuals*. If we look at the history of medicine, however, we see that it is individuals—specifically physicians—who have historically been regarded as the locus of health care quality and who have been held responsible for it. There are pronouncements throughout the history of medicine that reinforce this view. The American Medical Association's (AMA) first code of ethics states:

> A physician should not only be ever ready to obey the calls of the sick, but his mind ought to be imbued with the greatness of his mission, and the responsibility he habitually incurs in its discharge. Those obligations are the more deep and enduring, because there is no tribunal, other than his own conscience, to adjudge penalties for carelessness or neglect. (American Medical Association 1847, Art. I, §1)

In other words, the nineteenth-century American doctor was accountable only to himself. This assumption that the physician is the best guarantor of quality continues to be one of the hallmarks of medical professionalism. There is much to be said historically and sociologically about accountability in health care and the almost exclusive emphasis on physicians (Starr 1982; Sharpe 2000a). Most important for our purposes is the fact that these assumptions about accountability have shaped the culture of medicine such that a rethinking of accountability must be central to the "culture change" that is the rallying cry of reform.

If, as safety experts both within and outside medicine maintain, it is flaws in a *system*, rather than flaws in individual character or performance, that produce the vast majority of preventable errors (Maurino, Reason, and Lee 1995; Reason 1990, 1998, 2000)—a premise accepted in this essay—then the dominant strategy of blaming individuals will (continue to) be ineffectual and counterproductive in improving safety. This point was made early by leaders of the patient safety movement: "A new understanding of accountability that moves beyond blaming individuals when they make mistakes must be established if progress is to be made" (Leape et al. 1998). The dynamic between institutional and individual accountability is one of the most important and complex issues at the heart of patient safety reform. In this and other chapters in the volume, we analyze this concept and its practical implications.

Confidentiality—Keeping Information about Adverse Events from Public View

In addition to its recommendations regarding a nationwide mandatory reporting system, the IOM also recommends that voluntary, confidential reporting systems be implemented within health care institutions and encouraged through accrediting bodies.[4] Such systems, many of which are already in place in health care and other high-risk industries, are essential to safety improvement efforts insofar as they can encourage providers to supply information needed to identify and take action to address hazardous conditions. As many observers of high-risk industries have noted, it is the information about near-misses that provides the richest resource for safety improvement efforts (Deming 1986; Berwick 1989; Reason 1990). In its distinction between thresholds for mandatory and voluntary reporting, the IOM combines, under the voluntary reporting system, "near-misses" and errors that have caused minor or moderate injuries. Thus, voluntary reporting is intended to supply information not only on nonharmful errors but also on what Carol Bayley calls minimally or moderately "harmful hits" (Bayley, this volume).

In order for voluntary reporting to be workable, the IOM states, providers need to be assured that the information they report will not be used against them in the context of malpractice litigation. As such, the IOM recommends that "Congress should pass legislation to extend peer review protections to data related to patient safety and quality improvement that are collected . . . for internal use or shared with others solely for purposes of improving safety and quality" (Kohn, Corrigan, and Donaldson 2000, 10). Although the guarantee of secrecy has a political purpose—to gain buy-in from clinicians who would otherwise fear exposure to liability—from an ethical point of view, the guarantee of confidentiality is justified only by the principle of utility. A reduction in harmful errors across the patient population can only be achieved if frontline health care professionals are willing to supply information regarding specific health care delivery problems. The free flow of this information to create an epidemiology of error can occur only if secrecy regarding the information is assured.

As recommended, this proposal has been introduced into legislation under the Patient Safety and Quality Improvement Act, introduced in the Senate on June 5, 2002, and the Patient Safety Improvement Act, introduced in the House on June 6, 2002. In the bills, all information collected for the purpose of patient safety and quality improvement will be confidential and protected from sub-poena, legal discovery, Freedom of Information Act requests, and other potential disclosures.[5]

There are a number of ethical problems with this approach. The first is that the proposed legislation allows information about adverse medical events (the "lesser injuries") to be concealed from harmed parties (Gilbert, this volume). Importantly, it is not clear how the legislation squares with accreditation requirements for disclosure that are mandated by the JCAHO or that may be part of a hospital's institutional policy. Second, peer review protections formalize and reinforce the conflict between the provider's interest in self-protection and patients' legitimate interest in information about their care. In so doing, the restriction of access to information about adverse events undercuts fiduciary obligations and patients' right to know about information pertinent to their care. Third, the enhancement of peer review protection is premised on the assumption of the status quo with regard to the current malpractice system. Confidentiality is made to do all of the heavy lifting to circumvent what Troyen Brennan has called "the dead weight of the litigation system" (Brennan 2000). Brennan, like several authors in this volume, is critical of the IOM recommendations and other reform proposals that fail to address the ways in which the current malpractice system is ethically and practically counterproductive as a response to medical harms. As discussed below, the structures and incentives of the tort system are inconsistent with accountability for truth-telling and safety improvement (Dauer, this volume).

As I have pointed out, the notion of accountability is central to patient safety reform. It guides our expectations and judgments regarding the performance of health care providers. Moreover, the causal story now being told about medical errors from the systems perspective fundamentally challenges those conventional expectations and judgments, that is, the assumption of individual accountability that forms the fabric of medicine and law. So, in order to hold health care providers accountable under a systems approach, we have to reinvent not only our understanding of accountability but also the structures of accountability institutionalized in our legal and cultural approaches to medical error. We have to knit the sweater at the same time that we are wearing it.

Rethinking Accountability

In this section, I look at the notion of accountability as it relates to two different causal explanations for medical error. I examine some of the concerns that accompany the story of complex causation in a systems approach to error. As a way of addressing some of these concerns, I distinguish between accountability in the backward-looking sense and accountability in the forward-looking sense.

Finally, I examine the implications of these senses of accountability for both compensation and safety improvement. I use the terms "accountability" and "responsibility" synonymously.

Two Causal Stories

With the emergence of the systems approach to patient safety, a paradigm shift has occurred in the causal story of why errors occur and how they can be prevented. According to the conventional story, medical error, and specifically harmful medical error, is the result of individual actors and their individual actions—a slip of a scalpel, a wrong diagnosis, a failure to wash one's hands, a failure to check a hematocrit. As far as responsibility for such errors is concerned, the earliest modern codes of medical ethics by Thomas Percival in 1803 and the American Medical Association in 1847 state that the doctor's conscience is the "only tribunal" and his responsibility is to learn from his mistake and to make sure it doesn't happen again. As Kenneth De Ville has observed, after the late 1800s when medical malpractice emerged as a new public "tribunal," this causal story became the basis for negligence claims against physicians (De Ville 1990; De Ville, this volume). Tort law remains the dominant narrative of responsibility in the arena of medical error, and it operates on the basis of a notion of simple causation. Poor or unsafe care is attributable to the actions or inactions of individual health care providers who are cast as "bad apples" (Berwick 1989; Reason 1990). The shadow of liability reflects and reinforces a "shame and blame culture" within which people hide their mistakes.

In the last half of the twentieth century, W. Edwards Deming and J. M. Juran's work in human factors research and industrial engineering (Deming 1986; Juran and Gryna 1988), Charles Perrow's book *Normal Accidents* (1999), and James Reason's *Human Error* (1990) all offered a new causal story about quality and quality failure. That story, which has been told in the medical context by Donald Berwick (1989), Lucien Leape (1994), and the National Patient Safety Foundation (Cook, Woods, and Miller 1998), among others, is that human error should not be regarded narrowly as the *cause* of harm but should be regarded as the *effect* of complex causation. Why? Because the majority of errors do not produce harm but can reveal latent errors or potentially harmful failures within a complex system. Unless we look in greater detail at the causal web, we will be ignorant of the weaknesses in the system and powerless to prevent their causing future harm. The lesson of human factors research and cognitive psychology is that to understand error causation it is not enough to examine one's own actions or to look for the "smoking gun" or proximate cause of the active error; we must also examine the interrelationships between humans, technology, and the environment in which we work (see figure I.1). Applying this research to accidents involving the escape of radioactive material at Three Mile

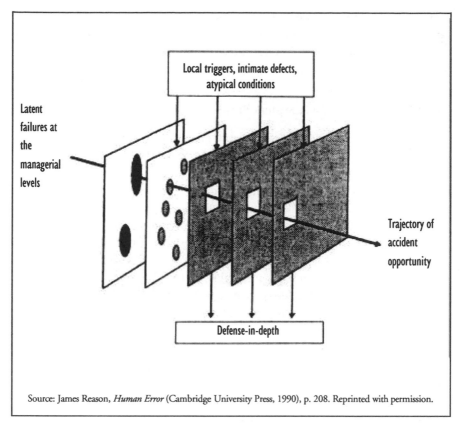

Source: James Reason, *Human Error* (Cambridge University Press, 1990), p. 208. Reprinted with permission.

Figure I.1 *The Dynamics of Accident Causation*

Island and the explosion of the space shuttle Challenger, psychologist James Reason determined that most accidents were caused by mismatches between the design of complex systems and the ways in which humans process information. In the medical context, a system failure in drug administration, for example, might involve look-alike packaging or sound-alike drug names— situations that are literally "accidents waiting to happen."

According to safety experts in aerospace, atomic energy, and other complex, technology-based industries, the most constructive approach to error reduction is the creation of a blame-free environment that sees every error as "a treasure" (Blumenthal 1994). There are at least two justifications for this counterintuitive approach to accountability. The first is, again, that error prevention depends on information that will only be forthcoming if individuals feel free enough from liability concerns to provide it. The second is based on the principle of justice. As Alan Merry and Alexander McCall Smith point out in their book *Errors, Medicine, and the Law* (2001), errors are by definition exculpatory because they are involuntary.[6] So, holding individuals responsible for errors is wrong on two counts. First, a true accident, whether act or omission, is not blameworthy because, by definition, its result was either unforeseeable or could not reasonably have been prevented. Second, most errors cannot be causally attributed solely to the proximate activities of an individual actor.

Don't Blame Me, It Was a System Problem

This new causal story has understandably given rise to a number of concerns about accountability for harmful mistakes.

The first worry is that a systems explanation gives people permission to pass the buck by saying that their own actions are so controlled by "the system" that they simply aren't free. In this sense, appeals to "the system" provide a convenient pretext for moral shirkers. In its most extreme form, this is the problem of free will and determinism in a new context. Appealing to "the system" in the broadest metaphysical sense, one's actions are seen to be determined by forces outside of all human agency. Responsibility is, thus, located outside the individual actor. This sort of defense against being held responsible is not really plausible in the case of health care practitioners, whose self-understanding includes the ability to influence the course of illness. In other words, it is not possible to reject the notion of free will while at the same time acknowledging that it provides one of the guiding justifications of one's work. That having been said, however, the literature on the history and sociology of medical law indicates that a fatalistic belief in divine providence was one of the key exculpatory factors in medical harm up until the early nineteenth century and continues to play an important, if sometimes disingenuous, explanatory role (De Ville, this volume). In her book *Wrongful Death*, Sandra Gilbert, whose husband died as the result of a medical error, recounts a story about the benefactor of a Catholic hospital who was repeatedly assured by his wife's doctors that it was "God's will" that she was comatose and later died after routine surgery. The woman's husband sued to find out what everyone had "known all along," namely, that the patient's coma was the result of an identifiable error (Gilbert 1997, 218–19).

A related worry about a systems approach is the "Dilbert problem" (named after Scott Adams's sardonic cartoon about the workplace). Unlike the metaphysical problem of determinism that implicates the human condition, the Dilbert problem implicates the conditions under which humans work and is manifest in the problem of learned helplessness (Reason 1998, 192). The worry is that the systems approach so minimizes the role of individual agency that it will choke off the motivation to sustain high-quality performance, encourage poor performance, and lead to an erosion of trustworthiness and professionalism (Pellegrino, this volume).

This worry is based on the assumption that individual actors are morally and practically disempowered within a system or that individuals can step "outside" a system and claim moral immunity. As we will see, however, the kind of responsibility envisioned within the systems approach is based on the empowerment of individuals to contribute to system improvement.

Another more practical concern about the systems approach to medical error is that it will make it difficult if not impossible to assign responsibility for preventable adverse events. This worry about the loss of an identifiable target of blame is fostered, in part, by the very human desire for vengeance (Dauer, this volume). The invocation of a "system" renders faceless and anonymous the perpetrator of harm, and victims are left powerless. Also at play here is the assumption that justice to harmed parties requires being able to point a finger at a wrongdoer. This is an assumption fostered by the evidentiary requirements of malpractice that link compensable negligence to an identifiable lapse in the standard of care. If a wrongdoer is able to take refuge in "the system," then harmed parties may be denied access to compensation.

This concern is directly linked to a worry that the practical demands of the systems approach—that is, the need to collect information about errors and adverse events—will be possible only at the expense of the patient's right to know. If protections against subpoena and legal discovery are extended to information regarding harmful quality failures, then accountability to individuals will be subordinated to the ostensible aims of safety improvement.

A distinction between two notions of accountability may help to allay some of these speculative and more practical concerns.

Accountability: Forward-Looking and Backward-Looking

When we think about accountability, its important to keep in mind that responsibility ascription depends for its sense on the purposes or ends to which we put it and the information that we take or do not take to be directly relevant. Said differently, when we talk about responsibility we need to be clear not only about the information that we take to be relevant, or not, but also about what we hope to accomplish in assigning responsibility. With that in mind, we can make a distinction between two types of responsibility ascription: responsibility in the backward-looking or *retrospective* sense, and responsibility in the forward-looking or *prospective* sense (Sharpe 2000b).

In the backward-looking sense, responsibility is linked to practices of praising and blaming and is typically captured in expressions such as "She was responsible for harming the patient," or "He made a mistake and he should be held responsible for it." When we speak of "holding someone accountable," we tend to do so after the fact of some action gone awry.

The forward-looking or prospective sense of responsibility is linked to theories and practices of goal-setting and moral deliberation. It is expressed in phrases such as "As parents, we are responsible for the welfare of our children," or "Democratic citizenship involves both rights and responsibilities." Responsibility in this sense is about the particular *roles* that a person may occupy, the obligations they entail, and how those obligations are best fulfilled. Whereas responsibility in the retrospective sense focuses on *outcomes*, prospective responsibility is oriented to the deliberative and practical *processes* involved in setting and meeting goals.

Currently, the dominant view of responsibility regarding medical error is grounded in tort liability, that is, in malpractice. The aim of responsibility ascription in this context is compensation to harmed parties and deterrence. Through the lens of malpractice, error becomes germane only as the *cause* of harm, and information about errors that *don't cause harm* is regarded as irrelevant. Responsibility ascription in this context is retrospective; its point is the assignment of blame.

A systems approach to error emphasizes responsibility in the prospective sense. It is taken for granted that errors will occur in complex, high-risk environments, and participants in that system are responsible for active, committed attention to that fact. Responsibility takes the form of preventive steps to design for safety, to improve on poor system design, to provide information about potential problems, to investigate causes, and to create an environment where it is safe to discuss and analyze error.

Although there is much disagreement in the medical ethics literature about the source of moral norms in medicine,[7] it is generally accepted that, at minimum, health care is guided by the imperative "To help, or at least to do no harm" (Hippocrates 1923–1988, 166).

Traditionally, this role-responsibility has been associated exclusively with clinicians—those who have a direct relationship with patients. In part, this stems from the historical origins of healing, which, until the emergence of the modern hospital, was largely performed by solitary practitioners. It also reflects the ethical standards established to legitimate professional self-regulation. Given the complexity in the dimensions of both financing and delivery of today's health care system in the U.S., a strong case can be made that this role-responsibility should also be extended to those who have indirect, but nonetheless significant, control over decision making that affects patient welfare. This includes health care managers and administrators who have not traditionally been held accountable to standards of medical professionalism.

Because prospective responsibility is linked to practices and roles, it applies to collectives as well as to individuals. To the extent that a group of people contributes to a practice and the goals that define it, they can, thus, be said to have "collective responsibility"—in the prospective sense. In health care, helping and avoiding harm is one of the primary bases on which physicians, nurses, and other health care providers find solidarity in their work. Collective responsibility in this uncontroversial sense has been largely overlooked because, like most discussions of responsibility in the philosophical and legal literature, discussions of collective responsibility have focused almost exclusively on the (retrospective) question of blame and whether and how collectives can properly be held accountable for harmful events (May and Hoffman 1991).

An emphasis on prospective responsibility is helpful because it forces us to reexamine, in light of the complexities of institutionally delivered health care, the content and scope of responsibility. This is something we have lost sight of in our narrow reliance on the malpractice paradigm as an explanatory framework for medical error. We literally need new structures to account for and be accountable for what we now know about the occurrence of error in complex systems.

In the context of health care delivery, the aim of prospective responsibility ascription is to orient everyone who has an effect on patient care (including clinicians, health care administrators, hospital managers and boards, technicians, computer data specialists, etc.) toward safety improvement. Through the lens of patient safety, error is germane as an indicator of vulnerabilities in a system and as an opportunity to prevent harm. The point of forward-looking responsibility ascription is to specify the obligations entailed in achieving a safer health care environment. From the point of view of a systems approach, these obligations entail a high degree of transparency about errors, the analysis of errors to determine their causes, and the implementation of systemic improvements. To the extent that current structures prevent health care providers from meeting these responsibilities, the structures are inconsistent with the ethics of professionalism.

Given this, what is the patient's *own* responsibility for safety? If, as Lucien Leape and others have argued, a system is "an interdependent group of items, people or processes with a common purpose" (Leape et al. 1995), and responsibility in the prospective sense belongs to all who contribute to the healing enterprise, isn't it reasonable to include patients in this collective?

For some, the suggestion is offensive because it can very easily shade into blaming the victim for harms that befall him. If the patient is responsible for assuring safety and she does not question a medication she knows to be unfamiliar, will we say that she somehow failed (Gilbert, this volume; Pellegrino, this volume)? On the other hand, if patients supply information and insights essential to their care, and indeed *must* provide information regarding their history, why shouldn't they be considered as members of the team (Goeltz, this volume)?

We can all agree that patients are de facto central to their care; however, does this translate into the claim that patients are morally responsible for the safety or quality of their health care?[8] Patients, unlike clinicians and others who deliver health care, have not committed themselves to the practice of health care delivery and the goals that define it. Most people do not freely choose to become patients. That having been said, the rise of the patient advocacy movement has been based on the call for patients to become more active in their care. Roxanne Goeltz—whose brother Mike died as a result of a medical error—argues forcefully that patients and their families should take active measures to assure that their care is delivered safely (Goeltz, this volume). This includes having a friend or family member with the hospitalized patient twenty-four hours a day, seven days a week. Bryan Liang also argues that patients are responsible at least for supplying health care providers with personal information that is as complete and accurate as possible (Liang, this volume).

An axiom of responsibility ascription is "ought implies can." In order to say that someone is responsible, he or she has to be in a position to act on that obligation. In the case of patients, taking responsibility for the quality or safety of their care will often be out of the question. For those patients who *can* be actively involved, their positive contribution to their health care delivery should be facilitated and commended, but it should be required only in the provision of information that is as accurate and complete as possible and in following, as much as possible, the treatment regimen. The onus of responsibility for patient involvement is on institutional and individual health care providers.[9] Respect for patient self-determination requires that providers involve patients in their care, and the lessons of safety improvement indicate that including patients (or their families) as members of the health care team (by asking them to confirm their surgical site, by paying attention to their self-reports) may be one of the most effective and commonsensical ways of improving care.

Again, if we accept the analysis of James Reason and others that most preventable harms are caused by complex factors involving latent failures at the managerial level, system defects, unsafe acts, and psychological precursors, and if we accept that an essential moral responsibility of health care providers is "to help or at least to do no harm," then meeting that responsibility will require conditions under which these causal factors can be brought to light, assessed, and improved. Currently, the system of liability for medical harms makes meeting that responsibility possible only through exceptional acts of courage (Hilfiker 1984). Likewise, it makes respect for patients through disclosure almost impossible, since it discourages honesty and openness on the part of health care professionals.

Justice

As part of our work in the project that is the basis for this volume, we asked project members to reflect on the ethical pros and cons of compensation schemes for adverse patient outcomes. We looked most closely at tort liability, no-fault liability, and mediation as means of achieving justice for harmed parties and as background conditions for safety improvement efforts. Overall, arguments for just compensation schemes that could succeed without inhibiting safety improvement favored either no-fault or mediation. For reasons described below, traditional tort liability was seen as the least ethically viable means of achieving these two goals, albeit the most deeply entrenched system, politically.

Tort Liability

Tort liability is a fault-based system of compensation for those who sustain injury as a result of their medical care. To qualify for payment, the injured party must prove that his or her injury was the result of negligence on the part of the health care provider. A second goal of tort liability is deterrence. The expectation is that the threat of legal action will keep providers from straying from standards of due care.

As David Studdert (this volume), Edward Dauer (this volume), and Bryan Liang (this volume) each argue, tort liability not only fails in respect of both compensation and deterrence but also inhibits safety improvement. As they point out, malpractice law falls short in at least six ways. First, it is a haphazard compensation mechanism. According to findings from the Harvard Medical Practice Study, one of the largest insurance industry–sponsored studies of medical error, only one in seven patients who are negligently harmed ever gains access to the malpractice system, with those who are older and poorer disproportionately excluded from access (Sloan and Hsieh 1990; Vidmar 1995; Weiler, Hiatt, and Newhouse 1993; Burstin et al. 1993). For those patients who do sue, there is evidence that the severity of the injury rather than the fact of negligence is a more powerful predictor of compensation (Brennan, Sox, and Burstin 1996). One consequence of such judgments is that physicians see liability correlated not with the quality of the care they provide but with outcomes over which they have little control. As a result, "risk management" has become an effort to avoid liability rather than an effort to avoid error. Second, malpractice delivers compensation inefficiently, with administrative costs accounting for more than 50 percent of total system costs (Kakalik and Pace 1986) and a successful plaintiff recouping only $1 of every $2.50 spent in legal and processing costs (Weiler, Hiatt, and Newhouse 1993). Third, malpractice claims offer only a monetary outcome, ignoring the harmed party's need for noneconomic remediation such as a guarantee of corrective action or an apology or expression of regret and concern. Fourth, the negligence standard, because it is embedded in an adversarial process, is inconsistent with attempts to learn from errors and improve quality. The malpractice claims process, including pretrial discovery, is shrouded in secrecy, with legal rules governing disclosure and protection of information. This means that institutions and individual providers typically forgo opportunities to learn from the problems that lawsuits can sometimes help to illuminate. Fifth, as Edward Dauer points out (this volume), the adversarial process is based on the belief that the presentation of relentless, one-sided arguments to an impartial judge or jury is the best way to discern the truth. This process necessarily rules out the prospect of information analysis as a collective way of discerning what happened. The malpractice system thus "externalizes" responsibility for truth by selectively taking information out of the hands of involved parties—a process that is emotionally brutal for patients and families trying to reconstruct their lives after a medical harm (Levine, this volume). Finally, regarding its deterrence function, there is evidence indicating that malpractice stimulates defensive medicine, rather than stimulating high-quality care (Kessler and McClellan 1996), and that the stress and isolation that physicians experience while being subject to malpractice claims may result in a degradation of their performance (Charles 1985; Passineau 1998; Liang 2000f).

The moral flaws of tort liability are embedded within these shortcomings. From the point of view of justice, the tort system fails to deliver compensation in a fair and timely way to harmed parties. Those with lesser claims are kept out of a prohibitively expensive malpractice system; those who are compensated may spend years of their lives obtaining this result; those who are older and poorer may be excluded from access. For those like Sandra Gilbert (this volume), who settle cases under the shadow of malpractice, the adversarial process guarantees that plaintiffs will never know the details of the case and will never receive apology or recognition from the defendant. The tort system creates incentives against truth-telling on the part of health care providers. Also, from the point of view of justice to clinicians, the tort system overlooks the system dimensions of error and thus may unfairly target individual providers for acts, omissions, and outcomes for which they cannot fairly be held culpable. From the point of view of harm prevention, the tort system stifles safety improvement and, by externalizing responsibility for truth, engenders a defensive rather than a constructive posture toward error prevention. From the point of view of utility, the tort process is inefficient.

No-Fault Liability

No-fault liability is a compensation scheme that does not base the award of damages on proof of provider fault. As David Studdert observes, "to qualify for compensation in these schemes, claimants must still prove that they suffered an injury, and that it was caused by an accident in a specific domain, such as the workplace, road, or hospital, but it is not necessary to demonstrate that the party who caused the accident acted negligently" (Studdert, this volume). No-fault liability is consistent with the prospective assignment of responsibility. It is predicated on a high risk of hazard in a particular industry and assigns absolute liability in advance regardless of contributory fault. In other words, no-fault is based on the presumption that harms will occur in a particular setting, and it builds in provisions for compensation.

Studdert cites empirical research indicating that no-fault has led to increases in average monetary compensation for injured workers as well as to gains in worker safety. Although more evidence will be needed, Studdert and others are optimistic that similar benefits will accompany the implementation of no-fault in the domain of health care. There are a number of potential moral advantages to no-fault. First, because it suspends the fault requirement, no-fault could remove incentives to conceal information, thereby supporting fiduciary obligations of disclosure and creating the conditions for the collection and analysis of error information. Second, no-fault has the potential to overcome some of the inequities in access to compensation under malpractice. Unlike the tort system, which distributes compensation haphazardly, no-fault, as an administrative scheme, could determine remedies in advance and distribute them according to the severity of injury. A potential problem here, however, is in the calculation of loss. If this is determined according to a person's current salary, for example, as occurred in compensation of victims in the attacks of September 11, 2001, age-based, gender-based, or income-based inequities could be reiterated in a no-fault scheme.

This weakness is also related to the health care financing system that we have in this country. As Haavi Morreim points out (this volume), in countries where no-fault schemes for medical harm have been implemented, there are also systems of universal health care coverage so that ongoing health care needs are already covered and need not be obtained through no-fault compensation. Without this and other social welfare programs to support the needs of the injured and infirm, the efficiencies of no-fault will likely not be realized.

Nonetheless, the potential for no-fault to remove barriers to information access both for patients and for safety improvement, and its potential for fairer distribution of compensation, make it a promising context in which justice, fiduciary responsibility to patients, and safety improvement can thrive.

Interest-Based Mediation

Interest-based mediation is a means of opening direct communication between the parties in a dispute. Its aim is to address the parties' interests and needs rather than their adversarial positions. Empirical research indicates that patients who suffer injury often have noneconomic motivations—such as the desire for information and communication—in bringing a claim (Dauer and Marcus 1997; Levinson 1994; Levinson et al. 1997). Likewise, it has been argued that what physicians want out of litigation (whether that means winning a malpractice suit or a subsequent defamation claim that they have brought as plaintiff) is not monetary repair, but repair of reputation (Sage, this volume;

Soloski and Bezanson 1992). Mediation is a means of addressing these interests in a "restorative" way that is impossible within the context of traditional tort litigation. Another potential advantage of mediation is that, though it takes place within the existing fault-based system, its confidentiality is ostensibly assured through statutory legal privilege in almost every state (Dauer, Marcus, and Payne 2000). Although the degree to which legal privilege does actually guarantee a "safe harbor" against subsequent litigation has been questioned (Liang, this volume), mediation has the advantage of "internalizing" responsibility for the resolution so that the parties are able to communicate directly rather than through legal intermediaries. As a result, the parties may all benefit from the resolution. Health care providers can avoid a costly lawsuit, consequent reporting to the National Practitioner Data Bank, and loss of reputation; patients and families can make a human connection following a loss; and patients can be brought into the peer-review process by requesting follow-up or remedial actions in lieu of or in addition to monetary damages. Although mediation does not offer a direct avenue to information collection about adverse events and errors, it may create a less adversarial context in which safety, rather than money, can be pursued as a mutual goal and the patient's experience can be explicitly used to improve care.

Mediation may also provide a much-needed context that supports truth-telling as an avenue to justice. Nancy Berlinger (this volume) outlines religious and cultural perspectives on error and forgiveness as a corrective against over-simplified expectations in the context of medical harm. In her research, Berlinger found that patients are routinely excluded from rituals of forgiveness in the medical context.

In Charles Bosk's description of forgiveness for the technical and moral errors committed by surgical residents, analogs of "confession" and "repentance" take place in the "hair shirt" ritual of the morbidity and mortality (M & M) conference (Bosk 1979). Here, physicians report to peers and superiors on the circumstances surrounding their involvement in an adverse event. Forgiveness is conferred by the superior, who assumes the traditional Jewish-Christian role of deity. The "hair shirt" is also a metaphor for self-criticism, which is then followed by "self-forgiveness." A third ritual involves peer-support for clinicians confronting the emotional trauma of harmful errors. The patient is absent from all of these contexts. Although, as Berlinger, Bosk, and others make clear, all of these rituals serve important purposes, justice to specific patients is not one of them.

Drawing on Dietrich Bonhoeffer's notion of "cheap grace," Berlinger (this volume) observes that the possibility of forgiveness or reconciliation in the service of justice to harmed parties—in this case, patients—involves repairing one's relationship with the patient. One's relationship with God, one's superordinates, one's peers, or one's self cannot be a surrogate for one's concrete responsibility to the patient or the patient's family. If it is to be achieved at all, Berlinger argues, forgiveness or reconciliation must be understood as a relational process in which actions of confession and repentance are directed to the proper persons. Specifying these actions, Berlinger recommends that "practices traditionally described as *confession*" in the Jewish and Christian traditions that have helped to shape Western cultural norms and expectations would include:

- promptly acknowledging error and disclosing to the patient a cogent and complete narrative of what happened;

- being personally accountable even in cases of systems error, bearing in mind that some patients may comprehend error in all cases as an individual rather than a collective or systemic failure;

- providing opportunities for clinicians to process incidents and receive counseling in a "safe," i.e., nonpunitive or demoralizing, environment;

- nurturing as a communal principle that withholding the truth violates patient autonomy and has a corrupting effect upon care providers;

- avoiding the scapegoating of subordinates; and

- avoiding the abuse of the unequal distribution of power between a physician and an injured patient, which may be further skewed by gender, race, income, age, culture, disability, or other factors. Relevant abuses of authority would include making a patient complicit in error by labeling her "noncompliant"; conflating known incidents of error with "complications" in general; and taking advantage of a patient's religious beliefs, e.g., "It was God's will," to hide or excuse error.

The practices traditionally described as *repentance* would include:

- apologizing and expressing remorse to injured patients—and allowing oneself to feel remorseful after harming a patient;

- not forcing the patient to interact with the person responsible for her injury if the patient does not wish to do so;

- appreciating the difference between appropriate feelings of guilt and destructive feelings of shame;

- offering injured patients and family members immediate access to pastoral care or other counseling services should they desire them;

- covering the cost of treating injuries resulting from error, and meeting other concrete needs resulting from loss of income due to injury or death resulting from error;

- recognizing that asking for "forgiveness" may be oppressive to an injured patient; and

- working to create conditions that may allow that patient, at some point in *her* future, to detach from this incident as a continuing source of pain, anger, and injustice.

The practices designed to promote *forgiveness* or *reconciliation* would include:

- inviting patients to be part of the hospital's quality improvement process, to allow them, *if they wish*, to take an active role in working with clinicians and administrators to create a patient-centered culture of safety by sharing their experiences of medical harm and their perspectives on hospital culture. This is *not* to suggest that injured patients are responsible for participating in quality improvement to prevent other patients from being harmed, or to solve systemic problems;

- using Clinical Pastoral Education and clinical ethics education opportunities to help chaplains, local pastors, counselors, patient advocates, clinical ethicists, and clinicians explore the psychological and spiritual aspects of medical error; develop their capacity to, as physician David Hilfiker writes, "see the world from the victim's point of view" (Hilfiker 2001); learn how to frame human forgiveness as detachment predicated upon justice; recognize non-Western paradigms of reconciliation; and work toward making justice for injured patients;

- offering a ritual or other forum for hospital staff to explore their emotions and responsibilities concerning medical error; and, finally,

- identifying and challenging any aspects of institutional culture that deny the fallibility, and therefore the humanity, of clinical staff, or that work against truth-telling, accountability, compassion, and justice in dealing with medical error and promoting patient safety.

As a specification of the obligation of disclosure, participants in the project on which this volume was based also discussed the scope of that obligation with regard to near-misses, that is, nonharmful errors. Albert Wu (this volume) examines whether health care providers have an obligation to disclose near-misses to patients. Assessing the potential risks and benefits of disclosure to patients, to physicians, and to the relationship between them, Wu concludes that disclosure of near-misses is discretionary but desirable. In its favor, the disclosure of an accident that almost happened (such as the aborted administration of penicillin to someone allergic to the drug) may provide a risk-free environment for practicing more significant disclosures; it may function as a "teachable moment" to impart useful information to the patients; and it might, in the particular circumstance, enhance the trust relationship between doctor and patient.

With this in mind, it is important to remember that the IOM report includes both errors that cause no harm (near-misses) and errors that cause "lesser [than serious] injuries" within its recommendation for voluntary reporting (Kohn, Corrigan, and Donaldson 2000, 101, 110). This recommendation should *not* be regarded as a substitute for the established professional obligation for disclosure of harmful errors, whether they be serious, moderate, or minor. Regardless of the *policy* recommendations, the ethical obligation for disclosure of harmful errors stands. The challenge, therefore, will be to create a context in which this obligation can be honored despite seemingly contradictory policy proposals.

As Berlinger's recommendations about disclosure make clear, delivering justice to harmed parties entails the institutionalization of new norms and practices of disclosure. Greater openness potentially afforded by no-fault or mediation and voluntary compensation in the context of existing tort liability may provide environments in which such norms and practices can take hold and harmonize with long-established fiduciary obligations of disclosure.

Safety Improvement and the Use of Information

As I have pointed out, the patient safety reform movement is based on a systems approach to error, the premise of which is that overall safety improvement depends on new forms of system "interrogation" (i.e., root cause analysis) rather than on old forms of individual interrogation (shame and blame). Another uncontested premise of a systems approach is that success depends on the collection and analysis of information gleaned from real-life health care delivery. In recognition of this fact, the IOM report recommends that information about error not associated with serious harm be protected from all uses not connected with safety improvement, including uses requiring access to information by subpoena, legal discovery, FOIA, etc. As just noted, the recommended protection of information about "lesser harms" is incompatible with professional obligations of disclosure. Equally disturbing, if not more so, the IOM recommendations and ensuing legislation to protect information (S. 2590, the Patient Safety and Quality Improvement Act, and H.R. 4889, the Patient Safety Improvement Act of 2002)[10] effectively make safety improvement contingent on patients being harmed—though the harms in question are of "lesser" severity. As I have noted, the legislation to protect information that is part of a voluntary reporting scheme is a "workaround" in the malpractice status quo. From an ethical point of view, this workaround effectively pits the value of safety improvement against the values of nonmaleficence and truth-telling. We acknowledge that the IOM sought to assure accountability through its proposed mandatory reporting of serious, preventable adverse events; however, not surprisingly, the dominance of malpractice has made this recommendation politically untenable. A reconsideration of the malpractice system itself, in favor of no-fault and mediation, may be a necessary step to overcoming the antagonism of safety improvement and the values of nonmaleficence and truth-telling, as well as to achieving accountability in the prospective and retrospective senses.

The Health Insurance Portability and Accountability Act (HIPAA) has also given rise to concerns about the extent to which data collection for safety improvement will be hampered by HIPAA provisions to safeguard the privacy of patient records (Department of Health and Human Services 2002b). At issue is whether patient records—primarily intended to support the health care needs of the patient—can also be used for the secondary purpose of safety or quality improvement activities. As Bryan Liang points out (this volume), HIPAA was not designed with safety improvement research in mind and, as a result, may present some obstacles to the use of patient information in this arena. In the original version of the regulation, before it was modified in August 2002, patient consent was required for the release of personal, identifiable information that may have been used for safety improvement activities in an institution. The modifications eliminate the consent requirement for the disclosure of personal information for "health care operations," which include quality improvement activities. Under the rubric of "quality," data collection for safety, without patient consent, appears to be allowable in the final rule. However, if quality or safety improvement activities rise to the level of "research," that is, the production of "generalizable knowledge," then the activities will fall under the requirements of human subjects protection, requiring Institutional Review Board approval or HIPAA authorization. Modifications to HIPAA also allow for researchers to have access, without patient consent, to a "limited data set," that is, information that has been partially de-identified. It is not clear whether this limited information will, in fact, be useful in fine-grained safety improvement work.

The final privacy rule goes some way toward harmonizing patient privacy and the promotion of safety improvement activities. Still, as I noted earlier, it will be especially egregious if safety improvement activities are conducted on the basis of information to which harmed patients themselves are denied access either formally through peer-review protections or because of provider reluctance to disclose due to liability fears (Brennan 1990).

One way around this conflict is, again, a shift to no-fault liability. Under such a system, existing obstacles to patient access to information about the delivery of their health care would be largely removed, and this secondary use of health information would not be contingent on depriving patients of their rights to know about problems associated with their health care. Although the HIPAA privacy provisions have been finalized and compliance is now required, it is likely that definitive answers to questions regarding privacy and "research" will only be obtained as the rule is tested or as advocates seek amendments to it.

Conclusions and Recommendations

In this volume, we hope to have gone some way toward setting an agenda for consideration of the ethical implications of patient safety reform. As policies are

debated at the federal, state, and institutional levels, we offer the following conclusions and recommendations.[11]

- Federal officials, privacy advocates, and advocates of safety improvement
  should work together to clarify the implications of the HIPAA privacy rule
  for the collection of safety data.

- Policymakers should look for alternatives to the tort system to serve the
  purposes of compensation and safety improvement.

- Institutional change depends on understanding how a cultural context
  shapes perceptions about why errors happen and how actors within a culture learn to think about and deal with them. Institutional leaders in health
  care will need to more self-consciously examine the "hidden curriculum" in
  medical and nursing education, that is, the practices that are taught and
  rewarded through example rather than through what is conveyed in the
  official curriculum.

- We can't eliminate errors: Human factors research and knowledge of our
  own humanity (to err is human) tells us why we can't. We can, however,
  reduce errors, learn from them, improve the way we handle them, and deal
  more justly with all parties (including clinicians) touched by them.

Acknowledgment

This chapter was made possible through the generosity of the Patrick and
Catherine Weldon Donaghue Medical Research Foundation. It was first pub-
lished as a special supplement to volume 33, no. 6 (2003) of the *Hastings Center
Report* (Sharpe 2003).

Notes

1. It is well known that the threat of medical malpractice has created a culture of silence
in medicine, discouraging health care providers from telling patients about problems associated with their care. Even claimants who settle a lawsuit may never know the events surrounding an injury. See Gilbert 1997.

2. Liang has indicated the multiple ways in which such confidentiality can, in fact, be
breached, by legal maneuvers (Liang, this volume).

3. See Joint Commission on Accreditation of Healthcare Organizations 2002. Standard
RI.1.2.2: "Patients and, when appropriate, their families are informed about the outcomes of
care, including unanticipated outcomes."

4. It is important to point out that confidentiality in this context refers specifically to the
restriction of public access to information on the quality and safety of health care delivery.
Ordinarily, when we speak of "confidentiality" as a professional obligation in health care we
are referring to the confidentiality of patient information and restricted access to that information except by patient consent. Thanks to Janlori Goldman for pointing out this important
ambiguity.

5. See the text of the bills, S. 2590 and H.R. 4889, on Thomas, the federal government's legislative information site on the Internet: http://thomas.loc.gov/.

6. It is also worth noting that in his *Nicomachean Ethics*, Aristotle observes that responsibility is only properly ascribed to actions that are voluntary (Aristotle 1999, 1110a ff.).

7. For example, are moral norms inherent to medicine, residing in the fiduciary nature of the healing relationship? Are they grounded in a pragmatic concern to produce "patient satisfaction"? Are they based in theories of democratic citizenship? Or is medicine simply like other market transactions that are based on contracts stipulating specific expectations and obligations?

8. There is a large literature on the extent to which people are responsible for their health and their health behaviors. Our question is much narrower and concerns only whether patients are responsible for the safety and quality of health care delivery.

9. This point is reflected in the Joint Commission's 2002 standards, specifically in standard number 3.7 on patient education. See Joint Commission on Accreditation of Healthcare Organizations 2002.

10. These bills can be found on Thomas, the federal government's legislative information site on the Internet: http://thomas.loc.gov/.

11. These recommendations are drawn from Sharpe 2003 and Berlinger 2004.

CHAPTER 1

Writing/Righting Wrong

SANDRA M. GILBERT

More than a decade has now passed since the sunny morning of February 11, 1991, when two orderlies arrived to wheel my husband of thirty-three years into the operating theater where he had a routine prostatectomy from which he never recovered. Though he was in robust health apart from the tumor for which he was being treated, Elliot died some six hours after my children and I were told that his surgeon had successfully removed the malignancy. But to this very moment, no one from the hospital has explained to us how or why he died.

"Dad's had a heart attack." That was the explanation my husband's doctor offered us as he strode grimly into the hospital lobby on the night of February 11, 1991. But the next day the medical center released a different story, alleging that the cause of death was "heart failure." And two weeks later, a death certificate signed by the chief resident who worked with my husband's physician gave still another account, asserting that death resulted from "liver failure."

Through painful investigation—first with the help of a close friend who was a pathologist, then with the aid of an attorney—we discovered that my husband had suffered a massive postoperative internal hemorrhage. In fact, he evidently bled to death because someone in the recovery room failed to get the results of a hematocrit that would have easily detected the problem.

Eventually, we filed suit for negligence—and our lawyer won a settlement just two days after he deposed the attending surgeon. Although, as in most settlements, the hospital admits no guilt, my husband had clearly been the victim of a "negligent adverse event": an event defined by one writer as "an injury caused by the failure to meet standards reasonably expected of the average physician, other provider, or institution" (Hiatt et al. 1989).

Eventually, too, I wrote a book titled *Wrongful Death* (Gilbert [1995a] 1997), along with a collection of poems titled *Ghost Volcano* (Gilbert 1995b), each focusing in its own way on the disturbing story I've just told. In doing so, I understood that I was writing (recording) as well as seeking to right (to rectify) wrong, and now, as I retell the tale, I realize that I am still writing and seeking to right a terrible wrong.

Many writers and speakers on the subject of medical error have considered the frightening prevalence of mistakes like the one that killed my husband: they have discussed the statistics showing that "[a]s many as 98,000 Americans die unnecessarily every year" from such calamities, more "than from breast cancer, highway accidents, or AIDS" and have considered the recommendations made by the Institute of Medicine's report *To Err Is Human* (Kohn, Corrigan, and Donaldson 2000, 31). Some have evaluated the preventive measures proposed by systems analysts, health care providers, and physicians themselves. Some have examined the deeply conscientious efforts many doctors have made to analyze and (sometimes) expiate their own errors (Hilfiker 1984; Fonseka 1996; Gawande 1999; Drayer 1999). Some have considered ways of guaranteeing accountability. Most address these issues, as is appropriate in this context, from the perspective of their own *professional* involvement, though some have begun to speculate on strategies for moving the patient from the periphery to the center of the "mistakes" dilemma.

I have a different mission: I write as both a witness—to testify to the experience of the patient who has endured the consequences of a catastrophic mistake—and as an informant—to help illuminate the complex sorrow that inevitably enshrouds such an experience. I speak as and for the one who is inexorably trapped at the center of the web of medical error, the unprofessional, often ignorant, and almost always innocent one who *suffers* the error—the patient who is the object of the mistake or mistakes.

Following several other writers on this topic, I use the word "patient" to signify not only the person who has been the direct recipient of medical treatment but also those associated with him or her who have also been profoundly affected by such treatment (Crawley, Shultz, and Weinberg 2000). It's interesting, in this connection, that my dictionary gives two meanings for the noun "patient": first, "one under medical treatment, and second ("archaic" but relevant to the pain of those whose loved one has been harmed by medical negligence), "one who suffers." Although I can only speak here *for*, not *as*, the patient in the first sense of the word, I do speak both for and as the patient in the second sense (*American Heritage Dictionary* 2000).

And that second, archaic but resonant sense of "patient" may also help me illuminate some of the pains and paradoxes that make the situation of the patient (or survivor) especially traumatic. Unlike, say, the French word for patient—"malade"—which is rooted in "mal" (meaning bad, wrong, and illness), our English word for the object of medical attention originates in the Latin *patiens*, meaning "to endure," and hence has affinities with the noun "patience" and its derivative adjective "patient," meaning "capable of bearing affliction calmly . . . capable of bearing delay . . . enduring or capable of enduring hardship . . . without complaint" (*American Heritage Dictionary* 2000).

Is it this cluster of not so secret linguistic associations that helps make it feel difficult for a patient to complain of errors in medical treatment? Do patients themselves internalize such meanings so rigorously that even to the one who has suffered drastic harm from medical error an *impatient* patient somehow seems like a contradiction in terms? I want to meditate on these questions first through a brief review of some psychological and cultural obstacles I encountered as I sought both to write (record) and right (rectify) the medical wrong I described in my book *Wrongful Death*, and then through more explicit analyses of the implications these obstacles to patient (or *impatient*) protest might have for professionals who want to deal sympathetically with problems faced by the victims of medical error.

Five Propositions

If it's hard—as it obviously is—for an agent who has erred (for instance, a doctor who has made a mistake) to contemplate the error, it's hard in a different, perhaps less obvious way, for one who has *suffered* error to contemplate the mistake made by practitioners she has trusted. In talking about *Wrongful Death* and the legal processes of discovery and complaint it narrates, I will offer (and repeatedly return to) five linked propositions about the problems implicit in the very process of writing or reporting (and complaining of) wrong, an activity that is, of course, as much a process of remembering and testifying as it is of striving to repair and readjust. As I'll try to show, such processes generate a range of fears and awaken a host of angers that are understandably hard to confront. And as I'll also try to show, such processes associated with writing and/or reporting wrong are especially painful for patients who have suffered from medical errors and wish to seek some sort of redress.

1. Perhaps most dramatic: Writing wrong is, or ultimately *becomes*, wrong— at the least problematic—because it's a hopeless effort at a performative act that can never, in fact, be truly performed. You can't, in other words, right wrong by writing wrong, even though you are engaged in the writing because consciously or unconsciously you believe that your testimony will reverse, repair, or undo the wrong you're reporting.

In a medical context, this means that complaining of and urging the investigation of error often feels wrong, or anyway pointless, because you can never right the wrong you're reporting. Whether (as in one notorious episode) you're a patient who had the wrong leg amputated, or (as in the case of a well-known San Francisco Bay area scholar) you're a patient who was paralyzed when a surgical sponge was inadvertently left in your body, or (as in my own case) you lost your husband when his massive postoperative hemorrhage went unnoticed, the harm you've suffered is irreversible. Complaining won't change anything— won't give you back your leg, your ability to move, your husband. Why exhaust yourself trying to remedy what is irremediable?

What was my own experience? I'll confide here that I began writing *Wrongful Death* on July 23, 1991, precisely the day—five months after my husband's death—when my children and I had our first meeting with the attorney who represented us in the lawsuit we brought against the medical center where he died. Although I wasn't aware of feeling this, I must have secretly believed that in some sense the "performance" of the narrative my children and I had just outlined to our lawyer would somehow revise or repair the script in which we were trapped. Did I feel that if I could *tell* the whole story it might end differently? Or did I suppose that if I got *that* story out of the way it might be replaced by another plot?

I certainly don't indulge in such speculations in the book itself. On the contrary, I offer a conventional expository paragraph in which I introduce my plans to write the book that the reader is now reading: "[T]hat night . . . when as usual I couldn't sleep—I went into the kitchen with a notebook, and began, weeping as I wrote, to try to write. Began to try to remember what happened to Elliot and me and the kids so people who get angry at supposedly greedy plaintiffs, and so maybe even doctors who self-righteously deplore the escalating costs of malpractice insurance, might understand the impact of medical negligence on one 'real-life' family" (239).

Earlier in the book, though, I wondered, speculatively, "Do I still believe that the lawsuit will, if only temporarily, resurrect my husband?" Did I, I'd now add, believe that by recounting the story of both the negligent, adverse event and the lawsuit to which it led, I could subtly, furtively, change its ending? Such a sense of authorial potency may be akin to the feeling some people have (I'm one of them) when watching films of great catastrophes—the assassination of John F. Kennedy, for instance—that if it were only possible to run the film backward or freeze a crucial frame, the inexorable plot of what-has-been might magically modulate into what-didn't-happen: the motorcade would take a different route, the rifle wouldn't fire, the young president and his pink-suited wife would return triumphantly to Washington the next day.

By the time I was ending the book, I have to admit, I was more moderate. "I know you, Mom," I report my son saying with a curious combination of weariness and trust. "You're going to write a book." "And my daughters agreed," I add. "Yes, that was what I should do. Because, sad as it is, there never was anything else to do."

Nothing to do, I seem to be saying, but bear witness to the truth of this account I hereby proffer to you, the reader. A sentence later, though, I can see that I must have been thinking in some part of myself of something different. If I couldn't inscribe a spell that would heal, then I wanted to spell out words that would curse those guilty of the crime that left my husband bleeding to death in the recovery room of a university medical center at this super-high-tech end of the twentieth century. Thus, and with deep passion, I quoted Elizabeth Barrett Browning's diatribe against slavery "A Curse for a Nation" (Barrett Browning 1900):

> Weep and write.
> A curse from the depths of womanhood
> Is very salt, and bitter, and good.

And though I then withdrew from my own rage—insisting in an open letter to all the doctors who seemed to me to be responsible for my husband's death that I don't "want to curse," I just "want to *talk* to you. I want you to hear me"—I nonetheless ended this meditation with the following sentence: "Says Barrett Browning, at the end of her poem, "THIS is the curse. Write" (Barrett Browning 1900, 341).

2. Writing wrong is wrong, or at least problematic, because it's not only painful but *writing* pain—pain that, as I've just claimed, can't really be righted, healed, or soothed. On the contrary, to write wrong is to tunnel into darkness, to drive oneself into the heart of fear, pain, rage. Barrett Browning's sentence to slaveholding America was also a sentencing *of* slaveholding America. "THIS is the curse. Write": consider the ambiguity of this phrase, which can surely be taken to imply *that the act of writing is itself a curse* inflicted as much on the accuser as on the accused, as much on the writer as on the target of the writing.

Of course, even to bring a lawsuit—that would-be performative motion of accusation always hurling itself toward the judicial words "I now pronounce this or that culprit guilty"—even to bring such a suit is to suffer the inscription of pain. You, the witness and accuser, do testify before the clerkly attorney-at-law who records your statements. The ancient formula has hardly changed: "Comes now before me so-and-so and *deposes*"—which is to say *puts down her word*—"and *says*."

Maybe I shouldn't have been surprised, then, at the number of people who wondered how I could stand to bring a lawsuit (*how can you keep on reliving it again and again*, they said) and worse, how I could stand to write a book about such grief and such anger. Perhaps especially in a medical context, complaining of wrong is wrong because it's too painful. As many victims of medical negligence have wondered to me (and others), "Why should I put myself through it again, when it won't do any good anyway?" Why relive the trauma of the moment when you realized you'd lost a perfectly healthy leg or discovered you were paralyzed or learned your husband had died? Rehearsing and reiterating the pain will only redouble your suffering!

Such pain is often particularly intense because it is suffused with fear as well as anger. I would be deceiving myself and others if I denied the anxiety that surrounded the very process of transcribing what I knew to have happened and, worse, *what I didn't know about what had happened.*

"That which you fear the most, that you must do." I said this sentence to myself over and over again, like a mantra, for several months in the spring of 1992. "That which you fear the most, that you must do." At this point, I was trying to imagine the contours of the story I have still never been told: the moments of my husband's death. In order to imagine something of that darkness I had to quell my fear of the hospital records I'd been given and struggle to reconstruct at least an approximation of the event. That which I feared the most, as I bleakly put it to myself, was what I had to confront; and I had to confront it precisely because in order to stand the pain of my loss I had to strive to stand *up* to the pain and loss, strive to *with*stand them by looking at them.

Of course I realized—and still realize—that this aspect of my procedure for grieving might be disconcerting to those who wanted to shield themselves as well as me from suffering. We live in a culture where grief is frequently experienced as at the least an embarrassment; at memorial services for the dead, many would prefer to "celebrate" the completed life rather than lament the irreparable loss. In daily life, mourners are often greeted either by silence or by circumlocutions. All too often grief is seen as an illness or a disorder from which one "recovers," as from alcoholism. The surgeon who came to tell us of my husband's death was accompanied by a woman wearing a badge that said "Carolyn, Office of Decedent Services"; she carried a large folder labeled "Bereavement Packet." Lacking traditional religious strategies for solace, we're so dumbfounded by death that we'd rather leave the pain to professionals.

Thus I know that in the years since *Wrongful Death* and *Ghost Volcano* were published I have probably embarrassed or distressed listeners at a number of readings from these books. To be frank, I myself am sometimes troubled by the words I have to say out loud when I tell the story that I tell. When I say these words, I go through a kind of performance anxiety very different from the nervousness ordinarily associated with public speaking. Have I required too much from my audience as I reiterated my script? In describing my writing of a wrong, as well as in the very act of writing this wrong, have I done something *socially* wrong—turned myself into a "loser," a "whiner," a "complainer"?

Without attributing such thoughts to my present readers, I can certainly testify that these judgments have been made by some. One, the well-known physician-author of best-selling books about medicine, praised the book privately but refused to make a public statement because he felt passionately that I was wrong to write the name of the real hospital where my husband died along with the name of the real surgeon who operated on him. And some people associated with that hospital have conveyed to me, via various colleagues, their view that I was somehow a "bad sport" [*sic*] to continue writing the wrong after their attorneys had settled our wrongful death suit.

3. Such remarks lead to a third proposition about writing wrong: Writing wrong may be wrong or at least problematic because you, the writer, might actually be the one who is wrong either in your perception of events or in your response to them. Perhaps people are embarrassed or distressed by your assertion that you've been wronged because you're asking them to judge the merits

of a case they can't evaluate. Perhaps you, the writer, are a wrongdoer who has leveled your *"j'accuse"* against an innocent person. What if writing wrong is really a confession of guilt on the writer's part, or in any case an evasion of responsibility?

Or, perhaps just as bad, what if writing wrong is an effort to exploit (and thus intensify) a wrong? This last notion, of course, is at the heart of public scorn for those so-called "ambulance-chasing lawyers" and greedy plaintiffs who are together held responsible for the escalating costs of malpractice insurance and thus the rising costs of medical care. But it is probably also at the center of the distaste some people seem to feel for any kind of public complaint or, more specifically, any kind of tell-all memoir writing that can be characterized as sensational and hence exploitative.

Grace under pressure, we're taught, is "cool." Complaint—*impatient* complaint—may thus be *uncool* as well as uncouth. "Revenge is *mine*," saith the Lord—not Job's or yours or any mere *writer's*. In the face of pain, one should be stoic, unflinching, *courteous.*

A few months after *Wrongful Death* appeared, my husband's surgeon was named director of a cancer research clinic at the medical center where he works, and I imagine that it was in connection with this promotion that he gave an extended interview to a local reporter, who produced an article that featured a prominent sidebar titled "When a Patient Dies," recounting the doctor's comments on what was clearly my husband's case.

Here's what the reporter recorded:

> Dr. X [that's right, at the moment I'm feeling too anxious to spell out the man's name] recently lost a patient for the first time in his career. "How do you deal with it?" reflects Dr. X. "You're there to look after people. You practice the best medicine that you possibly can. I don't think there's anything else that you can do. If you're talking in an abstract way about how you deal with the fact you may be sued, you thank God that most of the people you treat, and their families, *are marvelous people.*" (Emphasis added)

There it is. "Marvelous people" don't complain of medical error. "Marvelous" or just plain "good" patients are *patient*, forbearing, understanding. Marvelous people don't write wrong: they don't seek to rectify wrong, nor do they try to record the wrong. Perhaps, indeed, because they are marvelous people *wrong does not befall them!*

What gives this point special bite in a medical context is the possibility that the complaint may be wrong because *you* may not be the one who's been wronged, you may be in some obvious or some obscure sense the one who *is* wrong. In an obvious sense: maybe you just got the story wrong, maybe you're too dumb to understand what happened. Perhaps you inadvertently did something to make your "good" leg look like the "bad" one? Perhaps you foolishly elected an unwise surgical procedure? Perhaps you didn't help your husband choose the best doctor to operate on him? A major story in the March 2000 *Ladies Home Journal* speaks to just this point: under the headline "When Doctors Make Mistakes" and the subhead "How to protect yourself and your family," the editors group what they call "Strategies to avoid becoming a victim of medical error," including "Get informed," "Seek another opinion," "Track your medical history," etc. (Korn 2000, 100–105; Many 2000, 101). Well, you may think you did all these things—but what if you didn't *really*? Caveat emptor. It's your own fault if you were an uninformed consumer.

But worse still, your illness itself, the condition that was the *pre*condition for error, may be a sign of some inherent wrongness in *you* that destined you for this suffering. Poignantly telling, in this regard, is a comment by Marianne Paget, one of the most sophisticated analysts of medical mistakes, whose work became personal as well as professional when her own cancer was misdiagnosed (Paget 1993). As she reflects on her "abbreviated life," she suddenly muses—almost in passing and without much explanation—that she is not "a victim of error or even of chance. There is no simple perpetrator here. I am the subject of error. I embody it. Even my body has erred" (20). But to whom, then, ought one to complain of *such* error?

4. Writing wrong is wrong or anyway problematic because after all, as contemporary literary theory would tell us, if you can write it you've written it wrong.

This proposition, to be sure, can be applied to the writing of any memoir. Haven't I already confessed that what I feared the most was that I had to *imagine* (which is to say, I had in some sense to write *wrongly*) the for-me crucial moments of my husband's death, the moments whose truth I never had a chance to witness? "Art is a lie one tells in order to tell the truth," declared Picasso, who was, in fact, not just serene but seraphic about rearranging faces, bodies, curves, and angles (Ashton 1988, 21). But Defoe said—and his comment is darker, scarier—"Supplying a story by invention . . . is a sort of Lying that makes a great Hole in the Heart" (Defoe 1895, 99).

There is a hole in my heart where I had to supply the story of my husband's wrongful death by lying—that is, by imagining what I hadn't seen and thence by writing wrong.

And what of the "true"—supposedly real-life—episodes to which I declare I *have* borne witness? Have I transcribed them rightly or wrongly, wrong*fully*? Especially in connection with medical error, my fourth proposition—if you can write it, you've written it wrong—is closely linked to the third. If you're a patient, even if you're a *doctor*-patient or a *nurse*-patient, you're by definition not the doctor or nurse who's treating you, so therefore you can't formulate an informed complaint since you can't know all the intricacies of what happened, can't see yourself and your story from "outside," the way, say, the doctor can. Nor, certainly, can you understand what may be the extenuating circumstances surrounding the amputation of the wrong leg, the closing up of the wound with the sponge in it, or the massive postoperative hemorrhage. Which leads us to:

5. Writing wrong is wrong because it's writing pain, sorrow, grief, death, lack, absence—and in other words, complaining of error is futile because pain, sorrow, grief, death, lack, absence, and *error* are inevitable functions of the human condition. Or at least, to be less philosophically extravagant, writing or reporting wrong is wrong because some kind of wrong is inevitable: "To err is human" as not just the old saw but the title of the Institute of Medicine's recent report puts it. Which is to say, to formulate the point more vulgarly, "Mistakes happen" and to complain of them is naïve or petulant. Declares Paget about the series of misdiagnoses leading to her death, "There is no simple perpetrator here," no one cause of iatrogenic suffering that can be identified, isolated, and analyzed. No single narrative can be adequate to the complex sorrow of the underlying story. Why, then, even struggle to formulate *a* or *the* or *your* complaint?

I have devoted so much time to a meditation on some of the factors inhibiting patient protest against medical error—ending with this last, pathetic *Why bother?*—because I think it's important to try to explain what I consider one of the most striking statistics associated with the problem: less than 2 percent of people who are harmed by negligent medical care file malpractice suits (Weiler, Hiatt, and Newhouse 1993, 73), and given that there are few other channels for complaint, it seems clear that despite our society's reputation for litigiousness very few patients indeed find ways to protest their injuries. Why *should* injured patients and families seek redress, and what might such victims of medical harm consider appropriate remediation? What, in other words, do (or should) injured patients and/or their survivors want?

Astonishingly, although in the course of writing *Wrongful Death* I thoroughly investigated both the medical and the legal aspects of negligent adverse events like the one that killed my husband (and even provided rather an extensive bibliography of works on these subjects in the book itself), I can think of few researchers who have studied the wishes and needs of precisely the group that might be said to have the most intimate involvement with medical error: not those who have caused it or witnessed it, but those who have suffered from it. In fact, despite its eminently reasonable proposal to establish a Center for Patient Safety within the Agency for Health Care Research and Quality, the Institute of Medicine's *To Err Is Human* also suggests strengthening the walls of silence that surround American medicine's rightly named "culture of secrecy," recommending that "Congress should pass legislation to [further] extend peer review protections to data related to patient safety" (Kohn, Corrigan, and

Donaldson 2000, 111). Apparently, from the perspective of this report, information regarding patient safety ought to be the concern of everyone except the patient herself.

Any patient, though, who has suffered from medical error and confronted all or some of the five obstacles to complaint that I have outlined here, has basic needs that ought to be central to any discussion of negligence and malpractice. These needs, indeed, are encrypted in the very obstacles I have been discussing, so please bear with me while I revisit my five propositions.

1. Yes, following through on a complaint of medical error will not give you back your amputated leg, restore your lost faculty, or revive your dead spouse, but it will resuscitate your own sense of *agency*—a sense of self-possession, even autonomy, that was surely injured, if not shattered, by the harm that came to you from a situation in which you trustingly gave yourself up to the agency of others.

2. True, as you reiterate your story you'll relive or anyway revisit the details of shock, pain, and fear that were inextricably associated with the shock, pain, and fear of your injury—but arguably your rehearsal of these details will help release you from them. To repress the pain is not to be free of it, as many sufferers from medical error who *didn't* sue have told me in letters and emails about *Wrongful Death*. "My mother, a vivacious 57-year-old lawyer [died] of complications following a 'successful surgery'," wrote a fairly typical one of these correspondents, and "we have never learned exactly what caused her death." This woman noted that she and others in her family had considered suing but "could not face the prospect of endless depositions and having to relive it again and again." And yet, she remarked, "perhaps if we had allowed ourselves an outlet for the rage, the sense of injustice, I would not now feel this low-grade pain, as from unexpressed emotion."[1]

3. To be sure, your own anxiety about the medical choices you made together with the defensiveness of the health care professionals whose error you're protesting may well make *you* feel wrong and guilty—but all the more reason why you should try to get the story straight and figure out who or what *really* was to blame, since you yourself almost certainly were not. Despite the optimism of the *Ladies Home Journal*, you probably can't single-handedly "protect yourself and your family" from medical mistakes, even if you are a superbly "informed consumer." But when something goes wrong, you have a right to know when, how, and in what way it went wrong. Thus, although Why *me?* is often a question that can't be answered, Why *this?* should be explicable, whether the explanation is simple or complex. What you want, need, and should demand is *accountability*—here another word for "justice."[2]

And in fact, as one of the few patient-centered commentators on the subject explains in the 1993 British collection *Medical Accidents*, "it is the question of accountability which has proved to be [of most importance] to victims. Accountability from the victim's point of view means simply that something is done to ensure that those responsible . . . are required to give an account of themselves, that an explanation is given to the victim or family, and that steps are taken to try to avoid a similar accident happening again" (Simanowitz 1993, 209).

Questions of accountability and preventability, indeed, are further encrypted in my propositions 4 and 5 (4: If you can write it—i.e., formulate a complaint—you've inevitably written it wrong, since you only know your own side of the story, and anyway, 5: Wrong is in the nature of things, mistakes happen, etc.). Yes, you only know your own side of the story—and that's why someone ought to tell you the *other* side. And yes, mistakes happen, but they shouldn't, and if people investigate the other side of the story—the side that *accounts for* and *explains* the mistake—then maybe further mistakes, at least mistakes like this one, *won't* happen.

What would it mean if the administrators and staff of the medical center where my husband lost his life had taken these propositions—which I will now rename *imperatives*—as seriously as, with considerable struggle, I myself did?

In this final round with my five points, I will only consider what these health care professionals might have done—might in fact *still* do—for me and my children as representative victims of medical error.

1. How can caregivers who have erred bestow agency—or at any rate a minimal feeling of empowerment—on those who suffer from their mistakes? Although my husband's doctors and nurses, along with the hospital administrators, "bereavement counselors," and others couldn't give me back my husband and my children back their father, they could have acknowledged our existence as a traumatized and grief-stricken family. That would have meant treating us as real people—meeting with us, talking to us, offering us counseling and courage to confront the pain we were going to have to endure. Instead, the doctor walked away, the "bereavement counselor" from the "Office of Decedent Services" handed me a list of funeral directors, and the hospital administration released contradictory accounts of the cause of death. Is it any wonder that I've not only never been able to go near that medical center again, but I've also never, truly never, been able to reenter the city in which it's located?

In *The Vigil*, a poignant memoir of his cancer-stricken sister's last days, the poet Alan Shapiro meditates on the changing relationship between his sister and her doctor: "[I]f he were the benevolent deity when she was doing well," Shapiro notes, "he became the *deus absconditus* when the cancer had metastasized, and it was clear that she was going to die." To be sure, the writer concedes, for a doctor to maintain sanity, "some measure of detachment" is necessary. Yet "didn't he owe his patients what he or the nature of his profession had encouraged them to desire and expect? . . . [D]idn't his obligations toward them as a fellow human being . . . continue even after, as a doctor, there was nothing else that he could do?" (Shapiro 1997, 53–56).[3]

2. How can the ones who have made medical mistakes help those who suffer from their mistakes to cope with suffering? To be sure, if every reiteration of the terrible details of my husband's death was going to give us pain, it was also going to give the responsible physicians pain. My husband's surgeon not only conceded but in a way exaggerated this pain, when not long before he parted from us on the night of my husband's death, he said, "I know, for you this is unpleasant, awful, but believe me for me it's *shattering*." Yet in order to help release us (as well as, perhaps, himself) from the consequences of the error that killed my husband, he would have had to journey with us further into the tunnel of pain, fear, and shock in which I'm willing to believe he too may have found himself. And others who were involved in my husband's hospital care would have had to take that journey too.

Patients are of course frequently reassured that physicians regularly take such journeys at those closely guarded, highly ritualized mortality and morbidity (M & M) conferences of which we laypersons only hear secondhand tales. But that information is of little use to the wounded or grieving victim of error.[4] Not just for the patient's sake but for the doctor's sake, the erring practitioner should probably journey into the tunnel of pain and fear *with* the ones who have suffered injury, if only to understand more precisely the consequences of error and to grasp the elemental truth that my husband's surgeon got backward: For *him* as a doctor the calamity of February 11, 1991, was unpleasant, awful, but for *us* as survivors it was shattering.

3. How can health care professionals assume responsibility for their errors and demonstrate their own accountability while helping the patient *not* to feel guilty for having made bad medical choices, for complaining, for suffering, or for just plain being sick? Especially because the patient and/or his survivors may feel, with Marianne Paget, like the *embodiment* of error, it would seem particularly important for attending physicians to offer as detailed a narrative as possible. Stonewalling makes the patient feel crazy. Name-calling makes the patient feel sick.

Declared a woman whose four-year-old daughter suffered brain damage as a result of a series of medical mistakes, some made by the hospital where my husband died: "None of the doctors told me . . . what really happened to my baby. . . . I asked them crying and I asked them OK and I asked them mad. And they didn't tell me." But that this desperate woman wept and raged and begged for an explanation doesn't mean that she wasn't what my husband's surgeon so bizarrely called a "marvelous" person. It means that she was nearly driven mad by a traumatic event that dislocated her life and destroyed her daughter's future.

And it means that she needed, that she *deserved*, an accounting (Gilbert [1995a] 1997, 345–47).

4. How can health care professionals construct a narrative of a "negligent adverse event" that isn't merely partial, self-serving, or self-centered? And how can they help the victim of medical error produce an equally coherent and legitimate narrative? To begin with, we should remember that even though the only story the patient or survivor can tell as an at least initially ignorant but profoundly injured party may itself be riddled with mistakes, there are significant ways in which it may supplement the health care professional's story and thus help produce a clearer and more capacious account of what went wrong. Thus, although it is surely the case that the patient needs the doctor's or nurse's narrative in order to determine accountability more than they need hers, she just might have something to contribute that would be of interest even within the rarefied precincts of the M & M conference. The interests of justice are, after all, served by more witnesses, not fewer. If only to encourage the patient's account of the problematic event, the erring practitioner ought to produce an honest narrative for the one who has suffered injury.

And again 4 leads with inevitable logic to 5. How can—why *should*—doctors and nurses encourage patients to complain of medical error when we live in a world that is in essence, as it were, error-prone, even erroneous? How? Why? Obviously because—as I hardly need say—although the human condition is indeed riddled with error, though mistakes happen, every scrupulous effort to explain, analyze, and account for them helps prevent further mistakes and might even (though it sounds Pollyannaish to say this) in some small but important way improve the human condition.

The Nettle of Error

Yet even while I speak rather grandly about improving the human condition, I am going to close without using the all too popular but in this case meaningless word "closure." I won't use that word because for one who has through a medical mistake (or indeed any other accident of fate) lost a leg, or the ability to *move* his legs, or even worse the life of a loved one, there is no closure. The error is forever because the loss is forever. But surely, even at this hyper-skeptical and often terminally ironic postmodern millennial moment, we can agree that there *are* some few but precious gains to be won from losses. My husband was especially fond of a line from Shakespeare's *Henry IV* Part I that I think has some relevance here: "[O]ut of this nettle, danger, we pluck this flower, safety" (Shakespeare 1993, 843). At the very least, we can revise the line to be more moderate: "Out of this nettle, error, we pluck this flower, knowledge."

But one commentator's gloss on the line makes it even more apropos: "The nettle if touched tenderly will sting, if grasped firmly, will not" (Shakespeare 1993, 843 n. 1). Had my husband's surgeon firmly grasped and truly contemplated the nettle of error, he might have been less stung by it and would surely have become a better doctor. And had he helped me and my children firmly to grasp and truly to comprehend "this nettle, error," we might still not have become "marvelous people," but we would certainly be stronger, healthier, less traumatized survivors.

Notes

1. For these comments and other letters from victims/survivors of medical error, see "Introduction to the Paperback Edition: Carved in Stone" (Gilbert 1997, 1–11).

2. I am not here considering the vexed issue of financial compensation under the rubric of "accountability," yet clearly it has some place in the matter, and just as clearly the practice as well as the theory of compensating patients and/or their survivors is as confused and confusing as almost every other aspect of the "complex sorrow" of medical error. In *Wrongful Death*, for instance, I tell the story of a Bay Area man who was awarded $2 million in damages because of psychological injuries that he suffered when he was given the wrong eyeglass prescription. And in a fascinating, unpublished paper titled "The Cremated Catholic: A Tale of One Dead Body in Two Countries," anthropologist Stanley Brandes notes: "In recent years, in the San Francisco Bay Area alone, at least 62 people have won between $10,000 and $250,000 in lawsuits involving the careless mixing of ashes in local crematoriums. . . . In one case alone . . . plaintiffs' attorney Kevin McInerney was reported to seek more than $2.5 million in fees. 'You do these cases, and you hope to make a lot of money,' stated McInerney, whose earnings in class action suits against crematoriums already amount to $25 million" (Brandes 1997, 12).

3. In partial extenuation of the doctor's behavior, Shapiro draws on the theorizings of Sherwin Nuland in *How We Die* (1994) to speculate that many physicians "are driven by a preternatural fear of death. Each patient they bring back from the brink of extinction seems to confirm their own invulnerability. Those patients, on the other hand, who 'fail them' dramatize the limits of their power, the frailty of their illusion of immunity from death, which their professionalism helps them to sustain. Not to withdraw from their patients when they become a riddle that will not be solved is to confront their own mortality" (Shapiro 1997, 56). At the same time, Paget offers a conundrum about the doctor-patient relationship that also illuminates the behavior of Shapiro's sister's doctor: "He could not listen to her fear; she could not stop expressing her fear which he couldn't or wouldn't hear. He was the-one-who-would-not-listen and she the-other-who-was-not-heard, archetypes of an experience each of us knows" (Paget 1993, 23).

4. Although both Gawande (1999) and Drayer (1999) seek to justify the so-called "culture of secrecy," it has countless debilitating consequences for patients, ranging from doctors who "say they are peeved by the new demands being placed on them" (Kolata 2000) when patients seek to discuss information about their medical conditions that they've downloaded from the Internet, to doctors who insist that it's not in the interest of patients to "know about the degree [to which their physicians] may be impaired . . . by reason of physical or mental illness" (Bok 1993, 331). Many patients check out the Internet before they go to their doctors, deciding sometimes what they think their condition is, what drugs they need or what drugs they would refuse to take. Doctors can be taken aback. "Some doctors deal well with

it, some don't," says Thomas Reardon, president of the AMA (Kolata 2000). "[M]ost patients find out about such impairment the hard way. But what should they know beforehand, if at all possible? 'Nothing!' was the instant retort of one doctor upon hearing this question [—a response that echoes] the traditional approach . . . holding that the medical profession has the responsibility to safeguard the public against risks from physician impairment; persons seeking medical care should not be confused or alarmed by having to weigh such risks themselves" (Bok 1993, 331–40). See also the chapter by Nancy Berlinger in this volume.

CHAPTER 2

Life but No Limb:
The Aftermath of Medical Error

CAROL LEVINE

This is a story about living with, not dying from, the consequences of medical error. It began in January 1990 when my husband suffered a devastating brainstem injury in an auto accident on an icy highway in upstate New York. He was driving; we were both wearing seatbelts. The car hit a patch of black ice, skidded, hit a guard rail, rolled over, and landed in a deep gully. I emerged shaken but unharmed, but my husband was unconscious and unresponsive. In that brief moment our lives changed forever.

I have written about my experiences as my husband's caregiver, but I have avoided writing, even talking, about the medical error that occurred early in his hospitalization. It is only now, nearly thirteen years later, that I am cautiously ready to tell that part of the story. It is my story because the person to whom direct harm was done is unable to give his own account. The choice to write about such a painful experience brings up feelings of shock, disbelief, and even guilt. In some illogical way, writing about the medical mistake is an embarrassment, as if by doing so I will be exposed to the world as a person whom fate has singled out for a particularly nasty break.

Yet I have overcome these doubts in order to add a different perspective to the recent, oddly disembodied, professional discussion of medical error. Medical error is more than an engineering problem, amenable to technological and "systems" solutions. Policies put in place to reduce medical error must also address the needs of individuals and families who suffer great and often permanent harm.

"There Was a Mistake"

After the accident, my husband was brought by ambulance to a community hospital. The neurologist on call somberly told me that even if my husband survived, he would be seriously impaired, both cognitively and physically. I wanted another opinion. Despite bad weather and telephone outages, I managed to get my husband transferred to a major New York City tertiary-care hospital that same day. There the high priest of neurosurgery vigorously reassured me that my husband would be "one hundred percent OK." So, of course, I believed him, not the community hospital doctor, whose initial prognosis turned out to be right.

A week into my husband's stay in the ICU, when he still showed no signs of coming out of the coma, I received a call in the middle of the night from the neurosurgery resident. He said that my husband had a blood clot in his right hand and needed immediate surgery. At the hospital, the plastic surgeon called in on the case assured me that clots like this occur frequently; an operation would clear it out. He said they would give my husband a big dose of heparin to make sure the clot didn't recur.

The first surgery did not do the job, so back my husband went to the operating room in less than twenty-four hours. At that point, the neurosurgeon met me in the hall. He seemed very angry. "There was a mistake," he said. "The catheter used to measure arterial gases became clogged, and a new catheter was placed on the same hand instead of the other hand. You never put two sticks in one hand. When that catheter became clogged, circulation was blocked through his hand."

He then said, "It wasn't noticed for twenty-four hours," the passive voice subtly deflecting responsibility from a human agent. I can quote this verbatim because it was repeated many times by family members who were there. At the time, though, I saw only the doctor's mouth moving and his hand indicating where the catheter was placed; it was like watching a TV scene with the sound muted. He then said, and this I do remember, "They'll fix it. It's not life-threatening." I asked, "But it is hand-threatening, isn't it?" He only shrugged and walked away.

Only later did I remember that on the day before that first surgery, I had told the ICU nurse that my husband's right hand was very cold. She said, "I'll put on another blanket." That brief exchange haunts me to this day. Why didn't I insist that she look at his hand and call a doctor right away? Would it have made a difference? I will never know.

Several surgeries followed, each accompanied by larger and larger doses of heparin. Then came a final, middle-of-the-night surgery, after which the plastic surgeon told me, "We can't save his hand. He developed an overwhelming allergic reaction to heparin. Instead of clearing the clot, the heparin made his blood clot so quickly that we couldn't even begin to clear the vessels." I first asked whether this was a systemic reaction. Yes, he replied, but my husband would survive. I then asked whether his hand had been amputated. No, they wanted to wait to see how high up on his arm the damage went.

From Bad to Worse

For the next several days I sat by my husband's bed watching his hand and then his wrist and then his forearm turn black. Suddenly he developed a serious infection and needed emergency surgery, to which I consented. What else could I do? His right forearm was amputated an inch or so below the elbow. For the next several weeks I sat by his side looking at the raw, finally healing stump.

Four months later, my husband, still in a coma, was transferred to a rehabilitation facility. Gradually he came out of the coma, disoriented and confused, and incontinent. He was unable to sit up, eat, or move without assistance. The brain stem controls these functions; his was irreparably damaged. When he began to recognize me and understand a little of what happened, he repeatedly asked me to put his wheelchair in front of a mirror. He believed that his lost arm had been placed somewhere else on his body, and that I was not showing him where it was.

The psychologist on staff was sympathetic, but from the beginning the rehabilitation therapists dismissed any possibility that my husband could use his right arm in any functional way. In the acute care hospital, the specialists had assured me that with new prosthetic materials and therapy, my husband would be able to do almost everything he did before—go back to his job as a public relations executive, give presentations, everything. Upset by the rehabilitation therapists' appraisal, I called the original doctors and asked for a consultation. No one responded. My husband never got a prosthesis that provided any functional benefit, and he scorned the one that was supposed to look like a normal hand.

At this point—and only at this point—I started to get mad. Not only had my husband's prognosis for meaningful recovery been wildly overstated, but he had suffered a terrible loss and no one seemed to care. What would he have been able to do with a right arm intact? Hard to know. He was, in effect, paralyzed, but he was exquisitely sensitive to touch, which made physical therapy painful. His left hand was useless. Perhaps with a stronger right hand he could feed himself, turn the pages of a book, change the channels on the TV, help in transfers from bed to wheelchair, touch me, and hold our grandchildren. These are not meaningless actions in his life or mine.

Looking to the Law

A prominent corporate attorney I knew was trying to get our insurance company to cover some home care. He offered to talk to the hospital administration off the record and try to get a small settlement for us. No one at the hospital would return his phone calls, and then he too started to get mad.

As the deadline for filing a lawsuit approached, he urged me to think about this option. Our future was bleak. My husband's health insurer had paid for all the care associated with the medical error—amounting to several hundred thousand dollars—and we were rapidly reaching the cap on his policy. Moreover, as I was starting to learn, insurance coverage for home care would be very limited. To keep my husband at home and my life reasonably intact, I would have to pay for his care myself.

I had no idea how to find a responsible malpractice attorney, since all I had ever heard from my health care colleagues was the usual badmouthing of trial lawyers. I asked a friend who works in a different hospital to ask the risk managers who they would least like to come up against in a malpractice trial. With the *pro bono* lawyer by my side, I went to interview that firm. They took the case, warning me that the process would be long and painful. Was I up to it? I didn't know.

The firm filed the lawsuit, naming my husband and me as plaintiffs. Then began the excruciating experience of dealing with the hospital lawyers, their delaying tactics, and our depositions. Although my husband was able to participate in the depositions, I never knew exactly what he would say because of his brain injury, making the process even more anxiety-provoking.

Through their deposition questions and discussions with our lawyers, the hospital lawyers intimated that my husband was a reckless driver (even though several other major accidents, including a fatality, had occurred that morning on the same stretch of road). They focused on his brain damage, suggesting that the loss of an arm didn't make much difference. They asked questions about our sexual compatibility, marital disagreements, and personal histories. If doctors think trial lawyers are sleazy, they have only to look to their own advocates for evidence of ugly behaviors.

Months and months, and then a year, then two, passed. Delays and more delays. No settlement offers. I believe that the hospital lawyers were waiting for my husband to die, reducing the hospital's liability. At last the judge ordered the doctors' depositions to begin. And on the day before the first deposition (at which the extent and egregiousness of the errors would finally go on record), the hospital lawyers made an offer. Our lawyers said it was fair, and I immediately accepted. It was finally over, or so I thought. But it is not over and never will be.

Disclosure and Closure

Pain and suffering are real, not just legal fictions. Even after years of therapy I still have nightmares involving loss of body parts. My husband has adjusted better than I have, partly because he has no memory of the events. My grandchildren are now old enough to ask about Grandpa's missing arm. Where is it?

I do not want them to know just yet that doctors can make mistakes, so I say that the loss was part of the accident that put him in a wheelchair.

At present, individuals who have suffered medical harm have only one channel of recourse—the tort system. Lawyers take cases on contingency and their fees come out of an eventual award, if there is one. This system worked for me. But even so, the lack of a long-term care system that can manage complex cases like my husband's means that the award provided only the minimum financial resources needed to keep my husband at home and to allow me to cobble together a workable, though fragile, system. (My only alternative to suing the hospital was impoverishment so that my husband would be eligible for Medicaid. This would have ended my career and reduced the quality of our lives enormously.) But how many people can't get lawyers to take their cases, because attorneys feel that the evidence is too weak, the odds of recovery too low, or the recoverable amount doesn't justify the huge cost of going to trial or reaching a settlement? How many families give up because they can't stand the strain?

Beyond whatever tort reforms may be advisable, some nonadversarial system should exist to which people who have suffered financially from medical error can choose to apply. Some potential models are the federal no-fault schemes for children who have experienced serious side-effects from vaccines, or the federal compensation system for September 11 families. For some people, the benefits of certainty and speed may outweigh the downside of potentially lower compensation levels.

Nonetheless, lawsuits are filed not just for financial reasons but because people feel abandoned and aggrieved, in ways that better communication and acknowledgment might alleviate. Doctors and risk managers underestimate both the importance that families place on knowing what happened to loved ones and the frustration they feel when stonewalled. If there were more openness, including apologies, some lawsuits might be forestalled and others settled quickly, without so much emotional toll on families and physicians.

Our lawyers have reconstructed a fairly good but incomplete picture of what happened to my husband, but we do not know the details to this day. A single error, unnoticed and uncorrected, followed by a failed corrective strategy, led inexorably toward disaster. Was this an individual problem, a collective problem, a system problem? Probably all three.

Equally important, I have no idea what happened as a result of the inevitable hospital and, I assume, regulatory review. Good reasons exist to keep confidential a hospital's deliberations during a morbidity and mortality review, but I believe that it's essential to let patients and families know about measures that have been taken to prevent a similar error.

Despite this experience, I have entrusted my husband's care to the same hospital and even on one occasion to the same ICU, where the care was excellent.

But when he or anyone else in my family is hospitalized I am constantly vigilant, mindful of how little it takes to turn routine into disaster.

Acknowledgment

This chapter is adapted from a presentation to a meeting of the Medicine as a Profession Forum, a project cosponsored by the United Hospital Fund and the Open Society Institute. It was originally published in *Health Affairs* 21, no. 4 (2002): 237–41. It is republished with permission of Carol Levine, permission conveyed through Copyright Clearance Center, Inc.

CHAPTER 3

In Memory of My Brother, Mike

ROXANNE GOELTZ

A mistake in the profession of air traffic control can cause the death of hundreds of people at once. A mistake in the health care system can cause the death of hundreds of people one person at a time. What is the difference? Hundreds of people dying at once makes the front page of the newspaper as a disaster and requires answers and changes to prevent the same thing from happening again. But hundreds of people dying one person at a time does not make the nightly news—yet it continues to happen in a profession that has always been presented as one where mistakes are not capable of being made.

My family had to learn of this problem with our health care the hard way. On September 22, 1999, my thirty-nine-year-old brother Michael P. Lange died because of a medical error. He went into the emergency room of the local hospital with a gut ache. They admitted him and gave him morphine without knowing what was causing his pain. He was put into a room where, for reasons unknown to us, he was left unattended and unmonitored. In that void of care, he died. Why?

We may never have an answer, but I want to bring some meaning to my brother's death so we can prevent this question from continuing to devastate lives. I have to believe in my heart that no one deliberately let my brother die. The system in which these people work failed them and us. As consumers of health care we need to be informed so we can play a part in protecting ourselves. We must educate ourselves with the knowledge that our safety is sometimes compromised by human error. The more we educate ourselves, the better our chances of survival and the better care our health care professionals can provide for us. We are given safety speeches before takeoff in an airplane; we have safety warnings stuck on every appliance, power tool, and vehicle we purchase. Why aren't we given the information that would improve our safety and the odds of our survival when we enter the health care system?

I want to share with you the story of my brother Mike. Before September 22, 1999, I did not have a clue what the term medical error meant or that such a thing existed. Almost three years later, I still do not have a clear definition of what it means. What I do know is that needless harm is coming to people who enter the health care system.

The only thing Mike wanted from life was to have a family, spend weekends with them, cook great meals and watch the Packers. Unfortunately, Mike never found a person with whom to share his dreams. I last saw Mike in August, on his way through Minneapolis with friends going to the Sturgis Motorcycle Rally. We sat on the deck eating homemade pizza and drinking beer. Watching Mike, I was once again amazed at how much my son Derrick is like him. My heart filled with pride knowing that if my son were to become half the person my brother was, he would be a decent human being. The next morning I meant to get a picture of the guys on their bikes but forgot. I expected to get one later, but there was not going to be a later.

Mike was gone on his motorcycle trip for two weeks. It was a tense two weeks for my parents because my brother Craig had died ten years earlier in a motorcycle accident. They did not know that one month down the road Mike's life would be taken by something even more dangerous than riding a motorcycle.

Happiness filled the air when Mike stepped into my parents' living room at the end of the trip, in full riding gear, with a big grin on his face. "It was great, Mom, so beautiful." He gave her a big hug. A memory that now tears at her heart every day.

On September 21, 1999, my brother got up, showered for work, and as he was getting ready to leave, became light-headed and felt a severe pain in his stomach. He went over to my parents' house and asked if he could spend the day. He thought he had the flu. By 4:00 P.M., Mike was in so much pain he could not speak and agreed to go to the emergency room. My Dad took him and after Mike was checked in, Dad went home. That was the last time he saw his son alive, and my Dad will never forgive himself for leaving him there alone. He had always been taught that they care for you and you are safe in the hospital.

Dad called around 6:00 P.M. to see how Mike was, but he was still in so much pain he could not talk. Mike was eventually admitted to the hospital and given self-drip morphine for the pain without determining what was causing it. Mike called my Mom around 8:00 P.M. and said they wanted family history—would she call and talk to the nurse?

My Mom called the duty nurse and tried to tell her of the aneurysm history in our family and asked if they would do an ultrasound. I want to try and explain what this nurse did to my Mom. My Mom is not someone who is easily discouraged. When she wants something, she is a confident and forceful person. This nurse, with frustration and bother in her voice, said, "That information is not pertinent to the case." These few clipped words made my Mom feel stupid and incompetent. She responded with defensive, angry embarrassment and said, "I was only doing what had been asked and that was to relay family history." The opportunity for the professional to communicate with the family had been lost, and this became the foundation by which my parents judged future exchanges. Each time someone spoke to them they were defensive, angry, hurt, and distrustful. My Mom had been chastised into silence by this nurse, and she blames and questions herself daily as to why she allowed that to happen.

My Mom called Mike and told him that the nurse said the aneurysm history was not important and that she and Dad would be by in the morning to see him. That was the last time she spoke with her son.

My parents received a phone call from the hospital shortly after 3:00 A.M. on September 22, 1999, telling them Mike was not doing so well and asking them to come to the hospital. On the way there, my parents decided they needed to take Mike somewhere else. This conversation continues to haunt them with feelings of guilt for trying to take action too late.

When my parents entered the hospital, there was no one there to greet them. They took the elevator to the second floor. When the elevator door opened, the whole staff was standing there whispering. My Mom looked into the eyes of one of the nurses and knew. She turned to my Dad and said, "He is dead, Ray!"

What happened next has defined my parents' understanding of what health care is in our country and has motivated me to work so hard to change our health care system. It is the picture my parents have of their son every morning when they get up and every evening when they go to bed.

Screaming, my parents ran down the hall to Mike's room. They stood in the doorway and saw Mike lying in the bed, his arm hanging over the side with the I.V. still in it. My Mom and Dad traveled the space from the doorway to their son with a horrific feeling of failure, the failure every parent fears. The fear that they have not protected their child from harm. They felt guilt for trusting someone else with this task, and now they experienced the ultimate mistake that cannot be undone.

My Dad tried to put Mike's arm under the sheet but was unable to bend it. They leaned over their six foot, 200 pound son and hugged and kissed him. He was so cold, Mike was never cold, and he certainly could not be dead!

My Dad saw death in two wars but has suffered no greater trauma than seeing his healthy, loving son who had died alone, in a room, in a hospital, in a community he trusted. There is no emotional or physical pain greater than the loss of a child.

When people die in airplanes, their families are brought to the site where parts of the plane are gathered so they can attempt to begin the process of closure. They have grief counselors and supporting family members with them. An investigative process is begun immediately to try and find answers as to why the tragedy occurred. The families are kept informed and told what is found.

My parents were allowed to go to the body of their dead son with no one there to support them. They were made to feel they deserved no answers about what had happened to their son, as if dying under the care of the medical profession relieves the profession of any accountability. No one would talk to them about their son's last hours alive. My parents were treated with silence and compassionless statements. The death of my brother was a tragedy, but the treatment of my family is what makes the tragedy horrific.

My parents asked for an autopsy, and when they called the hospital about it, they were told the doctors were too busy to go over it. We wondered why the hospital staff found it necessary to continue putting us through such agony by not telling us how Mike had died. They continued to tell us by their actions that he did not matter, nor did we. Did they not realize that by not knowing we could not begin to deal with the loss? It is the hardest thing to understand: "How could they not care for him? Where was their compassion? How could they continue to treat us with such callousness?"

Do you know how difficult it was for my parents to walk up to that building again when the staff finally called them to the hospital for the autopsy results? To go through those doors and face people who had no compassion for them? The doctors told my parents that Mike died from blood around the heart. My parents asked how it got there. The answer was they did not know, and then they began with excuses. They had had people from a car accident come in that afternoon and the emergency room was busy.

The last thing a family wants to hear is that someone else was more important than their own loved one who therefore was not cared for. If they were so busy, why not tell the family so they could have a choice to take their loved one somewhere else?

Mike was misdiagnosed. The doctor made a mistake. A mistake! He never even tried to help him. Was any of the information my mother passed to the nurse even given a second thought? My parents left the hospital a second time still in shock over the fact that they had actually trusted their son to these people. Guilt, oh the guilt, anger, betrayal, disbelief. "Just give us one more chance, God. We will do better."

When I arrived at my parents' house, they were chastising themselves for leaving Mike alone, for taking him to that hospital. Of course a different hospital would not have treated Mike or them the way this hospital had treated them. They were unable to comprehend how the trust they had in the hospital to care for Mike could be ripped from them. It was a trust ingrained in them by their upbringing in a society that teaches people to blindly trust their doctors. This is with the people who had not cared for him. I had to move away from blaming an individual in Mike's death to looking at the system that failed all of us.

I tried to approach the subject of system failure with my parents, but they could not and cannot remove the last image they have of Mike in that bed—an image that was preventable if those involved had been trained by the system to handle such a situation with compassion instead of fear. My parents have a great deal of anger over the loss of their son, and I cannot deny them their feelings. I pray every night that their hearts can heal.

I was constantly dogging the National Patient Safety Foundation to let me get involved; to me, it was painfully apparent that the key player (the consumer) was not part of fixing the problem. I wanted to be part of the solution, as a tribute to my brother—to give his death meaning, because it had been so utterly useless. I started talking to my friends, coworkers, and email contacts about being partners in their health care.

One lesson I took away from my brother's death is that you do not leave your loved ones alone in the hospital. They are very vulnerable both emotionally and physically and need your support. They may not always believe that themselves, and it is very easy to talk yourself out of it, but I was to learn firsthand how important it was.

In June 2000, I went to see a specialist in internal medicine for symptoms I had been having. It had taken me several visits to Urgent Care and several phone calls to my insurance company's nurse line to convince me to set up an appointment with what everyone was calling a "primary care doctor." I did not have a clue I was supposed to have a primary care doctor. My obstetrician/gynecologist had always been the doctor I saw, and this time the nurse flat-out told me the doctor does not see people for headaches! To me, this just proved how uncaring and cold the health care workers were—no wonder Mike had died as he had!

I was very nervous about seeing a doctor. I knew something was wrong with me, but I also knew there was a good possibility I was suffering from depression. A wall had been put up between me and anyone in health care because of what had happened to Mike. I did not want this doctor to just write me off as depressed. I knew I had to tell him about Mike, and I was not sure what kind of reaction I would get by doing that.

He came into the exam room, washed his hands, and then sat down and asked me what was wrong. I looked at him and began crying, saying I had things to tell him and was not sure how he would react. This man very professionally but with complete honesty looked at me and said, "I am your doctor, Roxanne, and you can tell me anything you have to tell me." I was so relieved and encouraged by what he said; I took out a page-long list of symptoms. I have recently been told that this would have made many physicians turn ashen and begin to sweat profusely, but mine took it in stride. I told him briefly about Mike a system that fails doctors, too. My parents were educated the hard way price of the lesson, the death of their son. We can no longer blindly tru the health care system. We must become educated in our role as patient; the part we must play in ensuring our safety.

My parents tried to rationalize why no one cared for Mike. We found later that Mike had no insurance. Is that why they did not try to find out was wrong with him? Once again, my parents say, "Why didn't they ask us would have given everything to have Mike cared for."

The community was also in shock; Mike had so many friends who angry and wanted answers too. Those who could have given some answer; behind the hospital doors. The hospital administrator, who attends church my parents, offered no condolences. Is this the kind of person who is in ch of caring for their community's health? We are able to forgive mistakes but indifference, not denial and hiding. Why are the family members ignc shunned, and treated by the responsible facility as if they are at fault? Mike not need to die. In an age of medical miracles, he was not even given a cha He was quieted with a drug and left alone.

I began spending much of my time trying to find answers or to hel; dealing with the grief, injustice, and murder of our trust. I searched the Inte for "medical error" and came up with one hit. It was to the National Pat Safety Foundation (NPSF) website, and there I found that a regional forum going to take place in Milwaukee at the end of October 1999. I contacted organization via email and asked if I could attend. I told them I had recently my brother to a medical error and wanted to see what was being done about problem. They said yes.

It was a surreal experience. When the keynote speaker got up and be comparing the aviation profession to the medical field, a light of understand started to glow in my mind. I was in aviation, trained as an air traffic control I began to understand how what happened to Mike could have occurred, understanding and accepting were two different things. I ended up in fron the forum telling what little we knew of my brother's death and how we j wanted to be talked to honestly and for someone involved with Mike's death validate our loss.

During the drive to my parents' house after the forum, I started to realize h dangerous health care is and the struggle that was going on to bring errors light, to learn from them, and to do something about them. I started to thi about what happened to Mike and how to work with the hospital to correct t flaws in the system that failed him and those entrusted with his care. I slov began to realize that I was going to have to forgive so I could work with the individuals within the health care system to make a change. This was a gre struggle for me. I felt as though I was betraying my brother in my desire to wo and admitted that I could be suffering some depression but felt something else was wrong. He took notes and at the end of my list he said the symptoms could indicate many different things, including depression, but the plan was to check me physically first. Then he asked me if I agreed with that course of action! Someone in health care actually cared and wanted to involve me. The feeling of empowerment and trust I had for this doctor directed me in my quest to be a partner with my health care providers and no longer just a patient.

The last symptom I gave the doctor was shortness of breath, which I had been experiencing for the last two years. I was not going to tell him that it was probably due to the weight I had put on and my lack of exercise. I was embarrassed, but this man made me feel that I could tell him and he would not judge me negatively. It was the one symptom for which he ordered a chest X-ray, which eventually led to the discovery of my tumor.

On July 20, 2000, I was diagnosed with a malignant thymoma and underwent open chest surgery to remove a tumor next to my heart and lungs. I put into practice what I had been preaching since Mike's death: have someone with you twenty-four hours a day, seven days a week while in the hospital. My team of family and friends were great; they worked with the health care staff, knowing my medications and when I was to get them. They supported me emotionally, and anytime I opened my eyes someone I recognized was sitting there. I ended up suffering a pulmonary embolism my second day in the hospital, and many nurses have tried to convince me it was the fault of the registered nurse on duty that day. I do not believe that for one minute. I saw once again how the system failed her and me. She was covering twice the number of patients she should have been, and I had not been educated about the importance of becoming mobile as soon as possible after surgery. The appointment I had later with a doctor specializing in this area indicated to me that this clot had been waiting to happen and the surgery had just hurried it along. I was fortunate to be in the hospital when it happened.

The journey I have recently had in the health care system was very different from the one I would have had if Mike had not died the way he did. My little brother's death opened my eyes to the fact that we need to be partners in our health care, that our health care workers are not God or miracle workers. They are human just like us and need our help to do their job well and to make our journeys as safe as possible.

In my attempt to understand and, hopefully, do something about medical error, I started comparing health care to my own profession as an air traffic controller. I looked at the decisions that are made by controllers in the course of a normal day and how they could mean the life or death of many people. We do not work in a vacuum where our decisions and actions are completely our own. Instead, we work in a complex system where every decision made or action taken becomes part of a history that results in a particular outcome. There are times when we must distance ourselves from the image of our customers to accomplish the job and at the same time communicate with them in a professional, humane manner to instill confidence and trust in our abilities. As humans in both aviation and health care, we make mistakes and must learn from them to improve. That is where our two professions split.

The health care creed is "Do no harm." The controllers' is "Safety above all else." At first glance, they seem to mean the same thing, but when mistakes and errors happen they need to be brought into the light and looked at or they will continue to do harm. Presently, the health care system buries its errors. The aviation profession looks at its errors and adjusts and implements solutions to correct system flaws, making safety the number one priority.

I began to realize from this comparison with my own profession that the system health care workers function in was failing them and us. I asked someone at my facility who was recently involved in the evaluation of an error what he thought punishment accomplished in dealing with errors. He said, "Punishment does not prevent error; it prevents the reporting of it."

I am a firm believer in addressing the system and how it is failing. We have been blaming and punishing the individual, and it has not made health care safe. It has actually built a wall of distrust and misunderstanding between the health care workers themselves and their customers. It is this wall that prevents the communication and honesty that is needed to identify and correct the flaws in the system, which are contributing to errors.

I had a conversation with someone about a woman who had been given an epidural for knee surgery and all of a sudden was unable to breath. It was found that she had been given too much anesthetic and it had started to affect her lungs. The person I was talking to said that is a malpractice suit. I cringe when I hear that word as the first option we think about as consumers. I said to her, "Do you think that doctor deliberately gave the woman too much anesthetic?" Why don't we look at the system and how it failed this doctor and patient? The key to looking at the system is that we all must do our part to make it work. It needs to be addressed and supported from the top down, and that includes the patient and his or her family. There is concern that if we do not attribute blame for a harmful error to an individual, there will be no responsibility taken at all. If we work as a team, however, that concept actually increases the responsibility for each individual to do his or her part, both in error prevention and in humanely addressing the harms experienced by patients and their families.

When you are in a profession where mistakes take people's lives, it takes a lot of courage to admit you are capable of making those mistakes. I know. I am in the same type of profession. The difference that I have seen between my profession and health care is how we approach it. In health care, you are told you have to be perfect and cannot make mistakes, and therefore when they do happen, you hide them, deny them, and even ostracize those who have made them—as if you would never have made the same mistake. We, on the other hand, are told that we are human and can make mistakes, and we do our best to stay vigilant to that fact when doing our job.

As a family, we take part of the responsibility for Mike's death. We left him alone and should have been there to speak for him when he could not. Maybe he would have died anyway, but at least he would not have died alone. I envision that Mike, in the health care system of the future, would have taken a more active part as well. He would have known of the history of aneurysms in our family and how his own history of high blood pressure could contribute to his risk of having one. He would have been more aware of the risks and more educated about the symptoms.

When I began to understand the enormous task of patient safety, I became overwhelmed by it and had to decide what contribution I could make. I believe in the need to involve the patient and the family in whatever directions are taken by the industry. Patients and families are key players on the team, and all the efforts made to improve health care will be for naught if they are not educated in their role. We need to help the public and the health care workers themselves understand that it is the system of blame and secrecy that is failing us all.

CHAPTER 4

Error Disclosure for Quality Improvement: Authenticating a Team of Patients and Providers to Promote Patient Safety

BRYAN A. LIANG

Introduction

Tremendous attention has recently arisen regarding the social issue of medical error and its role in patient injury and quality of care. Traditionally, an individually oriented "shame and blame" conception of quality has been the standard, with the tort system focused upon individual actor blame for harm, accreditation standards based upon individual entity compliance and punishment, and medical culture reliance on an individual provider ethic of perfection (Hupert et al. 1996; Leape 1994; Liang 2001a; Liang and Storti 2000). Despite these mechanisms, over the past five decades, medical error and patient injury continue to plague the health care delivery system, and, indeed, this shame orientation and blame ideal have created barriers to practice change, quality improvement efforts, and improved health care (Davidoff 2002; Shekelle 2002). Such poor results have provided a significant impetus for reevaluating these traditional methods.

This reevaluation has resulted in the emergence of an understanding that the traditional methods focused upon a particular individual making a specific error are ineffective in improving performance within highly complex systems such as medicine (Leape 1994; Reason 1990). With the advent of new understandings and recognitions regarding the systems nature of error, and the success of other similarly complex industries such as aviation and nuclear power in using these lessons to reduce the incidence of error and to improve efficiency and efficacy, there is room for optimism that similar results could attend in health care (Liang 2001a).

Unfortunately, current legal and medical cultures continue to maintain the individually oriented perspective regarding error and injury (Liang 1999, 2001a). Further, accreditation organizations and others within the professions and the public, using the patient safety and medical error platform, now call for simple disclosure of errors to patients without reference to the systems nature of error, how these disclosures practically affect care, or how these disclosures could promote safety and quality;[1] indeed, such reactionary calls for indiscriminate disclosure reflect the shame and blame ethic. Moreover, they result in only *ex post* unidirectional information flow and do not authenticate the important role of partnership between patients, their families, and providers in medical care. Indeed, such mandates do not empower patients and/or families to directly impact care as part of the delivery team and to be another set of eyes to identify errors and reduce their consequences.

Thus, at present, although there has been a recognition of the fundamental basis of error—systems—the medical and legal communities as well as the general public have yet to embrace systems concepts to improve safety in health care delivery (Liang 2002a). Further, many who call for full disclosure of errors in the name of safety use patient safety jargon to simply promote the individually oriented, status quo "shame and blame" approach.[2] Unfortunately, such perspectives drive the knowledge and observations of error underground, fating others in the future to be subject to the same systems infrastructures and injuries that could have been corrected had they been discussed and addressed (Leape 1994).

Instead, following the successful model from other industries, to address the nature, incidence, and effect of error on safety, a systems approach must be undertaken that allows for all members of the system team to contribute to the safety enterprise (Liang 2000d, 2002a). In health care, this team includes providers and patients. By integrating providers and patients, each with rights and responsibilities, and by promoting communication between the two as equal partners, safety in health care can be advanced and a greater therapeutic relationship can be attained. However, such a partnership and relationship will require not only a recognition of the weaknesses that derive from current medical and legal systems, but also an adherence to an ideal of mutual respect that is often stated but little implemented (Liang 2002a).

Such an effort can begin with a system of medical error disclosure that takes into account current perspectives and educates providers and patients regarding medical error, patient injury, and systems processes. Further, in contrast to calls for disclosure that presume patients to have only rights, and providers to have only obligations, such an effort should be designed to indicate the essential role of both in promoting safety.

Error and Systems

Medical Error and Patient Injury

Medical error can be defined as a mistake, inadvertent occurrence, or unintended event in a health care delivery which may, or may not, result in patient injury (Liang 2000d). This definition in no way includes purposeful or reckless actions intended to directly or indirectly harm the patient. The distinction is critical. Purposeful or reckless actions are malicious and volitional—not the result of error; moreover, they are the source of a small minority of patient injuries in the health care system. Instead of focusing on bad actors, a focus on safety should be directed to the much more frequent problem of error by individuals who are in good faith trying to perform effectively, but are working in systems where mistakes can and do occur.[3]

The Basics of Error

Error occurs as part of the systems in which humans act to achieve a wide array of high-level social goals (Reason 1990). Importantly, "no matter how professional they might be, no matter their care and concern, humans can never outperform the system which bounds and constrains them" (Maurino, Reason, and Lee 1995, 83). Consequently, human error is both ubiquitous and inevitable.

Researchers have extensively studied the condition of human error and have identified the cognitive processes involved in error occurrence (Reason 1990). Errors arise from two major sources: unintentional actions made while performing routine tasks, and mistakes made as a result of mistaken judgment or inadequate plans of action. Humans are subject to two types of failures in this system: *active failures*—errors and violations of rules; and managerial or *latent failures*—those focused on the organizational or systemic processes in which the human operates.

Latent failures, those embedded in the design and structure of complex systems, are considered to be the most dangerous, particularly since they often remain unrecognized and extant in the system, increasing the potential for adverse events in the future and predisposing the system to failure. Under these conditions, latent errors are "accidents waiting to happen," with the human operator "'set up' to fail" (Leape 1994). It should be noted that active failures are ultimately part and parcel of and have origins within latent failures in the system (Reason 1990, 2000).

Complex systems have several layers of activity, each representing both a source of and a defense against error occurrence and associated adverse consequences. In the "swiss-cheese" model of error, each system layer has holes and solid areas—holes of active and particularly latent system failures and solid areas representing barriers against the occurrence of adverse events associated with error. When the holes of failure line up, an error penetrates through the entire system, resulting in an accident or adverse event (see figure I.1, this volume; Reason 1990). Of course, holes may line up only partially, allowing the error to penetrate all but a last barrier; these "near-miss" situations, thankfully, do not result in an adverse event and are much more common than total penetration.

Complex systems have a high potential for error. Generally, these errors result from common characteristics these systems share: for example, high-level technical requirements, the need for quick reaction times, twenty-four-hour-a-day/seven-day-a-week operations, team coordination, long hours, and trade-offs between service and safety. Also common to complex systems is the reality that one individual is not responsible for the outcome of the entire system and that very few errors lead to adverse events (Foushee and Helmreich 1988; Lauber and Kayten 1990; Liang 1999; Maurino, Reason, and Lee 1995; Reason 1990). The recognition that one individual is not solely responsible for error bears some emphasis. Using aviation as an example, it is not the pilot alone who is responsible for getting passengers to the appropriate destination without injury. The pilot, the stewards, the ground staff, the maintenance crew, and the air traffic controllers—each and every one of these aviation system members contribute to the outcome, positive or negative. Just as it is not the last person who touches the controls, it is not the last person who touches the patient who is solely responsible for the final outcome; it is the system that is the necessary and appropriate focus (Leape 1994; Leape et al. 1998; Liang 2000d; Voelker 1996).

Successful error reduction in complex systems has recognized and taken advantage of the systems nature of error, relying on both reactive interventions to error occurrence and proactive interventions for error prevention. A systems approach uses a continuous process involving several stages, with the goal of preventing errors and/or their negative effects. The stages of this error-reduction paradigm are in-process detection, process change/design, and process reassessment. They loop continuously for each detected error and intervention. Both the aviation and the nuclear power industries successfully instituted these systems-analysis and corrective-action efforts, so that errors and accidents were significantly reduced and productivity increased in both industries (Liang 1999).

This fundamental systems-based nature of error and its successful reduction clearly indicates that individually oriented, "shame and blame" mechanisms are antithetical to and ineffective in reducing human error (Leape 1994; Leape et al. 1998; Reason 1990). Because it is not the last person who touches the controls or patient that is responsible for the entire system outcome, shame and blame of that individual is counterproductive and serves only to drive knowledge and information on error underground; this recognition is particularly important due to the ease of hiding error in complex systems (Leape 1994). Such a focus neither induces the individual to perform at his or her best, nor the system of which he or she is a part to perform at its best (Liang 2000d). Fear of punishment simply does not promote mistake elimination, nor does it maximize system function; instead, a cooperative, nonthreatening, blame-free approach encompassing the entire system and its members is the primary tenet for effective error reduction in complex systems (Leape 1994; Moore 1998).

Problems: Medical and Legal Cultures

Medicine

The traditional method utilized by the medical profession in attempting to reduce medical error is based upon shame and blame of individuals—a "moral qualities" approach (Hupert et al. 1996). Because physicians and other providers are held to a standard of perfection, there is tremendous pressure for providers to never make an error—an impossible task—or at a minimum, never admit to one. Through attempting to shame an individual into believing that an error indicates a lack of professionalism, competence, and even the right to treat patients, this "gentlemanly honor" model (Sharpe 2000a) does not recognize the successful systems-based nature of error reduction and outcomes (Christensen, Levinson, and Dunn 1992; Hilfiker 1984; Leape 1994; Liang 2000d; Wu et al. 1991). Attempts to "correct" the error are entirely reactive, focusing on preventing the error from being repeated by the specific person who made it; systems assessments identifying underlying and root causes remain unexplored. As such, and particularly in combination with medical liability concerns, providers fear admitting mistakes;[4] thus, information is driven underground and key lessons that could have been learned from these situations are lost. This approach represents a tremendous failure in addressing medical error and patient injury.[5]

To make matters worse, providers more recently have placed significant reliance upon the concept of "risk management" to assist them in attaining this impossible level of performance. Unfortunately, this latter hope is likely to be misplaced. First, risk management, a concept derived from the malpractice crises of the 1970s and 1980s, is focused on managing risks of financial loss associated with malpractice suits, rather than on error analysis, safety principles, and corrective action associated with health delivery systems and care. Second, empirical study has indicated that there is no apparent reduction in patient injuries for those who engage in these activities, and indeed, there may be a counterproductive effect that could increase the chance of patient injury and lawsuit following recent participation in these risk management activities (Frisch et al. 1995; Liang 2000f; Walsh and Dineen 1998).

The medical culture does not recognize the fundamental reality that errors do occur, and to effectively address patient injury, providers must accept this fact and then work to design systems that take this reality into account. Indeed, a damning indictment of this lack of recognition is that there has been little or no educational attention in the professional fields on the student, postgraduate, and staff levels regarding systems, teamwork, and patients as members of the error reduction team.

Unfortunately, there is an additional barrier to effective systems analysis: the Joint Commission on Accreditation of Healthcare Organizations (JCAHO) sentinel events policy (SEP) (Joint Commission 2001b). The SEP mandates[6] that certain adverse events be reported to the JCAHO, that the hospital perform a self-critical, systems-based root cause analysis of these adverse events, and that the hospital submit this root cause analysis to JCAHO for review and approval. However, while this approach appears to recognize in theory the systems nature of error, in effect it is administered under the inappropriate "shame and blame" punitive rubric. For example, JCAHO may disclose to third parties, such as the lay press, that the particular entity is under sentinel event review. Further, if the adverse report is not made, or if the root cause analysis is not considered acceptable, JCAHO may place the provider on "accreditation watch," with the potential of revoking the provider's accreditation (Joint Commission 2001b).

This approach has raised valid legal concerns and created significant provider resistance to the policy (Liang 2000e; Liang and Storti 2000). Such a policy is also in direct contravention of the cooperative, nonthreatening, blame-free mechanism essential for reducing errors. Thus, as expected, the policy, and other similarly situated mandatory reporting systems such as state laws requiring reports of adverse events, have captured only a tiny fraction of adverse events—fewer than 1 percent of the errors associated with patient injury in hospitals, even under the best of assumptions (Liang 2000b, 2000e). Therefore, although the potential recognition of the systems nature of error may be a positive step, the shame and blame and potential punishment enforcement mechanisms are a step back to the traditional system (Liang 2000d).[7] Unfortunately, the practical effect of this policy may be to force medical error, patient injury, and the systems processes that cause them underground to avoid the potential punitive loss of accreditation.

Finally, the extant culture in health care inhibits open discussion of medical errors. Due to the "need" for perfection, the belief that an error represents a moral failure, and the practical reputational effects that disclosure of errors may cause, physicians are reticent to discuss them. Consistent with this, patients report that they frequently sue providers in response to their frustration over the lack of information regarding their care (Hickson et al. 1992, 1994; Shapiro et al. 1989). Moreover, beyond these patient communication concerns, other patient needs including resolution of uncertainty (Lester and Smith 1993), the need to vent and to be heard (Beckman et al. 1994), and acknowledgment of suffering (Vincent, Young, and Phillips 1994) create an impetus, beyond simple financial concerns, to sue providers.

Even within this culture, however, there is literature to suggest that patients and their families are much less likely to engage in lawsuits if they have a positive, open, and honest relationship with their health care providers (Levinson et al. 1997); there is also anecdotal evidence to suggest that full disclosure and honest admission of errors may result in smaller damage settlements and awards (Kraman and Hamm 1999; Levinson 1994). This information indicates the significant barrier that the current predominant medical culture represents, and one potential avenue for successfully moving past it.

Law

Traditional legal systems also assume the approach of individual shame and blame in an effort to reduce error and promote safety. The longest-standing social incentive structure reflecting this approach is the tort system—and specifically for health care, the medical malpractice system.

Unfortunately, civil suits under the tort system are perhaps the ultimate individually oriented, shame and blame mechanism. Such a system focuses upon punishing a particular individual for a particular error; it does not recognize the systems issues involved in health care provision. Indeed, lawsuits may result in additional risks for provider error and patient injury (Liang 2000f; Passineau 1998). As well, a lawsuit fractionates the members of the health care team—providers and patients—and creates a tremendous incentive to limit, rather than open, communication lines between these individuals (Liang 2001b). Under these circumstances, system failure conditions remain latent; and, adding insult to injury, most patients after enduring the high emotional and administrative costs associated with civil litigation are often never compensated, or must wait long periods of time before they receive any compensation (Brennan 1999; Liang 2001b). Patients who have been injured are perhaps the most vulnerable of individuals, and the least likely to weather effectively the legal machinations, personal scrutiny, and various maneuverings necessary to support litigation (Liang 2001b). Thus, traditional tort law not only thwarts the communicative environment essential for error reduction, it also results in only poor, significantly delayed compensation for a few of the countless patients who have been injured.

Further, on the provider level, for those individuals who wish to engage in safety activities through thorough systems assessments and corrective action, the legal system provides distinct disincentives for these willing participants to do so. Self-critical patient safety and corrective action assessments result in highly sensitive materials that discuss systems issues, sources of error, and potential failure locales within a health delivery entity. If these materials are not limited to their intended use for safety and corrective action purposes—in other words, if they are discoverable for use in a lawsuit—there will be tremendous negative incentives to prepare them, and for providers to participate in safety activities. Unfortunately, this very circumstance appears currently to be the case.

Generally, all materials that are not protected by legal privilege are legally discoverable. Even materials not admissible in court are discoverable if these materials are "reasonably calculated" to lead to admissible materials (Liang 2000e; Liang and Storti 2000). Further, the U.S. Supreme Court has issued discovery rules that indicate all "relevant" materials must be *automatically* provided to the opposing party without request (Liang 2000e; Liang and Storti 2000). Thus, with such significant legal favor to material discovery, it is essential to assess the scope of legal privilege protections for materials created in the safety realm.

Unfortunately, legal privilege does not appear to be effective in limiting safety information to safety use. The major legal privilege protections touted by accreditors and others as protecting safety information are the peer review/quality assurance (PR/QA) privilege and the attorney-client privilege (Liang 2000e; Liang and Storti 2000). However, these legal privileges are quite limited in protecting safety information. Although there are several difficulties with assessing such privileges, including their basis in state and federal law and their variations across jurisdictions, some major themes emerge upon review. First, the PR/QA privilege does not appear to apply to materials collected and created "in the normal course of business." Because safety information and assessment in an enlightened health care enterprise would likely be collected as part of its standard operations, such information could easily fall outside the PR/QA privilege (Liang 1999, 2000d, 2000e; Liang and Storti 2000).

In addition, attorney-client privilege does not apply to information discussed in any manner *other than* in preparation for litigation. Thus, if collected information were discussed for the purposes of improving patient safety and reducing medical error, the attorney-client privilege would not protect these discussions or any resulting information (Liang 2000d; Liang and Storti 2000). Thus, building on these major legal privileges appears to be building on a soft foundation at best.

Furthermore, this state of affairs is also made difficult by the nature of the rules of the U.S. court system. If a patient injury suit is brought in federal court (rather than state court), no *state-based* privilege law generally applies. Hence, reliance upon state-based privileges such as PR/QA, even in the most protective of states, is misguided, for these privileges do not generally apply in federal court (Liang 2000e; Liang and Storti 2000). And in any event, even in the best of circumstances—strong state PR/QA privilege and suit in state court—due to the extensive nature of systems analysis and the broad array of persons who are engaged in systems assessments, most of this information can be elicited by standard subpoena and testimony. Indeed, some courts refuse to break the PR/QA privilege for plaintiff's attorneys, simply because they can elicit the same information from standard subpoena and testimony mechanisms (Liang 2000e; Liang and Storti 2000).

Other legal problems inhibit participation and discussion of safety and quality issues. For example, when Medicare patients lodge a complaint against a Medicare provider, generally a Medicare Quality Improvement Organization (QIO) investigates the complaint. Note that no actual injury need occur for purposes of instigating a complaint and an investigation. Due to the sensitive nature of such an investigation and in order to promote participation and frank discussion by providers of the relevant clinical activities, the information gleaned by the QIO is necessarily confidential. However, a federal court has recently overturned these regulatory rules, and has held that Medicare QIO investigation findings must be provided to the patient and/or his or her representative/attorney within twenty days of completion (Liang 2001a). Although quality findings should be disclosed to patients, such a blanket holding of disclosure in the current legal environment will severely chill participation in these quality activities and the full and frank discussion of the circumstance by those who may be directly or indirectly involved. Further, such a holding will provide an opportunity for legal maneuvering to obtain sensitive information that may not have been subject to normal disclosure; it may also serve as a vehicle to obtain the names of potential parties to sue in order to maximize the opportunity to obtain settlement or judgment amounts (Liang 2001a).[8] Indeed, because injury need not occur and information disclosure is not limited to those dictated by the discovery rules, the potential for access to safety information to support lawsuits may be quite high.

Further, public mandates under the law may also chill safety activities and efforts. For example, between one and two dozen states in the U.S. have adverse event reporting statutes (Kohn, Corrigan, and Donaldson 2000; Liang 2000d). Under these statutes, specific adverse events must be reported to the state Department of Health or equivalent agency, under the provider's name— emphasizing the blame ideal. Further, such mandates have significant legal risks for unintended use rather than for safety activities. First, this information may in fact be used against the provider for purported poor quality of care—the reasoning being that "because" an adverse event/medical error occurred at the facility, quality at that facility "must be" poor. Second, the information may be discoverable under general discovery rules as indicated above. And third, under the state's freedom of information act, since the information is supplied to a public entity such as the state Department of Health, the information may be disclosed through a citizen's/attorney's freedom of information act request.

It should be noted that JCAHO SEP materials may be subject to discovery through legal maneuvers. These highly sensitive, self-critical materials have been subject to discovery in malpractice lawsuits (Liang 2001a). Further, since the JCAHO has "deemed" authority by the federal government that allows those accredited by it to serve and charge Medicare beneficiaries for services, provision of SEP materials to the JCAHO is equivalent to provision of this information to the federal government. As such, these materials may be vulnerable to disclosure under the federal Freedom of Information Act (Liang and Storti 2000; Liang 2000e). Finally, as a practical concern, since these highly sensitive materials were authored by the facility/provider itself, they may be seen by the agents of the legal system—judges and juries—as an admission of fault (Liang 2000d).

In relation to lawsuits, another major and practical concern attends: the vagaries of medical liability insurance. Generally, these insurance contracts contain a standard clause: the "no statements/no actions" clause. Under this provision, the insured agrees to take no actions and to make no statements that could impede the insurer from defending against the claim. Such a provision has tremendous implications for patient safety work. If patient safety activities and assessments are deemed discoverable, not only are providers subject to a lawsuit, they are subject to a lawsuit with highly sensitive information in the plaintiff attorney's hands; indeed, this information may be considered "relevant" and therefore must be disclosed automatically under U.S. Supreme Court rules. Further, by participating in patient safety activities—including the creation of discoverable materials—these providers certainly have taken actions and/or made statements that would impede the insurer from defending the claim. Thus, providers who participate in safety work may be in breach of the liability insurance contract and may face suit and potential liability without liability insurance (Liang 2000d, 2001a). As such, there are significant incentives against participating in safety activities due to the likelihood that these activities may be used against those who engage in good faith in this quality improvement effort.

Solidifying this risk, insurers themselves are sometimes resistant to any change from the litigation process, therefore reinforcing these negative provider incentives to engage in safety work. As Dauer, Marcus, and Payne (2000) have reported, litigation serves to inhibit relatively low-level claims that might otherwise be pursued if the high cost of doing so were reduced, say, through alternative dispute resolution. Such a litigation threshold keeps claims costs down for medical liability insurers. Further, litigation provides a well-defined role for insurers, thus allowing them to preserve their role and existence in the process. These interdependent concepts result in a circumstance where "[t]he legal system is acting properly within its frame of reference; insurance organizations are operating properly within theirs. It is [this] symbiosis that results in resistance to change" (185).

This state of affairs is particularly important because the vast majority of physicians in the United States are considered to be independent contractors. In the United States, independent contractors are generally alone on the liability hook for all patient injury—even when they are subject to health plan patient lists, exclusive contracts, call schedule, utilization review requirements, clinical practice guidelines, and method of payment. Consequently, physicians may be reticent to report errors and participate in delivery system patient safety activities when they bear the full economic and emotional costs of liability (Liang 1997a, 1997b, 1998, 2001a). Further, on the basis of standard independent-contractor contract law, independent contractors may be terminated, or in medical care parlance, "deselected," for any or no reason at all, even in bad faith, as long as civil rights laws are not implicated. Thus, providers who continuously request organizational commitment to patient safety activities, aggressively advocate for patients through promoting programs on medical error reduction and awareness, and/or report errors that may in fact potentially put the health plan in a negative light (or be perceived by management to do so) are at significant risk for deselection. It is eminently logical from a business perspective, but not from a patient safety perspective, to eliminate these high-cost providers (Liang 2001a). Since, practically speaking, independent contractors cannot be so brazen as to ignore their financial lifeline, such legal realities may put a significant damper upon broad-based participation in error reduction activities (Liang 1998, 2000d, 2001a).

Finally, even assuming away difficulties associated with the tort law, legal privilege, and independent-contractor law, there may be a significant practical problem in performing patient safety work at all. The source of this difficulty is HIPAA: the Health Insurance Portability and Accountability Act, and specifically, its medical privacy provisions. This law and its accompanying regulations cover all forms and uses of patient-identifiable information: oral, written, and electronic.

Formerly, written HIPAA "consent" was required to be obtained by providers and other covered entities from patients for all routine treatment, payment, and health care operations functions. However, changes to the regulations in August 2002 have obviated the need for such administrative HIPAA consent to use or disclose patient information for these purposes (Department of Health and Human Services 2002b); instead, providers and other covered entities must provide patients with notice of the patient's privacy rights and the privacy practices and policies of the provider or entity and must make a good-faith effort to obtain written acknowledgment of this notice from patients.[9]

However, for all nonroutine treatment, payment, and health care operation functions, it appears that HIPAA "authorization" will most likely be mandated.[10] Since patient safety researchers need access to patient information in order to assess health delivery systems, HIPAA privacy rules apply to these activities. However, at the outset, there are no provisions in the regulations that explicitly discuss or allow for patient safety work. Further, although health care operations distinctly include "quality improvement," the regulations specifically note that such activities performed *cannot* result in "generalizable knowledge"—any such activities must be performed under the research exception (see below). Hence, it would appear that qualitative patient safety research cannot be performed under HIPAA consent provisions, since one primary goal of this work is, in fact, to obtain generalizable knowledge of health delivery systems in order to reduce medical errors (Liang 2001a).

Patient safety researchers and participants may instead consider obtaining HIPAA authorization from patients in an effort to gain access to patient-identifiable materials so as to perform safety work. However, beyond the significant issue of precluding larger population studies, there are extensive requirements to obtain valid HIPAA authorization (Code of Federal Regulations 2000). As such, it may be highly impractical, expensive, and administratively cumbersome to draft specific authorizations for each unique safety circumstance and investigation, even assuming the information sought could be specified in advance, which in qualitative safety work may be impossible. Simply put, with such authorization requirements, providers and patients may perceive creating and considering, respectively, its contents to be too costly to contemplate in time, energy, and resources (Liang 2001a).

There are three exceptions to the authorization requirements, and safety workers may consider these as an avenue to perform this work. However, two immediately do not apply: the health oversight activities exception and the public health activities exception. The former focuses upon fraud and abuse and licensure activities of the state; the latter focuses on traditional public health activities. And, perhaps most importantly, both apply only to public facilities and agencies rather than community providers. The final exception is research; however, the research exception contemplates clinical trials type work where specific information can be requested before the study begins, rather than qualitative patient safety activities, which require deeper and deeper analysis of the system and continuous identification of variables as system analysis progresses (Liang 2001a).

There is a safe harbor that can be used to fulfill the research exception: de-identification of patient information. This can either be shown through a person with "appropriate knowledge and experience" in statistics who indicates that the "risk is very small that the information could be used . . . to identify the subject" and through documenting this analysis; or through removing a laundry list of nineteen patient identifiers, including "[a]ny other unique identifying number, characteristic, or code." However, it is difficult to ascertain how "statistically" risks could be deemed "very small" for "inappropriate use" in research activities, and particularly for patient safety work; and moreover, because dramatic adverse events are rare, the event itself would have to be de-identified to fulfill the requirements of the rule, making the resulting information worthless to safety researchers.[11] This difficulty is exacerbated in nonurban communities and rural settings due to their smaller patient bases—the very providers who need to be engaged in this work for substantive progress to be made (Liang 2001a).

Finally, HIPAA compliance will be expensive: both government and private estimates have placed the cost of implementation in the tens of billions of dollars (Nolan 2001; Office of Management and Budget 2002). Further, harsh civil and criminal penalties—civil fines up to $25,000 and criminal penalties up to $250,000 and ten years in prison for each standard violation, which are not mutually exclusive (Liang 2000c)—ensure that providers err on the side of too little disclosure rather than too much. Unfortunately, since noncompliance with medical privacy provisions (as well as other compliance-based activities such as fraud and abuse) carries such heavy penalties, while organized, broad-based patient safety activities are voluntary, providers in a world of limited resources may have no choice but to focus on compliance-based requirements rather than safety. This is particularly true in nonurban communities and rural areas where the rule affects the vast majority of health care providers, but where providers have experienced long-standing financial difficulties and receive only a disproportionately low share of health care reimbursements (Liang 2001a). Unfortunately, these are the very frontline providers affected by the rule but whose participation and leadership are essential for patient safety promotion and implementation.

Disclosure: Addressing Medical and Legal Issues

A New Paradigm of Obligations and Rights

A systems approach to disclosure of medical error is essential to ameliorate the difficulties associated with misunderstandings regarding the genesis of error in the medical community, to educate and integrate patients in the safety effort, and to avoid the damaging effects and poor compensation function of litigation. Without such an approach, simply forcing disclosure of errors will improve neither understanding of safety principles nor the causes of error and needed system corrections and will propagate "shame and blame" approaches while inculcating further the current health delivery system's latent failures.

To fully integrate and realize the potential of members of the health care team in reducing errors and improving safety, it is vital to clearly define the obligations and rights of the members of the health delivery team. A foundational precept must reflect a true partnership and team of patient and provider consonant with the safety context and systems approach. The health care team has the following obligations:

- All members of the health delivery team have an obligation to assist in improving the system; this is the appropriate focus due to the systems nature of error and outcomes.

- Providers have an obligation to have appropriate medical knowledge, to be part of the systems process of care delivery, and to improve outcomes to result in an acceptable level of health.

- Patients have an obligation to maintain and communicate personal medical information and to be part of the systems process of care delivery and improvement that results in an acceptable level of health.

Accompanying these obligations are rights. The rights of the provider/patient health care team include the following:

- All members of the health care team have the right to point out, and discuss openly and honestly without sanction, errors that occur within the system, as well as to participate in corrective action to address the errors in a systems manner.

- Providers have the right to engage in error assessment and improvement of those process accidents of which they are a part or which affect their activities.

- Patients have the right to vent, communicate their perspectives regarding error, participate in corrective action, and obtain compensation for medical process accidents of which they are a part or which affect their activities.

Note that the inclusion of patients as partners in the health delivery system includes family members as well, since highly debilitated patients may not be in a position to be effective observers to promote safety.

These rights may or may not be legal rights; patients within Western jurisprudential boundaries are not always entitled to disclosure of all information (Hebert, Levin, and Robertson 2001; Liang 2000c). However, important ethical concerns surrounding mutual respect and partnership should mandate that shared responsibility reflect shared information between the parties—a concept not reflected by current disclosure mandates.

It should be noted that although there are extant medical ethics perspectives that indicate that providers, particularly physicians, should take all responsibility for errors, and that full disclosure of errors to patients should be the ethical standard, this perspective does not recognize the systems nature of error and outcomes (Liang 2002a). The idea of "taking responsibility" and blanket disclosure, without more attention to systems, simply represents a move back to traditional, individually oriented "shame and blame" approaches. Critically, as noted earlier, physicians can neither claim full credit for a positive patient outcome nor full responsibility for an error and a negative outcome; rather, it is a team effort involving, at a minimum, physicians, nurses, administration, and the patient him- or herself. This is a fundamental understanding vital to the success of systems-based error reduction methods and disclosure efforts.

This systems basis does not mean that providers forgo individual responsibilities. The system is now the focus of quality, and therefore all members of the health care enterprise must be vigilant regarding all aspects of care and must note all actual or potential sources of error, going beyond traditional activities, observations, and/or turf. As well, they must be flexible in learning and compensating for these errors and must use these observations as an opportunity for corrective action. As in aviation, corrective actions may include individually oriented activities; however, the difference between traditional medical methods and a systems approach is that such actions look to improving the system and its outcomes, occur in an environment of cooperation and continuous improvement, and focus on system performance, not on individual punishment.

Accountability

Consistent with these concepts, and in concert with the systems nature of error and outcomes, when error occurs because of failures within the system, the system is accountable to those who are affected by the failure. And if the terms of patient care obligations are to be taken seriously, operationalizing them means that system errors should be disclosed to those who have been adversely affected as a matter of mutual respect, trust, responsibility, and partnership (Liang 2002a). Such rights do not arise merely from legal rules or quasilegal accreditation rules that reflect a traditional medical care ethos and gentlemanly honor system, but instead from important ethical bases of obligations that health care team members have toward each other in the highly complex endeavor of health care delivery.

However, it bears emphasizing that disclosure and accountability rest with the system, rather than with an individual. Simply requiring the last person who touched the patient to take on a persona of humiliation and forcing him or her to disclose represents an iteration of the ineffective, individually oriented "shame and blame" approach. Instead, disclosure that takes the system as its basis and takes patient care philosophy to heart can result in opportunities to improve quality and enhance safety in the medical delivery system.

A System of Disclosure

Laying the Foundation

Due to the reality of systems having tremendous influence upon error and injury, the first step in creating a system of disclosure that promotes safety is to educate providers regarding this appropriate focus. Providers must be involved, first, in understanding the role systems play in error reduction, and, second, in instituting means by which these principles can be applied to daily practice. Leaders from "above and below," i.e., administrative personnel, clinical staff, and other support staff, must be engaged in this education, understanding, and application (Liang 2002a). Without such engagement, health delivery systems will not reap the benefits associated with an enlightened group using established error reduction means as experienced in other industries.

Next, integration and education of the other essential member of the health care team—the patient—must be accomplished (Liang 2000d, 2002a).[12] This is particularly important since many patients do not feel empowered to be part of the health delivery process (Editor's Choice 2002). Most medical care systems have an underlying philosophy and ethic regarding patients, including an ideal of partnership between patient and provider. Unfortunately, this partnership is not always implemented or respected. A philosophy of true partnership between these two as a team in the health care enterprise mandates that both engage jointly to ensure that appropriate care is provided at the right place at the right time to the right person in the safest and most efficacious manner possible.

Hence, beyond educating physicians regarding the systems nature of error and outcomes, patients, too, must be informed about and understand their role in promoting safety. Since there are many more patients than providers or administrators, patients represent a tremendous resource for system information. Further, their experience with the full spectrum of health care providers is unique among team members and therefore highly valuable (Liang 2000d). In order to engage the patient, a clear understanding between the provider and the patient should be entered into at the outset of all encounters (Liang 2002a)—an understanding that has been described as a "health care partnership agreement." This agreement would seek to have the patient not merely see the care and delivery system around them, but instead actively observe and report on it. For example:

> Medical care is complex and sometimes complicated. We believe that patients and their families are equal partners in the delivery of care and essential in improving the system. We will do everything we can to provide safe and effective care. As our partner, please ask any questions you have about care, please inform us of any information you think would assist in providing care, and in particular please let us know if you observe *any* mistakes and/or "eyebrow-raising events" in your care so we may use this important information as an opportunity to improve how we treat you and all patients. We want to work with you to make the best health delivery system for everyone! Thank you for your help and participation!

As relevant to the particular entity, the agreement should indicate that such information can be given to providers directly and/or to a well-identified patient care liaison or office if patients and/or their families feel uncomfortable in speaking with the provider. The period after such education may be an opportune time to discuss patient and family information use for patient safety activities. Further, to maximize information from patients consistent with this effort, patient and family surveys should be administered and collected on discharge that ascertain whether patient questions, information provided, and errors and/or "eyebrow-raising events" noted were appropriately answered, utilized, and addressed, respectively. Moreover, any additional concerns regarding these areas as well as a section on errors not reported by the patient and/or family during the patient's stay should be included.

This partnership agreement thus asks the patient and/or family to be an active partner in safety and empowers them to assume a direct role in the outcome of care. This approach also reflects the ideal of mutual trust, respect, and shared responsibility. It may also result in an improved therapeutic relationship based on open and encouraged communication between providers and patients.

Policies and procedures must be drafted that are faithful to these concepts. Disclosure of errors at the present time in most facilities is haphazard. Currently, there are many ad hoc methods, varying published approaches, and vague standards promulgated by accreditors. Yet few or no extant approaches result in learning from errors, particularly in an uncertain legal environment. A clear approach that provides information to the patient and encourages information flow, but avoids the ever-present risk of shame and blame retrenchment, is essential. Disclosure of hospital errors resulting in adverse events is the focus of this approach since they are often the most difficult; however, these principles can be applied to other provider locales, to errors that were unpreventable (such as drug allergies that arise on first administration), and to near-miss errors.

The entity's policies and procedures should provide for an "error investigation team" and a "system disclosure team" acting in parallel. The error investigation team should have "on call" members so that the entity may, upon determination of an error (and particularly an error that causes an adverse event), immediately engage an appropriate person to begin assessment. This includes sealing off the site and pathway of care for the purpose of maintaining the environment for appropriate detailed investigation as is done in aviation accident investigations (Liang 2002a).

The "system disclosure team" should be comprised of a high-level representative of the administration, a patient care liaison, and a clinically trained individual in the relevant specialty relating to the potential error/adverse event. The provider who last touched the patient should not be part of this system disclosure team, at least initially, for his or her presence may cause the disclosure effort to devolve into an unhelpful fingerpointing exercise. Moreover, the provider is much too close to the circumstance and may be experiencing tremendous emotional turmoil due to the error (Brazeau 2000; Christensen,

Levinson, and Dunn 1992; Leape, Swankin, and Yessian 1999; Wu et al. 1993; Wu 2001); at this time, the provider will be likely to be ineffective in discussing it. Of course, the patient and/or his or her family will also be experiencing tremendous turmoil, and a baseline rule of avoiding provider participation initially in disclosure should not imply a lack of concern regarding the patient and his or her family's feelings. Instead, the goal should be to provide information to the patient systematically so he or she and the family are given disclosure promptly and with understanding, empathy, and compassion from those who are trained and skilled in this endeavor. The provider should be part of the error investigation, however, which may allow him or her to sublimate the significant emotional anguish experienced after a medical error into positive corrective action efforts (Liang 2002a). This may also include later discussions with the patient/family.

It should be expressly noted that the individuals affected by the error will likely be angry and may be seeking to identify culprits. It is essential that individuals on the disclosure team understand that there will be significant emotional, and possibly hostile, reactions by patients/families to the error disclosure, although of course not all patients and/or their families will react in this way. Given this reality, the individuals who represent the system in the error disclosure must be specially trained in communication and empathy. They must exhibit the "three C's": concern, commitment, and compassion; above all, they must not act defensively. Critically, these individuals must take into account that it is often not merely what is said, but how one says it, that determines the listener's reaction (Liang 2002b). Thus, language, cultural values, and other specific factors defined by the individual circumstance (e.g., communication aids for those with physical handicaps) should be noted and addressed to facilitate complete comprehension and open discussion between the disclosure team and the patient/family. Finally, it is essential that this team communication to the patient/family reflect the immediate and unceasing investigation of the event by all relevant parties until the situation is understood (Liang 2002a).

Importantly, policies and procedures should expressly indicate that the patient care liaison will communicate regularly with the patient/family regarding the progress of the error investigation. This patient care liaison's responsibilities should include being the contact for the patient/family for any and all information regarding the error and its investigation. Keeping the patient/family within the communications loop is essential as a matter of mutual respect, and this approach establishes a consistent communication and information line between the patient/family and the provider entity. Perhaps more importantly, it also avoids the anger of patients/families in not being able to discuss the error, its investigation, or other matters with the provider entity. Finally, the patient care liaison should assist the patient/family in obtaining any remedial care for the patient, regardless of whether the negative outcome was a result of error or not, consistent with the philosophy of the organization. This also includes whatever external needs might be necessary (such as temporary housing, contacts with relatives, transportation, and other practical concerns).

There are relatively clear situations where disclosure is not appropriate. For example, those situations include: when there is a suspicion or even actual knowledge of abuse or neglect by a member of the patient's family that may be continued and/or intensified by the disclosure; investigations by formal authorities such as the police; and psychological concerns for the patient. The first two are generally rare; and the third should not be used as an excuse to avoid disclosure (Liang 2002a).

Finally, a "disclosure record" should be described within the policies and procedures. The standard "when, where, who, what" of the first disclosure meeting, as well as a description of the objective information discussed, should be documented in this record. As well, all future communications between the disclosure team and the patient/family should be documented and maintained here. It bears emphasizing that this record should include only objective, descriptive information; no conclusions, accusations, and/or assessments of fault should be made (Liang 2002a).

Perspective and Risks

Once providers and patients are educated, the perspective of the entity or institution shifts. Acceptance of disclosure, education and integration, and infrastructural policy and procedure components all become part of the health delivery process so that disclosure as part of quality promotion can occur. Unfortunately, at this juncture, tremendous legal risks arise as well as the common tendency to blame and to draw unsubstantiated conclusions. These latter actions are inconsistent with the systems nature of error and may result in adverse legal consequences, including a finding of liability admission; therefore, they should be avoided.

Objectivity should be the theme of disclosure and all subsequent discussions with the patient and/or his or her family. A descriptive approach is appropriate because a full systems assessment and root cause analysis has generally not been completed by the provider entity. Thus, any "conclusions" regarding the error are at a minimum premature and potentially misleading.

When an adverse event occurs, the error investigation policy should be immediately invoked, and the on-call investigator/investigation team (including all relevant providers) and system disclosure team should begin their activities. The disclosure team should meet with the patient/family as soon as practically possible after the event occurs. The disclosure team should indicate that there may have been a systems problem, and that this may have adversely affected the patient/family member. The team should communicate to the patient/family that the on-call investigator, providers, and team are undertaking the investigation even as they are speaking and will continue until all root causes are identified. The team should then describe to the patient/family the steps that are being taken. At a minimum, this should include:

- a determination if the adverse event is a result of a medical error or complication associated with the patient's clinical condition; and

- the means by which the investigation team are studying and assessing the event (including a description of systems assessments and root cause analyses as relevant to the clinical and administrative circumstance).

The patient care liaison should notify the patient/family that he or she will be communicating with them regularly regarding the error investigation, and that the patient/family should feel free to contact the patient care liaison at any time with any questions or suggestions they might have. Further, the patient care liaison should also indicate that he/she can assist the patient/family in any additional care access or other supportive means relevant to the situation that might be needed (Liang 2002a).

In addition to these activities, as part of the partnership between the members of the error reduction team, the patient/family should be asked to assist in the error investigation. This request can be made by the disclosure team during initial contact if suitable, or by the patient care liaison during later contact. The request can range from asking the patient/family to discuss with the error investigation team or representative any factor, problem, and/or witnessed error that may or may not have contributed to the negative outcome, to a full debriefing on all stages of care from before entry into the facility to the event itself (and even after, if appropriate). Such open communication efforts with the patient/family again are consistent with the systems nature of error and outcomes and are faithful to the philosophy of partnership between provider and patient; importantly, such efforts may also provide the patient/family with a vested interest in corrective action at the facility.

It should be noted that certain actions should not be performed because of the high risk of appearing and being insensitive or inappropriate. These include sending the patient or the patient's family a bill for services, at least before a resolution of the investigation (or even after, if appropriate); putting the patient/family on hold during telephone conversations; and delaying communication with the patient/family after they have requested it (Liang 2002a).

The Role of Apology

Apology is a valuable signal of empathy and is often desired by those who have been injured (Cohen 2000).[13] However, apology is laden with legal risks, particularly its potential interpretation by the legal system as an admission of liability and blameworthiness (Campaigne et al. 2000; Ness and Cordess 2002).

Apology should be provided as a sincere expression of empathy from system representatives reflecting system accountability. Statements such as "I'm sorry that I made a mistake that injured you" or "It's all my fault" should be avoided, since they are inconsistent with the systems basis of outcomes. Instead, statements such as "We are so sorry that this event has happened to you" or "We will do all we can to make sure it never happens again" are much more appropriate expressions of empathy and reflect system accountability for the event.

However, these kinds of appropriate empathetic statements should only be made after a thorough review of the law of the provider's jurisdiction. There are some jurisdictions where such an expression of empathy or offer of assistance after an injury may be considered appropriate and not an admission of liability (California Evidence Code 2000; *Deese v. Carroll City County Hospital*, 1992; Demorest 2001; *Phinney v. Vinson*, 1992; Massachusetts General Laws 2000; *Senesac v. Associates in Obstetrics and Gynecology*, 1982; Texas Civil Practice and Remedies Code 2000). These laws and general laws on the legal interpretation of apology and, particularly, their relation to party admissions, should be reviewed by competent counsel in detail to determine the practical means by which apology can and should be used. Empathy should always be expressed, but apology as a means to show empathy requires careful attention to legal detail before it is used.

Avoiding Lawsuits as Patient Advocacy

As part of a system of disclosure that seeks to promote communication and quality as well as to advocate for the patient, a system of alternative dispute resolution should be offered to the patient and/or family. Litigation may not be resolved for as long as a decade and has tremendous administrative costs deducted from the award (if any) (Brennan 1999; Meadows 1999; Dauer, this volume).

Further, alternative dispute resolution is a viable means of mitigating the emotionally damaging effects of litigation for all parties, litigation's incentives to prevent communication between provider and patient, and the extensive pecuniary and nonpecuniary costs associated with lawsuits (Meadows 1999; Metzloff 1991, 1992). Beyond the high costs for those presently injured, litigation is a poor avenue for quality improvement in the health care system—improvement that could benefit future patients. Because the very conditions that resulted in the error and injury remain undiscussed, latent, and unaddressed, the litigation sets up another provider and patient in the same system to experience the error and injury that could have been corrected through an appropriate systems analysis of relevant information (Liang 2001a, 2001b).

A method that addresses patient/family concerns and their need for effective and open communication is mediation (Dauer and Becker 2000; Liang 2000a). In this forum, not only are the parties themselves encouraged to vent, discuss, and review the circumstances surrounding the injury (in contrast to litigation, where attorneys control all communications), a wide variety of settlement solutions can be offered to the patient/family for consideration beyond simple monetary transfer (litigation's sole remedy). Such solutions could include a prominent and/or additional role(s) for the patient/family in corrective action efforts, naming a corrective action policy after the patient/family subject to the error and/or assisting in its assessment, public thanks to the patient/family for their assistance in improving the health delivery system if they participated in corrective action efforts, and/or apology and corrective action training (Liang 2001b). Finally, in contrast to litigation, providers and patients have reported high levels of satisfaction with mediation (Dauer and Becker 2000), and thus the use of this dispute resolution tool benefits both parties while resolving the conflict in a much shorter time so that all may move beyond the incident to heal physically and emotionally.[14]

Conclusion

Patient safety is now on the policy agenda on all levels. However, the medical and legal professions as well as the public have had little education on the appropriate means by which safety is promoted—through systems assessments and actions. Calls for blanket disclosure of errors to patients reflect a similar lack of understanding. By implementing a *system* of medical error disclosure and recognizing that providers and patients have important obligations and rights in the health delivery enterprise, providers and patients can work together to understand and improve patient safety through reducing medical error on a systems level. Such a system would also provide many more patients with much more rapid compensation for medical injury. Overall, if we can fulfill the often-stated philosophy of partnership, mutual respect, and trust between provider and patient, then patient safety can be promoted and its benefits can inure to ourselves, our communities, and all who follow us. As such, it is indeed a goal worth striving for; for we, and they, deserve no less.

Acknowledgment

This chapter originally was presented at "Promoting Patient Safety: An Ethical Basis for Policy Deliberation," The Hastings Center for Biomedical Ethics, Garrison, N.Y., July 12–13, 2001. I thank the members of this forum for their insightful comments. I also gratefully acknowledge the comments and substantive assistance of Virginia A. Sharpe, Ph.D., Ed Dauer, LL.B., M.P.H., Roxanne

Goeltz, Mary Anne Bobinski, J.D., LL.M., and Shannon M. Biggs, J.D., M.A., M.Ed., in improving this work.

Notes

1. Standard RI 2.90 (previously 1.2.2) mandates that "[p]atients and, when appropriate, their families are informed about the outcomes of care, including unanticipated outcomes" (Joint Commission 2001a).

2. For example, although error disclosure should be "objective," reflecting systems concepts, it should occur to allow patients to see that the individual physician is "remorseful" (Hebert, Levin, and Robertson 2001); individual providers should be held "accountable": "Healthcare is not a science. But, this does not excuse our system of not holding the [individual] healthcare provider accountable to errors" (PULSEAmerica.org—Persons United Limiting Substandards and Errors in Health Care, available at www.pulseamerica.org, accessed April 16, 2002). Here, "accountable" appears to be replacing the concept of moral blameworthiness but means the same thing. Note also that organized medicine retains such an approach; although medical errors "should be understood to refer to errors committed within a health care environment," physicians should disclose "even if it places the physician at risk of humiliation, blame, or legal liability" (Paul Barach, personal communication, 2001).

3. Because medical care is highly complex, even when providers are working at a 99 percent level of proficiency—and medical personnel "are among the most careful professionals in our society"—this performance level is still less than the level that exists in other similarly complex industries, and even a 99.9 percent level of proficiency may not be enough in complex systems (Leape 1994).

4. This factor is particularly important since providers generally do not accept the legal system as a legitimate purveyor of patient care standards, only of punishment (Liang 1997c). Thus, there is little incentive to change behavior on the basis of liability.

5. Note, however, that anesthesia is the exception to this lack of systems focus. Through simulation and systems analysis, anesthesia has reduced errors and associated injuries by at least an order of magnitude (Cooper, Newbower, and Kitz 1984; Cullen et al. 1992; Gaba 1989; Gaba and DeAnda 1988).

6. Although there are claims by representatives of the JCAHO that adherence to the SEP is merely "voluntary," accreditation, and thus the ability to provide services to at least Medicare and Medicaid patients, hinges upon adherence to the policy (Liang 2000b).

7. There may also be a significant conflict of interest in the SEP itself. The JCAHO not only decides the acceptability of the root cause analysis and, critically, accreditation status, but also offers "consultant" services to perform this very analysis. This situation provides highly difficult decisions for providers subject to the SEP (Liang 2000b, 2000d). In addition, under standard RI 1.1.2, now renamed RI 2.90 (see note 1), the JCAHO under its hospital accreditation standards requires physicians to disclose "unanticipated outcomes" to patients, which has been seen to require physicians to "tell patients when they received substandard care" (Joint Commission 2001a; Lovern 2001). Providers have expressed concerns regarding provider liability for this new policy: e.g., every admission has unanticipated outcomes; the standard will create awkwardness between hospitals and medical staffs; and "the hospital, by definition, is now intruding into the patient-physician relationship if there is a [JCAHO] documentation process required" for these disclosures (Lovern 2001).

8. See, in particular, text in note 29 in Liang 2001a.

9. Note, however, that there have been efforts to reintroduce the original HIPAA consent requirements (iHealthBeat 2002).

10. Note that the efforts to reform HIPAA may not practically address safety research concerns. HIPAA authorization will still be required for any nonroutine use or disclosure of patient-identifiable information, although the new regulations would allow a single combined form to be used for informed consent and HIPAA authorization. The HIPAA authorization will still require an extensive statutorily mandated list of information to be provided to the patient if it is to be legally valid, however. In the event that patient safety participants obtain a research/IRB/Privacy Board waiver obviating patient authorization, the use and/or disclosure of patient information will continue to be subject to the minimum necessary rule as before. No changes were made under the new regulations to the relevant de-identification provisions.

11. Note that under the new federal regulations, another exception has been allowed. If researchers wish to create "limited data sets," which cannot include direct patient-identifiable information, it is permitted and deemed "research" without the need for patient authorization or accounting. However, the privacy rule requires that disclosure of the limited data set of a provider or covered entity to another party requires the execution of a "data use agreement," where the receiving party agrees to limit the use of the data set for the purposes for which it was given, to ensure security of the data therein, and not to identify the information or use it to contact any individual. The creation of the limited data set must also fulfill the minimum necessary rule. Of course, first, the costs associated with yet another agreement to be executed without formal regulatory guidance may be prohibitive; and more substantively, qualitative patient safety research may require much more than is available in a limited data set, and brings the difficulties of accessing patient safety information back to a circumstance of obtaining individual HIPAA consent and/or the problems of de-identification.

12. Education is important, particularly due to the trend of "irrational" decisions by the public (Smith 2002).

13. Note that such apology should be provided when appropriate, rather than as a placating measure "smacking of sophistry" (Burke 2002).

14. Of course, although this system would potentially deflect many claims from litigation, alone it certainly will not deflect all of them. Further, although there exists some potential for confidentiality under a "mediation privilege," such a privilege is also subject to use in lawsuits due to discovery efforts (Deason 2002; Liang and Small 2003). Preferably, as part of any legal reform, discovery rules should also be altered not only to limit unintended use of patient safety information for lawsuits, but also to include mediation discussions so as to promote information flow to improve the delivery system.

CHAPTER 5

Prevention of Medical Error: Where Professional and Organizational Ethics Meet

EDMUND D. PELLEGRINO

Introduction

The report of the Institute of Medicine (IOM) on the prevalence of medical error has engendered widespread attention to a human problem as old as medicine itself (Kohn, Corrigan, and Donaldson 2000). Physicians, patients, and the public have always recognized the fact of medical fallibility. Few physicians can claim that they have never made an error of judgment or procedure. Few have not observed the errors of their colleagues. All are cognizant that the claim of the profession to police itself has never been responsibly actualized. To date, no comprehensive program of error prevention has ever been actualized. It is the possibility of such a program that the IOM report, its shortcomings notwithstanding, has brought into public and professional consciousness.

Past efforts at prevention of error relied exclusively on the moral restraints of medical ethics or the deterrent effect of punitive laws. Like modern tort theory, the Law of Hammurabi (circa 1900 B.C.) and the Roman Lex Aquilia and Lex Cornelia imposed harsh penalties for medical harm (Castiglioni 1941, 40). The Hippocratic oath and similar codes in many cultures centered on the moral obligation of nonmaleficence. In the last century, autopsy reports, morbidity and mortality reviews, pharmacy and therapeutics committees, as well as quality control and risk management policies have had small but definitive effect. But as the IOM report and other studies show, these measures have not on the whole been sufficiently effective (Sharpe and Faden 1998).

Against this background of ineffectiveness, the report and many of the chapters in this volume turn away from blame and moral censure of individual physicians and health workers toward systemic changes in every level of the health care system. Models of accident prevention taken from air safety, the nuclear power industry, and occupational safety are being fitted to the organizational context of contemporary health and medical care. Central roles are also given to cooperation between administrators, health professionals, patients, and accrediting agencies as well as individual health professionals. The locus of confidence is being consciously shifted from individuals to systems, institutions, policies, and regulations.

These are obvious responses given the prevalence of medical error and the institutionalized and organized context of today's medical care. Such changes should be encouraged, but with caution. Social crises always spawn enthusiasm for "salvation themes"—new ideas that are expected to revolutionize seemingly decrepit traditional practices. In our enthusiasm for the new we must remember that system change has its own failings.

The more complex a system of any kind, and the more finely articulated its elements, the more vulnerable it is to failure. Humans are unavoidably elements in a system; individual performance is still crucial. In spite of systemic safety practices in aviation and the nuclear power industry, human error in these areas has not been eliminated.

In this chapter I argue (1) that a properly organized organizational and systemic context is essential to reduce the prevalence of medical error, (2) that its effectiveness and efficient working depend on a parallel affirmation of the moral duty and accountability of each health professional in the system, (3) that each individual health professional must possess the competence and character crucial to the performance of his or her particular function as well as those of the system as a whole, and (4) that the major function of a system is to reinforce and sustain these individual competencies and virtues.

Systems Are Not Enough

Systems cannot make the professionals within them virtuous, but they can make it possible for virtuous professionals to be virtuous. Correspondingly, a defective system can discourage even the conscientious individual or reduce his or her aspirations to nothing higher than the level of the average. The moral sensibilities of each health professional must be preserved lest the system for error prevention itself become part of the problem.

All of this is especially relevant to health care systems. Medical error takes place in a nexus of intricate human relationships. Health "care" is channeled ultimately through persons in unique relationships far less subject to formularization than air travel, nuclear power production, or the manufacture of automobiles or complex pharmaceuticals. No system of error detection or prevention can confine these intricate human relationships within a set of preordained algorithms.

There are also rogue systems, as there are rogue individuals and nations. The ingenuity of humans to distort, bypass, or subvert any system has been demonstrated all too often. Overreliance on a systems approach can be as illusory as past overreliance on the moral integrity of individuals. Even while systemic responses are being designed, it will be necessary to reaffirm the moral nature of medical error, and to retain the notions of blame, accountability, and responsibility. Any system designed to protect patients must sustain and nourish the ethical obligations inherent in professing to be a healer, helper, and caretaker for humans in distress (Pellegrino 2001). In fact, the "system" (team, hospital, policy) will need to make the same "pro-fession" of commitment to the welfare of the patient.

This line of argument will require integration of professional and organizational ethics, as well as the relationship between them. Each domain has its own set of obligations. Conflicts between, and among, domains will arise. In an effective "system" of prevention and detection, these conflicts must be put into the right moral order in accord with some order of priorities.

This balancing can only be effected by an architectonic "first" principle fundamental to what medical and health care are all about. That principle, in both the system and the individual clinical encounter, must be the primacy of the good of the patient. The patient is the presumed beneficiary of the individual clinician and the system as well. Detection and prevention of medical error has its ethical foundation in the duty to act for the good of the sick and to avoid harm to patients. Every action of individual professionals and every organizational policy and regulation must be measured by this gold standard of traditional medical morality (Pellegrino 1983).

Individuals and Systems— Some Philosophical Notes

The moral interdependence of individuals and societies was a subject of major import to Plato. In the *Republic*, he proposed that a good society was one that acted for the good of its citizens (Plato 1983, Book IV, 420b, 519e). On the other hand, social good depended upon each person in a society performing that task for which he was best suited and qualified (Book II, 369b–e; Book IV, 423d). This interdigitation of individual and collective virtue, according to Plato, makes for a well-ordered and well-functioning republic.

This same ethical reciprocity is applicable in an analogous way to a well-functioning system of medical error prevention. This is different from the utopian social engineering schemata of Charles Fourier or Karl Marx (Fourier 1829). Their hope was to design social systems that would reshape human moral conduct and perhaps even human nature. The malignant social engineering of totalitarian states had the same goal. Their common failing was to substitute social for personal virtues in violation of the Platonic ideal of a balance between them (Simon 1986, 3–15). This is the danger an overly enthusiastic embrace of any "system" must avoid.

This is not to deny the potential for modifying and sustaining professional virtues in a system whose end is truly the good of the patient. One might then be able to speak of "virtuous" organizations and systems for error prevention. In such organizations the individual and the system reinforce each other in the pursuit of the good each purports to serve. Systems do not have a blank slate on which to write a prescription for human behavior. The "blank slate" conception of human nature is a recurrent fallacy, whether the proposed designing agent is genetic on the one hand or environmental or social engineering on the other (Pinker 2002).

Individuals can be inspired by the ideals of a morally sound organization. The best always rise above the satisfaction with mediocrity that systems can induce even in ordinarily well-intentioned professionals. Witness the lassitude of even good clinicians in the face of the injustices of today's "health care system," or the subversion of professionalism in managed care organizations. Systems are no more immune to moral corrosion than the individuals within them.

Medical Error Morally Defined

In its report, the Institute of Medicine provides a topography of definitions of medical error (Kohn, Corrigan, and Donaldson 2000, 28, 36, 54). It settles on the following: "the failure of a planned action to be completed as intended (error of execution) or the use of a wrong plan to achieve an aim (error of planning)" (54). The Institute focuses for the most part on errors of execution.

Under its preferred definition, the Institute of Medicine includes "adverse events," i.e., injuries caused by medical management. When the adverse event is attributable to medical error, it is considered "preventable." A preventable adverse event due to negligent care becomes malpractice when it meets the legal criteria by violation of the prevailing "standard of care" (28). Later the report distinguishes "slips," "lapses," and "mistakes," as well as latent errors (those at a distance from the "front line") and active errors (those on the "front line") (54–55).

In each of these definitions, the meaning of "error" much depends upon how error is measured. Methodological limitations and differences in interpretation that may affect the significance of the report have been mentioned already (Thomas, Studdert, and Brennan 2002; Brennan 2000; McDonald, Weiner, and Hui 2000). Whatever more reliable measures of error may later reveal, the report has sounded an alarm that challenges our complacency and commands a critical appraisal of causation, remediation, and prevention of error.

Finally, the very term "medical error" is misleading. It seems to suggest that all error is physician-generated. As the report itself makes clear, this is not the case, particularly if its recommendation of a systems approach is valid (Kohn, Corrigan, and Donaldson 2000, 54–55). I believe that "patient care error," which includes everyone that participates in health care, is a more suitable term. However, "medical error" is used so widely that I shall retain it in this discussion, despite my preference for the more inclusive term.

Error and Blameworthiness

The ethical desiderata outlined below can apply to all forms of error at the front line, i.e., errors attributable to the direct encounter of a patient with the health professional or an organizational policy or procedure. A blameworthy error is one in which there is a failure for which moral accountability can be assigned, one that was preventable if obligations had been fulfilled, if competence had been maintained or properly designed procedures had been consciously followed. Blame can be attached to individuals, teams, organizations, system designers, institutional trustees—to those who act in a system on the "front line" or to those at a distance who authorize others to act in the name of a system or organization.

The degree of blameworthiness will vary with the degree of negligence, the amount of harm done to the patient, the degree of collaboration with the harmful action, and the level of responsibility and authority. With respect to blameworthiness, errors of execution and planning are not as neatly separable as the Institute's report suggests. It is helpful to focus on the stages of care at which the error occurs, i.e., history taking, diagnosis, prognosis, selection of treatment and laboratory examination, performance of interventional procedures like surgery, cardiac catheterization, prescription writing, etc.

By focusing on specific elements in the patient care process, the relative contributions of the individual health care professional, the technical assistant, the system, the procedures, and the organization to the error can be better differentiated. Any culpability for the error will depend on the degree to which it is preventable in the expected operation of each of these agents, frontline or distant.

Errors can occur in what has been termed the "inherent" fallibility of medicine (Gorovitz and MacIntyre 1976). This term refers to the limitations of medicine as a science of the particular in which the application of general rules and laws may not fit particular cases precisely. Thus, adverse outcomes at certain levels of occurrence can be expected even in the "best hands" following the best procedures. A certain level of morbidity and mortality, for example, can be expected in complicated or delicate procedures. If all has been done properly, error due to the inherent fallibility of a system or the state of the art may be the only acceptable, really "blame-free" error, at least from the ethical point of view. As the profession's and the professional's knowledge and experience grows, the excusable level of these "inherent" errors may decrease.

A preventable adverse action is a moral failure that cannot be exculpated by the "blame-free" approach advocated by proponents of the system-dimensions of error. Whether it is committed by an individual, a team, or an institution, culpable error is a violation of the implicit promise each of these entities makes when it offers itself as an instrument of help and healing. By offering to help, the physician and nurse, the health care team, the hospital, and even the managed care organization implicitly promise competence and good judgment in the interest of the person who seeks help. This is their "act of profession," their commitment to the good of the patient.

The professional, the team, or the hospital is morally required to be faithful to this trust. Preventable or negligent harm as the result of error is a moral failure, whatever its legal status may be. Moral blame and culpability are therefore unavoidable. Removing individual blame could conceivably encourage better reporting of errors or more readiness to accept rehabilitative measures. It might also simplify litigation and standardize the tort system. It could mitigate the punitive atmosphere and enhance collegiality and interprofessional communication (Liang, this volume).

However, despite these beneficial possibilities, there are the associated dangers of complacency and dulling of the moral sensibilities of the humans in the system when either a "blame-free" approach or a "blame-the-system" approach is adopted. The power of individual guilt can be constructive as often as it is destructive. Personal accountability is owed to the person injured. The deterrent effect of fear of shame and blame is not safely ignored.

However well-organized and finely tuned the system may be, it must leave room for discretionary space in so human and uncertain an enterprise as medical care (Pellegrino 1977). The health professional needs that space if the care she provides is to be personalized, individualized, and humanized. That space is also necessary to provide for the unforeseen, unique, or unpredictable event in clinical care. It is within that space that the health professional can prevent the systemic shortcomings of the system itself from injuring the patient. It also allows the individual to detect the ill-conceived or poorly designed element in a systems approach. Of course, it is also within the region of discretionary space that the possibility of error may be increased. Within that space, the character of the health professional is the patient's last safeguard.

The blame-free approach advocated by many in the patient-safety movement cannot erase the individual moral onus of preventable error. The physician or other health professional cannot blame the system for his or her failings. Organizational conformity cannot take the place of moral responsibility even if the system follows a no-blame rule. The physician or the nurse, in their respective realms, are the pathways through which harm or good comes to the patient. They are responsible for what they order, or the way they follow an order or procedure. They are responsible for monitoring the health care process, at least in the steps immediately proceeding and following their personal function in that process.

The blame-free approach is most properly applicable when the harm done is the result of a chain of small errors or the concatenation of such errors inherent in a complex system involving many steps and many persons. This is somewhat parallel to the inherent fallibility notion of Gorovitz and MacIntyre (1976) applied to the system of patient care rather than to the procedure itself. It is, in effect, the "inherent fallibility" that may be built into a complex system meant to prevent error that paradoxically produces opportunities for error itself by the way it is structured. This is the case at times in air, rail, or nuclear power industry failures, in which a long history of error prevention has lulled everyone into complacency.

But even here the human factor remains. Just two examples from newspaper stories appearing as this chapter was being written will illustrate this point. Both are from the two industries singled out as models of systemic change of the kind health care should adopt. Neither vitiates the need for system control, but both illustrate the necessity for parallel attention to traditional notions of professional responsibility.

One story tells of an airport control tower in Sweden left unattended because the air traffic controller on duty failed to return from his vacation on time. Nobody noticed until a passenger aircraft sought landing instructions (Associated Press 2002a). The plane landed safely at another field. The other story concerns erosion of a nuclear reactor head, reportedly the most extensive erosion found yet in the United States. The Nuclear Regulatory Commission judged that the defect should have been detected at least four years ago. Now there are allegations that the operator of the utility, FirstEnergy Corporation, backdated videotapes, falsified documents, and withheld photographs (Associated Press 2002b). The "cover-up" is a classical ethical violation in corporate and government operation.

Who was to blame in these instances? The humans responsible for failure in their duties? The corporation or authority operating the airport or the reactors? On the facts presented it is reasonable to blame both. Professional and organizational ethics were both violated. We need not multiply examples like these. They are all too familiar, not just in systems of air and nuclear reactor safety, but in police departments, fire departments, sanitary systems, and in every walk of life in a society as complex and highly organized as ours. A no-blame system could too often be a travesty of social and commutative justice.

Blameworthiness and the Moral Spectrum of Error

Assigning individual or system responsibility is a difficult task sometimes admittedly impossible to accomplish with any degree of certitude. Bright-line distinctions are also difficult to make with respect to the moral gravity of an error. Yet if individual blame is to be attributed to a certain person or persons, some measure of moral culpability will be required to render justice to those injured. Both punitive and rehabilitative measures will bear some relation to the degree of moral failure in a particular instance.

All negligent error, that is, error that violates generally accepted standards of knowledge and skill, is morally blameworthy. This is true even if an error produces no harm or only slight harm, or is a "near-miss" automatically corrected by some system safeguard. The degree of blame will depend on a number of variables, singly or in combination.

In his study of two surgical services, Charles L. Bosk made a distinction between technical, judgmental, and moral error (Bosk 1979). Technical error he ascribed to conscientious physicians who met their professional obligations but erred due to lack of knowledge or proficiency. Judgmental errors are the result of a faulty strategic decision despite conscientious attention to professional obligations and requirements. To be blameless, these lapses are expected to be infrequent, not follow a repetitive pattern, and remain within the norms of professional obligation.

When these limits are exceeded, when there is a lack of conscientious attention to expected obligations, or when performance and knowledge deficiencies are allowed to persist, then the error is a moral failure. It is of course difficult to assign a number to the times one may licitly make an "honest" error. Moreover, "conscientiousness" in fulfilling professional obligations is often a subjective evaluation of one's professional peers. The distinctions Bosk suggests are heuristically helpful. They are, however, dependent on assessments of the character of one's colleagues. This is a notoriously flexible yardstick often influenced by friendship, kinship, hospital, and school ties.

The central moral issue is the degree of culpability an individual, i.e., a truly conscientious physician, may feel about this error. In the realm of conscientiousness, the character of the physician is the only measure that assures that blame is appropriately assumed. This should include steps taken to eliminate the underlying deficiency of information or skill as soon as possible, even if one's colleagues label the error an honest one. Not to do so is to compound the moral onus of further error.

Here again the interaction of a system of error prevention with preservation of a sense of individual responsibility and culpability is essential. Technical and moral error too easily overlap, even with "conscientious" physicians. Ideally, a virtuous physician in a virtuous organization would take even "honest" mistakes to be serious moral issues. Moral conscientiousness can be more demanding than simple fidelity to prevailing professional obligations. The prevailing mores of a blame-free system can all too easily exculpate failures of professional accountability.

The nature and content of professional ethics have been markedly altered in the last thirty years. Its normative content and thrust have become diluted and problematic (Pellegrino 2000). One may now fairly ask not only if a physician is conscientious but also what specifically he or she is "conscientious" about. With the gradual erosion of a universal ethic specifically defining professional obligations, professional conscientiousness can cover a wide variety of obligations.

We need only list changes in what is acceptable practice—financial conflicts of interest, limitation of practice to a "boutique" mode (Brennan 2002), refusal to care for Medicaid patients, unwillingness to see patients at night, etc. In all these instances, error can occur as often as neglect and even as a result of neglect. As a result, the putative line between technical and moral error has become seriously blurred.

In complicated medical procedures and cases, especially in acute intensive care units or when multiple disorders affect the patient, the so-called "cascade effect" may make detection of causation, responsibility, accountability, and remediation particularly difficult. T. P. Hofer and R. A. Hayward (2002) report an illustrative case of a patient subjected to a series of diagnoses and procedures. Different attendings, residents, radiologists, cardiologists, and other specialists sometimes successively, and sometimes simultaneously, treated a series of life-threatening complications. These authors show that in such cases of overlapping judgment and execution, the precise localization of error is uncertain and assignment of responsibility is accordingly difficult. At the end of their paper, Hofer and Hayward state: "Although carefully evaluated error-reducing systems are an important and essential part of health care delivery, for many problems in medicine fostering individual professional skills, expertise, values, responsibility, and accountability remain the best available approach to patient safety" (Hofer and Hayward 2002, 331).

Patient Care Error and Team Care: Ethics of the Microsystem

Up to this point, I have emphasized the moral accountability of the health professional, principally the physician, though the same spectrum of responsibility can be constructed for all the other health professionals. Modern medical care, of course, takes place in team settings. We must factor in the intricate interdependence of a group of health professionals who are essential to any complex procedure. If the surgeon is to accomplish his task, he must depend on the bypass pump operator, the anesthesiologist, the surgical nurses, the laboratory, the technicians who check, repair, and standardize the physiological monitors, the cardiologist who saw the patient preoperatively, the pharmacist who prepared the preoperative and intraoperative medications, the intensive care unit staff responsible for postoperative care, etc.

All varieties and magnitudes of error may occur between and among team members. Assignment of accountability, and therefore of blame, is more complex than in the one-to-one healer-patient relationship. Ultimately, of course, all group decisions and individual actions do channel back to the individual patient. But the collective nature of the team dynamic opens up the problem of individual versus group moral agency and underscores the need for an ethics of collective human acts as well as an individual ethic (Pellegrino 1982).

The team is a microsystem in which adverse actions of execution and judgment may occur—on the part of individual team members or in the articulation of their particular functions with each other. Morally, the microsystem of the team is something more than the numerical sum of the actions of its individual members. Team decisions require a common consent. Team actions share a common purpose, and team error becomes a shared responsibility. In that sense the team is a moral agent—a body of humans collectively capable of communal praise, or of communal blame for their collective errors of judgment or execution.

Each member of the team is responsible for the competent performance of his or her own assigned and peculiar function in the team activity. At another level, each member bears some responsibility for the performance of the team as a whole. To varying degrees each team member is therefore implicated in team or system error. This complicity can be expressed in different ways.

For example, a nurse may perform her part for the care of the patient well but may observe and fail to report, or do anything about, a pharmacist's medication error. The internist may interpret the electrocardiogram correctly but may fail to object to surgery he thinks inadvisable on the basis of that cardiogram. The surgeon may complete his operation successfully but may fail to note the inattention of the anesthesiologist or pump technician at a critical point in the procedure. In each case, the patient might have been endangered, or even injured. Under these circumstances the interdependence of team members imposes a certain measure of complicity in any adverse outcome.

A systems approach to avoidance of patient care error must attend simultaneously to each member doing her part well and to the shared responsibility of each member for assuring that the team's responsibilities are conscientiously assumed as well. No team member, on this view, could claim innocence if she participated in a wrongful group decision or overlooked the failure of other individual members to perform their specialized tasks well.

Thus, the team member who, for reasons of friendship or a desire to avoid conflict or save face, fails to object to a group judgment she thinks erroneous is complicit in whatever harm may come from that failure. So while the "cascade effect" is a reality, it is a summation of errors both in the system and on the part of individuals in the system. When the relative weight of each item in the cascade might be extremely difficult or impossible to ascertain, the idea of a "blame-free" system gains validity.

But when the loose link in the concatenation of events is clearly identifiable, the collective moral agency of the team as a team is lessened. Thus, the pilot who takes off with assurance from the mechanic that the engine repair is complete cannot be held responsible if that engine fails, nor can the "team" as a collectivity be held responsible. When the part is defective in manufacture, however, and the mechanic unknowingly uses it in his repair work, neither he nor the pilot is accountable. Rather, the manufacturer incurs the blame. The same is true when the system or policy is at fault.

Whatever safeguards a systems approach may provide and however well they are conceived, someone in team care must be prepared to "throw the switch," so to speak. Emphasis on the system is essential, but so too is the retention of moral accountability of the team as a whole and of each of its members. At some point in every system, there is need to bypass the system if the system's true purposes are not to be frustrated. The responsibility for the discernment and courage necessary for this kind of action is shared by team members. These responsibilities can be preserved only if individual accountability is retained. Those who follow a defective policy may rightfully blame the system if its design is faulty. But it is also necessary to maintain a sense of accountability that will motivate each team member personally to monitor the system and to feel responsible for the way its human components interact with each other.

Social and Organizational Ethics: The Macrosystem

The health professional as an individual functions within the microsystem of the health care team that is itself part of two larger "systems": the institution and the society. Any approach to systemic change will inevitably involve the impact of policies, procedures, or laws promulgated in these "macro" systems on the care of patients. Macrosystems are answerable for the way their policies modify the discretionary space, and action, of the individual practitioner, as well as the actual care for the sick.

Even at the macro level, and perhaps especially at this level, the issue of personal accountability remains. Boards of trustees, members of executive committees, and other board members of hospitals or hospital systems can only delegate authority to act; they cannot delegate final responsibility for what is enacted and approved. Administrators and trustees are indeed "entrusted" with the organization, legally, fiscally, and morally. This means they must monitor its fidelity to its mission and those it purports to serve. They act collectively and they share responsibility collectively for what has been done, decided, or approved by those they have appointed as administrators or professionals (Sharpe 2004).

Therefore, organizations as a whole have moral obligations to those they purportedly serve. Hospitals, for example, have obligations to serve the welfare of those they presume to treat. They usually say so in their mission statements. If a procedure or policy ends in harming rather than helping, the institution as well as the responsible individual cannot escape culpability. A "systems" approach to preventing medical error cannot absolve executives, decision makers, or those who carry out their directives. To say, as so many do, "We have a procedure for that. In this case it failed," or simply, "We take responsibility" and "move on," can hardly claim to satisfy any satisfactory criterion of accountability.

The current rash of cases of corporate malfeasance is a cautionary tale for anyone considering systemic approaches to prevention of medical error, or patient care error. That sad tale need not be repeated here. It is not new, as the history of corporate America so amply testifies. The corporatization, commercialization, and the entrepreneurial cast of health care are already well advanced. We have reason to worry about overreliance on a systems approach and especially a blame-free approach in health care. Despite supposed checks and balances, lines of authority, accounting boundaries, etc., the venal purposes of corporate executives and boards of directors were not prevented. Some if not the majority of these corporations had "ethics" committees. Organizational ethics itself is a dubious enterprise without a cadre of persons of character to detect and correct the tendency of profit to distort even the highest motives.

To acknowledge the failure of corporate ethics and the frailty of the safeguard supposedly built into its systems of surveillance is not to abandon hope for morally responsive organizations. Such organizations do exist and, like morally upright individuals, receive no public notice. Indeed, it is the belief of many virtue ethicists that there can be "virtuous" organizations, those whose habitual disposition is to act in such a way as to protect the interests of those they serve. We all know of local businesses, auto repair shops, merchants, and service organizations whom we trust to act well, even while others do not.

Virtuous organizations usually propound mission statements promising ethically responsible conduct. These missions will not become a reality unless they permeate the life of the organization. Needless to say, this must be sustained from the top—from the example and witness of the chief executives and boards of directors. This is not the place to delineate how one generates a sense of ethics and virtuous conduct in organizations.

It is important, however, to emphasize that for all members of a micro- or macro-system to act in a morally responsive way, a sustaining culture of morality is necessary. Of course there are persons who will be virtuous and upright no matter what milieu they function within. But all persons do not have the same strength of character to be virtuous without a morally responsive work environment to sustain and correct them.

Having said this, it is again important to recognize that even when character formation, honor codes, and fostering a culture of virtue are present, individual virtues are still the bedrock. The military academies in our country emphasize honor codes, character, and virtue. Yet all too sadly, we know they have been the sites of egregious violations of cheating and other reprehensible behavior. Again the necessity of a balance between individual accountability and organizational safeguards is obvious in the prevention of medical error, as it is in every other life arena.

With specific reference to health care administrators and executives, we must not forget that the organizations they head are health care organizations. They are thus charged with the welfare of sick, dependent, anxious, vulnerable, and exploitable human beings. These humans are patients primarily, not consumers, customers, or subscribers. Nor do they fit any of the other metaphors derived from business, industry, or commerce. Health care trustees or administrators, like it or not, must be judged on the impact of their decisions on the patient in the clinic or the bed. Health care organizations may be corporate entities, but they cannot be excused if their level of ethical sensitivity does not rise above that of the ordinary corporation.

While the executives of health care "systems" may see themselves as primarily corporate officers, they cannot avoid the fact that they too are bound by the norms of clinical ethics. Of course their responsibility is not the immediate responsibility of the doctor or nurse. But the more they recognize the notion of the primacy of the welfare of the sick, the more clearly will they set the proper moral tone of the institutions they direct. We used to hear the claims of certain pharmaceutical companies to be "ethical" and to set a higher standard for themselves. This notion has been dissolved in the corrosive acid of competition and profit so that the pharmaceutical industry is now on the ethical defensive. But the return of the notion of an "ethical" health care organization is as important as a new system of rules, algorithms, policies, checks, and monitoring mechanisms in preventing medical error.

The same set of considerations applies to the broadest systemic approach of all, the macro "system" of social and political change. Here the need for restoration and indeed accentuation of personal accountability is ineradicable. Societal legislation and policy are not self-justifying, no matter how great their majority appeal. Certainly democratic societies must elaborate laws, regulations, and the like. But like all the levels of systemic change, however well-intended, we cannot dispense with the concept of personal accountability, or with protection of the whistle-blower and the alert individual who detects danger to patients.

By all means a systems approach should be elaborated. Examples from successful systems of error control outside health care should be translated into the ethics of medicine and health care. These borrowed systems will be most successful if we retain and refine the sense of individual moral responsibility within them as well.

Individual and System Accountability: Synergy, Not Opposition

Some of the defects attributable to the current focus on providers are: lack of recognition of the interdependence of team care; suppression of error reporting and information; discouragement of open communication and partnership between patients, families, and providers; and some of the defects of compensation litigation (Leape 1994; Leape et al. 1998; Liang, this volume). Yet there is no assurance that a blame-free approach and displacement of responsibility from individuals to systems will remedy these defects. The "system" can be just as reluctant to admit error as the individual. The temptation to cover up, minimize, or deny system error will not be erased. Anyone who has tried to elicit an admission of error or recover compensation for harm done by an institution, business, or corporate entity knows how difficult both justice and satisfaction for harm done can be.

The confidence some bioethicists place in a transfer of trust from physicians to the health care organization is wholly without justification in fact. The ethics of organizations are not necessarily more reliable than those of individuals. We need think only of the corporatized impersonality of managed care organizations to doubt whether a "system" of apology, appeal, or system compensation will be effective in preventing error. We may speak of the ethical obligations of the system to provide quality care, but systems are just as eager to minimize complicity as individuals. In fact, organizational loyalty and complicity all too often make a mockery of appeal systems.

Blaming the system may diffuse accountability so widely that no one feels responsible. Organizations and systems are collectively accountable, to be sure, but this does not assure that each member of the collectivity or team will feel responsible enough to report errors made by friends or associates. It takes as much courage to blow the whistle on the system as it does on an individual in the system. The system is still dependent on the ethical sensitivity and courage of each of its members as individuals. Traditional medical ethics remain an essential element of a patient's safety.

Expecting patients and families to be "partners" in a system-oriented error prevention system is a dubious recommendation. This asks people in distress to bear some of the burden in detecting error. The possibility that such an invitation will worsen the situation is not trivial. Patients and families are already involved in micromanagement at the bedside. They may actually hamper the best care by seriously limiting the professional's discretionary space. It takes courage today for physicians to do what they think right medically when it is thought to violate the autonomy of patients and families to choose otherwise.

Rather than being a sign of respect and empowering patients and families, this partnership in error detection asks them to carry a burden in addition to the ordinary burdens of a serious illness. Does this mean that they share the blame for an untoward outcome? Clearly patients and families should be informed, told about lapses in the system or errors made by an individual caregiver, and encouraged to communicate. But this cannot be "sharing" in any genuine sense. We cannot ask the patient and family to beware of medical error as we ask buyers to beware (Goeltz, this volume; Liang, this volume).

The team functions by coordinating the functions of many persons, each of whom has a specific responsibility for an essential part of the team effort. The system can only succeed if each member is faithful to the trust invested in her special function by the patient and the system. Each individual can only function well if the others also do their jobs well. Once this reciprocity is accepted, retention of the ethical accountability of individuals need not be punitive. The system can be designed to emphasize personal accountability yet assist the responsible persons in disclosing error and do so in a supportive environment. The anguish of a conscientious professional for an error, blameworthy or not, is not to be discounted as just punishment for wrongdoing. The emphasis in a system can be on prevention, re-education, and rehabilitation of individual actors.

Overemphasis on the anguish of the caregiver, however, can lead to laxity in removing an inadequate team member. Unfortunately, some cannot be successfully rehabilitated. Others may too readily transfer their personal responsibility to the team. Others may be protected by friends reluctant to hurt them. The primacy of the welfare of the patient must not be diluted in a mistaken effort at compassion for the error-prone caregiver.

In any case, in the processes of error detection, investigation, or disclosure, individuals will unavoidably be identified. That information will often become known. It is unlikely in reality, therefore, that the systems approach will entirely shield the individual from blame. Nor will it assuage the anguish and anger of the patient, who may know or suspect the person responsible. It is wiser, therefore, to acknowledge when an individual is responsible. This will clear away unwarranted suspicion and provide opportunity for personal apology when there is actual fault.

Disclosure: Professional and Ethical Obligation

Principle II of the code of ethics of the American Medical Association imposes two duties of disclosure, one based in "honesty with patients and colleagues," and the other based in exposing "physicians deficient in character or who engage in fraud or deception" (AMA 1999, section 8.12).

The findings of the IOM report underscore the need for a more rigorous application of this principle and the associated guidelines. The urgency for such reaffirmation and further elaboration of these standards of conduct is further underscored by the standards now being set by the Joint Commission on Accreditation of Healthcare Organizations (JCAHO 2001a). These standards call for organization-wide disclosure practices with executive involvement and implementation.

If the AMA principles and guidelines and those of the JCAHO were to be cooperatively applied, the desired integration of individual and organizational ethics could be realized. Two "systems"—the AMA and the JCAHO, and the individual physician's professional and ethical obligations—could act synergistically to reduce the prevalence of error.

A fuller exposition of the ethical foundations for disclosure is provided elsewhere in this volume (Berlinger, Gilbert, Wu). It suffices to say here that the moral obligation of disclosure lies in the trust relationship that binds patients to physicians and health care organizations (Pellegrino 1982, 2001). Patients submit to care by physicians and hospitals because they must trust them to be competent and to use that competence in the patient's interest. Fidelity to these promises of trust is at the root of professional and institutional ethics. Medical error, however caused, blameworthy or not, is a violation of this trust. That is why patients have a moral claim on disclosure.

Several aspects of this moral claim are linked to the questions of commutative justice that disclosure entails. Patients, in seeking justice, should know when an error is blameless, and thus not a violation of trust, and when it is blameworthy and therefore a violation of trust. Knowledge is needed by the patient to understand and cope with whatever impact the error might have made on the course of his disease. Disclosure also allows patients to change physicians or hospitals. It also permits a more just appraisal of whether or not suspicions of error are based in fact, along with the chance of personal apology, which is more likely and more satisfying than an organizational apology. Finally, disclosure allows for more genuine and less frivolous litigation for compensation.

In all of this, the need for a conjunction between individual and organizational ethics becomes clear. The Institute of Medicine has alerted the profession and the public to a serious problem. While its data and conclusions have certain shortcomings, they merit the serious response they are receiving (Brennan 2000). What is clear is that both a systems approach and an approach that reinforces the traditional ethical obligations of individual practitioners are necessary. Individual patient-oriented medical ethics and the new domain of organizational ethics are required to act synergistically if the welfare of the patients is to be optimized.

CHAPTER 6

Medical Mistakes and Institutional Culture

CAROL BAYLEY

Introduction

This chapter outlines the role of a hospital system in the way medical mistakes are handled. Much of the recent writing on medical error has either concentrated on the individual clinician and his or her responsibilities in disclosure of medical error or, like the watershed Institute of Medicine (IOM) report *To Err Is Human* (Kohn, Corrigan, and Donaldson 2000), has drawn attention to industry-wide problems and their potential solutions. Here I look at the nexus of these domains, at the ethical responsibilities and motivations of particular health care institutions.

The first section of the chapter situates this work within a three-tiered model of ethics. Just as the behavior of an individual springs from values that person holds, so institutional behavior expresses the values that characterize that institution.

Since institutional behavior with regard to mistakes is the focus of this chapter, thinking about an institution as a system is important. Therefore, the next section describes two meanings of an institutional view of a "systems" approach, and suggests why the "system as culture" is more fruitful than the "system as business entity" for bringing about change in the way institutions handle mistakes. Finally, the third section illustrates the way in which one large West Coast health system, using its core values as the engine, undertook such a change.

I write this as the vice president for ethics and justice education at Catholic Healthcare West (CHW). My role is parallel to the role of ethicist in other health systems, but my focus is on education of physicians, nurses, staff, and boards rather than more exclusively on crisis intervention or ethics committees. I am a member of the Mission Integration Department and report directly to a member of the senior management team. With the senior legal counsel and the vice president for risk management, I developed the materials referred to in this chapter, and I drafted the philosophy statement set out below for the board's approval.

Three Realms of Ethics

Jack Glaser (1994), a theologian and ethicist, describes three realms of ethics by employing a model of concentric circles. The smallest, innermost circle is the realm of individual ethics. The individual patient is often the subject of our thinking in biomedical ethics. Should we take this patient off the respirator? Would this incompetent patient have wanted what her daughter is now asking us to do? In the case of the ethics of error, we may look instead at the individual clinician who made a mistake. Did she cover it up? Did he confess it honestly at the morbidity and mortality conference? Did she apologize to the patient?

That individual, as Glaser's model goes, finds himself or herself within an institution. In the case of medical mistakes within the hospital setting, the erring physician or other professional practices within the institution of a hospital, an organization with policies, procedures, practices, reporting relationships, credentialing systems, and ways of doing things—in other words, a "system."[1]

This institutional realm of ethics is situated within the larger societal realm. At this level, the larger social and legal picture sets the stage for what happens to individual persons within an institution. This societal level contains, among other things, social attitudes toward blame, forgiveness, and lawsuits; ideas and practices regarding medical malpractice, torts, and tort reform; and mechanisms for justice. Although these societal factors influence and shape the context for what happens within the other two realms, analysis and change at this level are easy to generalize about but difficult to effect. During otherwise serious conversations about medical mistakes, we hear that "patients who are harmed just need someone to blame—even if it was no one's fault," or "Doctors are treated like gods in our society; no wonder they find it hard to admit mistakes." While these observations may surely contain a grain of truth, they do not advance change. In fact, we may be wrong to hope for comprehensive change beginning at this level.

The Hospital Institution

The "systems approach" to understanding medical mistakes is gaining ascendancy in the philosophical and medical literature, as well as in the way many in the health care industry have begun to think about error. Advocated by theorists such as Leape (1994), Reason (2000), Liang (2001a, 2001b), and Berwick

(1989), systems theory points out that errors are often the result of a badly designed system in which multiple factors combine to produce ideal conditions for error. An error in the administration of medication, for example, may be the result of a number of factors, from the way orders are written to the procedures used in the pharmacy to the staffing patterns on the unit. Simply censuring the nurse who administered the harmful dose as a response to the error will miss the opportunity to correct the error upstream—the way the orders are written, pharmacy procedures, or staffing. Assigning blame, according to systems theory, is not helpful in reducing error, since it discourages admission of error and a frank scrutiny of the conditions that lead to it. As Virginia Sharpe (2000b) points out, the usual way we look at error is after the fact, when a patient has been harmed. In this system, harm becomes a necessary component in prevention since there is no system to identify errors that do *not* cause harm.

Using systems theory to more adequately address the handling of medical error in a hospital requires a particular view of "the system." There are at least two ways to view the hospital system in thinking about opportunities for resolution following a mistake. One way is to look at the hospital as a business entity, with policies, procedures, staff, and management whose "product," so to speak, is optimal outcomes for patients. By outcomes, we could mean purely statistical health outcomes—successful valve replacements, fewer nosocomial infections. For a richer sense of outcomes, we could also include those harder to measure, such as peaceful death when extended life is no longer possible or desirable, trust, confidence in the hospital, etc. But no matter how the outcomes are characterized or defined, the hospital is an organization of individuals working together to produce them.

On this view of a hospital as a system, a sensible approach to medical error is to analyze it with regard to the process of which it was a part. If a set of instruments was incompletely sterilized, putting patients at risk of infection, what is the process used for sterilization? Who designed the process and who uses it? Are those who use it adequately trained and reminded about it? When does the sterilization take place—at the end of shift, by the last one to leave, or at a better time? Does the process contain built-in sources of confusion, written in shorthand by someone who performs it routinely? Has the process been designed to be "idiot proof" (or exhaustion proof, or distraction proof)?

This kind of thinking underlies the directives of the Joint Commission on Accreditation of Healthcare Organizations (JCAHO) for analyzing the root causes of mistakes and taking steps to ameliorate them (Leape et al. 1998, 1446). The JCAHO, which can take away a hospital's accreditation, has, up until recently, embraced this less comprehensive systems model. A hospital that (1) self-reports the error and (2) completes a thorough and credible root cause analysis with an action plan for change in a timely manner is not subject to the same censure by JCAHO as an organization that does not do these things.

This kind of approach, at work in many hospital settings, conforms nicely to the requirements of current management theories in process improvement (known as Continuous Quality Improvement or Total Quality Management)—theories that direct managers to dissect each process (emergency room visits, hospital admissions, and the like) in order to see the whole flow of work. Only in the context of the desired outcome (reduction in wait times, for example), and situating the process within the larger processes of which it is a part, can quality outcomes be improved. This approach to medical error—simply concentrating on outcomes—springs from this view. It might be viewed as a "systems approach" because it contrasts with one that simply blames individual actors, but it does not embody a rich enough view of a hospital as both an environment of care and an environment of work.

This view of a hospital system contrasts with another view that is more comprehensive, but is considerably more complicated. This more comprehensive idea of a system may still view the hospital as a business entity, with quality outcomes for patients as its product, but must also account for the factors that are not reducible to parts of a process or items on a flowchart.[2]

Putting the issue of medical errors into this more comprehensive approach to the hospital as a system requires that we recognize that a hospital is more than a collection of processes and procedures operating (relatively) efficiently to produce good patient outcomes. A hospital, because it is a place where people work together, is also the locus of a particular set of social practices enforced or legitimized by traditions, rituals, and customs that promote certain values. That is, a hospital is the locus of a certain culture. Changing the way the hospital handles mistakes, then, is a function of a change in the hospital's culture. This begins, in part, with an understanding of the institution's core values.

CHW's Project to Change the Culture of Medical Mistakes

Predating the publication of the IOM report by a little less than a year, Catholic Healthcare West (CHW), a large, West Coast nonprofit health system, undertook a project to change the way its member hospitals handle mistakes. CHW was founded in 1986 as a collection of twelve hospitals belonging to two congregations of Catholic Sisters. The Sisters' original intention was to form a system to which other Catholic sponsors would be attracted and gradually to expand the system to include other nonprofit, values-based hospitals, even if they were not Catholic or faith-based. The system grew quickly during its expansion period, and at of the beginning of the Mistakes Project, there were forty-seven participating hospitals, approximately two-thirds of which were Catholic.

As every culture is, hospitals are the locus of a set of power relations that affect what changes and what stays the same. Hospital members of CHW, like other hospitals, have internal sets of such power relations, but by virtue of membership in a system, they also are subject to the power of that larger system. The history of the system (Catholic Sisters inviting like-valued hospitals to become part of a large network) combined with the power in the larger system gave the project its effective start. The senior executives for risk management and legal services (with me, the system's ethicist) recognized that the way mistakes were being handled across the system was out of sync with the values of the organization. This experience underscores the need for careful selection of executive leadership by organizations that purport to act out particular values. Unlike the ethicist, the risk manager and senior legal counsel were not hired primarily to wonder whether certain behaviors evidenced the system's espoused values, but unless they had so wondered, this project never would have begun.

This group, following much of the literature in other areas of quality improvement (e.g., Berwick 1989) also recognized that the most effective way to correct the situation would be to start at the top. For this reason, the corporate members were advised of several situations that had triggered the realization. One such situation was the following. On a step-down unit, two patients were being cared for after cardiac surgery. Patient A was doing well; patient B was not. A nurse at the desk saw a blip on A's monitor, went to check A and saw that A was fine. Shortly afterward, B died. The monitors had been cross-wired, so that the blip the nurse originally saw was an indication of B's condition. Although the CEO was advised immediately of the issue and her first impulse was to arrange for the disclosure of the event to the family, when she called the physician to ask him to be present, he convinced her that disclosure was wrong. He said it would not bring the patient back, that the patient was so sick he might have died without the mistake, and that the CEO was risking an enormous lawsuit by telling the family of the error that they would otherwise not be aware of. The several cases, including this one, of a mistake being handled in a way that seemed out of character for CHW, given its core values, convinced the corporate members of the need for a change, and they expressed interest in receiving a white paper, based on the organization's five core values, describing the way people at CHW should behave in the wake of a medical mistake. That document became CHW's Philosophy of Mistake Management.

Although disclosure of medical error to patients attracted much of the attention the document subsequently received from physicians, it did not start as a disclosure policy, or even as a disclosure philosophy. Rather, it went the other way: because the values of dignity, collaboration, stewardship, justice, and excellence are the foundational reasons the system was formed, its behavior as a system must be shaped by them or it risks forsaking its identity. "Values" that do not affect actions are hardly worthy of the name. Disclosure was the bloom, not the root.

The philosophy statement regarding CHW's attitude toward mistakes is structured around the five "core values" of Catholic Healthcare West: dignity, collaboration, justice, stewardship, and excellence. Unlike a mission statement, which most organizations have and which tells in broad terms the goals of the organization, the core values are meant to be characteristics of CHW as it pursues its goals. Broadly speaking, these are human values that many persons, Catholic or not, share. In the context of a ministry of the Catholic Church, however, most of them have a particular meaning.

The value of dignity reflects the traditional Catholic view that every person is beloved by God and worthy of respect because of his or her membership in the human family. Treating people with dignity includes patients as well as workers, managers, vendors, and others who come within CHW's orbit.

Justice as a value is a feature of the way CHW wishes to treat persons whose dignity is thereby respected. In the Aristotelian sense, justice means treating like cases alike, but in a Catholic health care system, justice also takes on a biblical imperative that in some cases contradicts the Aristotelian sense of fairness or at least gives it a particular spin. In this biblical sense, justice is not blind, but has a preference for the poor and disenfranchised. Like cases may be treated alike, but only after they are adjusted for the imbalance of poverty or marginalization.

Stewardship as a value in a Catholic health care system also has biblical roots. This value promotes the prudent use of resources for the ministry, including both spending and saving appropriately. More than simple frugality, stewardship contains the notion that good things are to be carefully nourished, grown, and shared.

Most Catholic health care systems, because they are rooted in the traditions of religious sisters and Catholic Church teaching, appeal to these three values in some way. The remaining two have their source more in the ambient business culture in which American health care is delivered. The value of "excellence" in particular became part of the named values at the time when "exceeding customers' expectations" was the mantra of many businesses that served the public. Its inclusion in the five core values of CHW helps emphasize dedication to clinical quality and continuous improvement.

Collaboration is probably the value most unique to CHW, in that, unlike other Catholic health systems founded and sponsored by a single congregation of religious sisters, CHW was founded by two congregations with current sponsorship by eight. Collaboration with others who shared a vision of health care was part of the founding identity of the organization, and it has continued to mark CHW's character. No other Catholic health system in the United States has so much identification with hospitals that share dedication to similar values but are not Catholic or faith-based. At this writing, about half of CHW hospitals are non-Catholic.

With this general understanding of the values in the background, it is appropriate now to review the actual philosophy statement as the Sisters and the CHW board of directors approved it.

CHW's Philosophy of Mistake Management

Catholic Healthcare West strives to provide the highest quality of care to patients and is committed to developing and maintaining excellent relationships with the physicians, nurses, and others who render that care. The CHW Philosophy of Mistake Management challenges us to accomplish our goals by implementing management practices that are driven by the CHW core values of dignity, collaboration, stewardship, justice and excellence.

Inherent in CHW management processes, including good faith claims management, effective loss prevention and care management, is the recognition that sometimes, in spite of our best efforts, systems fail, individuals make mistakes and patients are harmed. Most often this injury will be the result of multiple factors; in some cases, doctors, nurses or other caregivers will be responsible; in others, the failure of our systems and processes may contribute to the mistake. Dedication to our core values requires that we work diligently to identify practices that may pose harm to our patients, and to implement systematic improvements that will ensure consistent, safe patient care. In the unfortunate event that a person under our care experiences harm, devotion to the CHW core values requires a full and honest disclosure to the patient or other appropriate parties. CHW is committed to full and timely disclosure in a manner that expresses our values and fair compensation to a patient or the family by the responsible parties, whether that is CHW, one of our partner health care providers, or both.

Quality improvement, fair and honest claims management and effective loss prevention can be achieved only through constant reflection on the meaning of the CHW core values and their impact on our daily actions.

DIGNITY

Everyone we touch—patients, family members, physicians, other health care workers, and our own CHW team members—possesses an inborn dignity as a person worthy of respect. We respect each person when we realize that everyone is different, and that different cases may require us to seek creative, alternative resolutions of claims.

Respect for a person's dignity means that we are honest and direct in communicating to a person who may have been harmed while under our care. Together with the physician, we must promptly supply all information to a person that is rightfully his or hers, including his/her medical record, the circumstances which resulted in the harm, the extent of the damages and the right to fair compensation. Respect for the dignity of the person and good faith claims management compels us to advise an injured party about his/her right to obtain advice from legal counsel, and other information appropriate to the case. Respect for dignity means that, acting through our administrative and clinical leadership and as soon as the facts are fully known, we take responsibility for any mistake made and apologize for any harm that has resulted.

COLLABORATION

Working together with physicians and other team members is at the heart of our service to patients. We are successful because of the work of an entire team. We strive to foster an atmosphere of trust, honesty, and transparency. We try not to blame one another. We work together to get to the bottom of problems and solve them. Our value of collaboration fosters the development of healthy relationships between system resources, such as the Risk Services, Legal, Ethics and Care Management Departments, and the divisions. Together we strive to deliver high quality health care in which the right resources are directed to the right persons at the right time. In the spirit of collaboration we will work with physicians to ensure respect for all individuals.

JUSTICE

In the context of risk management, justice has a very particular application. First of all, it means that we treat everyone fairly and equitably regardless of rank or status. Whether a patient is well educated and assertive or is someone whose native language is not English or is someone who is simply not confident within the medical system, all are equally deserving of fair treatment. With physicians and other partners, justice requires that we take our fair share of the burden of a claim and expect the same of our partners. Moreover, despite the perceived or actual difference between the status of physicians and nurses, both will be treated equitably by CHW. CHW will seek justice in honoring the larger public systems and rules for reporting errors, whether to boards or to departments of the government charged with protecting the public.

STEWARDSHIP

We hold precious assets of CHW—our human resources, our finances and the trust the public places in us. Sometimes protecting one may seem to jeopardize the others. In the management of mistakes, we believe no such conflict exists. From a risk management standpoint, it is axiomatic that patients are far more likely to seek legal representation if they believe that information has been concealed from them. Hence, timely disclosure of mistakes is cost effective. The trust the public gives to us, placing their health and often their lives in our hands, requires that we steward all of our resources with integrity. This means that we fairly compensate an injured party even when that involves the expenditure of CHW funds. At the same time, we are careful to share the burden of claims and suits fairly with those institutions and individuals that bear some responsibility for them. Faithfulness to the value of stewardship compels us to explore every avenue for a just settlement.

EXCELLENCE

Always striving to do better requires a frank admission that we can always improve. With humility and determination, we seek constantly to improve the manner in which we provide care to avoid injury to patients, families or caregivers. In some instances, an individual is primarily responsible for a mistake. In many other cases, we know that errors occur because of the failure of systems to prevent them. As such, we seek to improve our care in an environment of learning rather than of punishment. Our dedication to improvement requires that we share claims information and other patient care data among all of our facilities and with other appropriate partners so that we can study the causes of our failures and effectively structure systematic opportunities for improvement.[3]

As is evident, the "philosophy" of mistake management of CHW is neither a policy for disclosure nor a project description for improvement in procedure. It is not even a statement of commitment to improved patient safety. (CHW has undertaken separate, though related, efforts in each of those areas as well.) Instead, this statement of philosophy is structured around the core values at the heart of the self-identity of CHW, and it is an effort to set out expectations of behavior demonstrating those values when efforts at patient safety have failed and we make a mistake.

Beyond Inspiration to Brass Tacks

Once the very top levels of the organization had made a clear statement of the desired behavior, it remained to saturate the organization with that expectation and to learn what kinds of barriers to it existed. The plan of the project leaders was to address key constituencies within CHW to educate them about the project, to listen to what they would need to implement the philosophy, and to take their feedback into consideration before addressing the next group.

Three examples of the need for further refinement are illustrative of this give-and-take process. The first was the rough-and-ready taxonomy of mistakes used to narrow the first stage of the project. In our initial conversations with physicians about the philosophy, we heard criticisms of the disclosure expectation of roughly the following sort: "You mean you expect me to *tell* a patient when a small mistake I made did not harm her and had no effect on her recovery? That will just make her worry more!" Comments of this sort made us realize that some refinement of "mistake" needed to be made, particularly with regard to the expectation of prompt and honest disclosure. This was more a practical decision than a philosophical one.

So in subsequent conversations about that part of the philosophy, we talked about four "kinds" of mistakes in the following way. One is the kind no one, including those who made the mistake, ever knows about. A further distinction is made between "near-misses" and "harmless hits." In CHW's terminology, a "near-miss" is a departure from the standard of care that never gets delivered, and so cannot affect the patient. An example is the nurse who mistakenly brings the green pill to the patient for her 8:00 P.M. dose, instead of the blue one. In this example, the patient is vigilant and suggests that the pill she is supposed to take at this hour is blue, not green. The nurse checks and sure enough, she has brought the wrong pill, a mistake she corrects by bringing the right one.

The "harmless hit" is not the same as a near-miss, although some taxonomies lump them together. A harmless hit is a mistake in which the departure from plan is executed, but with no appreciable effect on the patient. For example, the patient above thinks it strange that she is getting a green pill but says nothing and takes it anyway. Thirty minutes later, the nurse discovers her error and brings the blue pill, an antibiotic. Absent any contraindication for the first pill, and if there is no reason the two shouldn't both be taken, the nurse's error is without consequence to the patient. It is a "hit," but a harmless one.

The final category of mistake is the "harmful hit." These are mistakes that result in harm to the patient, in the form of the need for more or different medication, a longer stay in the hospital, more tests or invasive procedures, disability, or death. In these situations, where a clinician suspects that a mistake may have caused or contributed to the harm a patient has experienced, appropriate disclosure will not "just make her worry more."

These distinctions are an example of learning from the "front line" about the barriers to implementation, even at the cost of the morally more satisfying philosophical answer to the question of disclosures of all mistakes. As noted above, the project leaders agreed that requiring a system to produce harm before improving the system was not a sound way to proceed. On the other hand, practically speaking, we made the distinction between a mistake that causes harm and one that doesn't (or couldn't) in order to reduce the number of excuses clinicians could use for not treating victims of mistake with the appropriate respect.

A second important learning came in response to challenges of this sort: "My medical malpractice carrier told me *never* to admit liability—and now you're telling me I should?!" This criticism resulted in two helpful advances. One was to help clinicians and others understand the difference between admitting a mistake and admitting liability.[4] The other was that we scheduled interviews with the main medical malpractice insurers that cover CHW physicians. In three cases, we were able to learn directly from the industry representatives that their philosophy of disclosure is very similar to ours, and that early appropriate disclosure actually minimizes awards rather than increasing them.

One of the most important requests that came from practicing clinicians was that we develop a kind of flowchart of disclosure, about "who says what to whom when." Since some physicians expressed concern that CHW was going to "tell on them" against their will, it was important that we develop a clear pathway, with assumptions about who would be present at disclosures. This necessitated further distinctions, not about harm this time, but about who was involved in the mistake.

Because the financial interests of physicians and hospitals are not aligned, there is a perception that hospitals out to preserve their own assets could unfairly blame a physician for a mistake and vice versa. This complicates the picture of most hospital-based errors, which are, in fact, made neither by physicians nor by agents of the hospital such as nurses or pharmacists, but by all of them together. It is easy enough to say that when a CHW employee (a nurse, a technician, a therapist, etc.) makes an error, our CHW philosophy will dictate our behavior. But physicians are not employees of the hospital, and there was some sense that a physician's mistake could end up being disclosed to a patient in spite of the physician's protest or even in his or her absence.

These concerns prompted the "Pathways for Disclosure" flowchart (appendix B), accompanied by the simple assumptions that a physician (either the physician who made the error, a department chair, or the chief of staff) would always be present at the disclosure of an error a physician participated in, and that a hospital representative would always be present at the disclosure of an error in which hospital personnel were involved. The obvious corollary was that when a mistake was contributed to by both, both would be present at disclosure. The flowchart also included assumptions about timing.[5]

These were three of the important aspects of the project that unfolded as we heard from key constituencies. Space does not allow me to describe the others, but they included an information sheet of frequently asked questions (appendix A) and a series of skill-building exercises for risk managers and others.

Is the Culture Changing?

It would be nice to have data sets that could illustrate the success of this project, but we do not. Because of the unfolding and interactive nature of this project, it is not possible to ascertain a clear "before" and "after" between which to measure change. It is also not entirely obvious what would indicate that change has occurred. Because behavioral conformity to core values was the target, and not a reduced number of suits, claims, or settlements, measurement of the latter would not indicate whether we are achieving our goal. Furthermore, culture change is glacially slow, and must constantly be reinforced by new means, such as orientation, standards for mission integration, and other opportunities to make the values of an organization present. These efforts are just starting or in some cases have not yet begun.

However, anecdotally we do seem to be seeing fewer claims arising from medical mistakes, and workers in risk management believe this is due, at least in some part, to this different approach. We have also heard, again anecdotally, that physicians and other clinicians are discussing these issues more often (this is likely due to increased attention to the subject elsewhere). Probably the most frequent comment from nurses in direct relation to this project and the values that underlie it is along the lines of "At last this is out in the open." This is also an indication for us that there was ripeness for change.

Furthermore, the values that impel us to more honesty, greater fairness, better stewardship of public trust, etc., in the realm of mistakes also reach into other areas of hospital behavior. How physicians and nurses demonstrate respect for each other, the need to inform patients carefully before securing their consent, and the recognition that "harmless hits" are a rich ore of information to be mined in subsequent projects will eventually all profit from such culture change.

Getting it right at the level of institutions has, I believe, the greatest likelihood of perceivable success when it springs from the values that give meaning to the organization's work. Change may happen at a societal level—slowly and as a result of Herculean efforts to solve large, complex problems such as tort reform. It may also happen, one by one, in the hearts and minds of those individual clinicians who make mistakes. Institutions, though, are where people actually do the work of health care. Here they carry out the interventions that sometimes result in mistakes, and here they influence each other's behavior through relationships and structures, policies and procedures, accountabilities of professional authority and collegial friendship. These are the real avenues of change. When individuals in their communities of work learn together, those individuals change. And when those communities of work organize their voices, society will change.

Notes

1. We might also say that the practice of medicine is influenced by the institution of medicine itself, which also has standards and norms. The institution of medicine ("the profession") may tolerate some departure from these norms, but altogether the profession is a powerful force for conformity and, to a certain degree, quality. For my purposes, the institution of medicine will be examined *in situ*, that is, in the practical context of the hospital.

2. Quality improvement techniques appear to have greater success in processes that contain a smaller proportion of "human factor" elements. For example, hospitals have used Continuous Quality Improvement techniques effectively to improve admissions and discharge processes, where attitudes and emotions are not featured prominently in the perceived problem. They are less successful in improving, for example, processes to improve the way patients die in the hospital, unless the techniques manage to address fears about death, resistance to "giving up," myths about addiction to pain medications, etc.

3. This statement was drafted by me, the system's ethicist; the corporate members of CHW approved it.

4. Admitting an error is not the same as admitting liability. Analysis of a tort (the determination of liability) requires a finding of three things: (1) negligence, i.e., departure from the standard of care; (2) harm, i.e., the patient must have been harmed; and (3) proximate

cause, i.e., harm must have resulted from the departure from the standard of care. It is this third element of causation that is not known with certainty until an investigation has been completed. Admitting an error, even in the presence of harm to the patient, does not necessarily mean that the error caused the harm, which is why it is important that disclosure is made early, carefully, and without promising that more is known than really is known. If disclosure is made appropriately, the truth unfolds for the patient or family, and for the institution, as the analysis goes forward.

5. This pathway flowchart was eventually replaced by an actual disclosure policy. Both are included as appendices B and C.

Appendix A: Frequently Asked Questions

1. I heard that CHW now has a policy of being more honest with patients when a mistake is made in their care. Does this mean I should go directly to a patient to apologize when I think I made a mistake? Shouldn't my supervisor go with me?

CHW has documented its approach to sharing information with patients and their families in the Philosophy of Mistake Management (a copy of which you can obtain by accessing the Risk or Care Management Intranet website). This Philosophy clearly articulates CHW's commitment to our values in the context of disclosure of information about mistakes. The Philosophy of Mistake Management is compatible with your hospital's current process for disclosing medical information.

When you believe that a mistake occurred, you should immediately report the incident to your supervisor on duty at the time. You should complete the required documentation, i.e., an event/incident report, medical record documentation of the objective facts in the situation, etc. Your supervisor will make sure that the appropriate individuals, such as the attending/involved physician, risk manager, pharmacist, and/or administration, are informed and participate in a discussion as appropriate on a case-by-case basis. After the discussion, your supervisor will decide what should be the next steps. For example, your supervisor may ask that you talk to the patient, if you feel you are able, or others may take the lead in talking with the patient and perhaps also the patient's family.

We understand and expect that mistakes will occur and are sometimes unavoidable. One of the purposes of the Philosophy is to assure that our patients experience the CHW values in relation to the management of information about their care, condition, and course of treatment. Your collaboration and participation is a key element to our success in this process.

2. It seems to me that when mistakes happen on my unit, it frequently relates to the action or inaction of several people, including physicians. How do we inform the patient under those circumstances?

The physician, healthcare workers, and the hospital all have relationships with the patient. Therefore, the responsible physician or his or her designee (such as the nurse supervisor) will clearly explain the outcome of any treatment or procedures to the patient and, when appropriate, the family, whenever those outcomes differ significantly from the anticipated outcomes.

For example, whenever an error has occurred, the patient's physician will be promptly informed of the error and the circumstances. If the error involves only the hospital, we encourage the physician to be with hospital personnel when we discuss the error as support to the patient and to have him/herself available for questions the patient may have regarding the impact of the error on the patient's care. However, there are situations where the physician cannot be part of the conversation, and both the physician and hospital personnel are comfortable with disclosure to the patient without the physician's presence.

However, in cases of medical mistakes that occur because of physician error, then a physician will always be directly involved in discussion with the patient and when appropriate, the family. The nurse supervisor and the medical staff leadership will ensure that the patient's rights are respected at all times.

3. This statement says we will talk to patients and their families with information "in a timely manner." What does this mean?

The patient and when appropriate, the family, should be informed of an error as soon as we can productively do so. Sometimes, the facts are clear and the consequences are evident. In those circumstances, the patient should be informed without unreasonable delay. Sometimes, however, more information is needed. We can still inform the patient of the facts that are known at that time (using the process described above) with the promise of further discussion with the patient, as more information is available. Patients are entitled to all pertinent information about their medical condition. The appropriate persons should disclose facts about medical errors significantly impacting the patient, as they become known. When it is more likely than not that a medical error contributed to an adverse event, disclosure should be made as information is obtained. Disclosure of this likelihood should be made long before the last pathology report or the final autopsy report is available.

4. How should a caregiver act if he/she is genuinely uncertain whether a particular adverse outcome is due to a mistake?

When there is an adverse outcome and it is not clear whether a medical mistake caused or contributed, the usual hospital procedures should be followed. Ordinarily, those procedures require reporting to a supervisor and completing an event report. An investigation by appropriate individuals will determine whether mistakes occurred. As a matter of course, the investigation will evaluate whether or not the standard of care was met.

5. Does this mean it is appropriate to provide copies of event reports or medical records when a patient or family member asks for all the information?

Once again, the Philosophy and our obligations under the Philosophy are not meant to replace current practices and policies. Current policies regarding medical records should be used in providing access. In most facilities, patients are allowed to review their records upon request. If possible, the physician or other healthcare worker or his or her designee is involved to provide explanation for terminology and procedures. If an error occurs, offering such a review, consistent with hospital policy, is one service to support the patient or their family.

Likewise, you should follow current procedures for handling incidents. You should not make copies for distribution outside of the peer review process.

6. You are encouraging us to report our errors. Does this mean we won't be disciplined for an honest mistake?

If an honest mistake is made, the provision of education and information will occur. If a pattern of issues emerges despite retraining, education, and coaching, we do have an obligation to responsibly manage the competence of our employees. These situations will be managed in the context of human resources policy and our core values.

If mistakes are not reported in a timely way (or at all) or a determination has been made that the facts were misrepresented, there will be consequences consistent with policy and core values.

Other industries have embraced confidential, non-punitive approaches to reporting after accepting the notion that, while human error might be the immediately observable reason for an incident, the "root cause" is generally a flaw in the systems governing human action.

The first difficult step is making the transformation to seeing medical systems and processes as the critical source of most error, not individuals. That requires moving away from a culture of fear about admitting error and blame, and both the leadership and individuals within the systems must make this journey. When other industries have successfully made the leap, they have not abandoned the traditional ethic of personal responsibility but rather transformed it so that individuals take responsibility for reporting error and fostering improvements.

7. Our mistake rate has sky-rocketed since all the cutbacks. Fewer of us are doing more work and are fatigued more often, which is when accidents happen. How is that being tracked?

Redesign initiatives have required us to reevaluate processes to improve efficiency and productivity. Since processes are being evaluated in this context, we are working with leadership to incorporate methods which have been effective at reducing error rates in other industries. These include simplifying, standardizing, reducing unnecessary reliance on memory, implementing forcing functions (reengineering a process to prevent a specific error, such as requiring a foot on the brake pedal to put a car in reverse), improving information access, reducing reliance on vigilance, and reducing the number of handoffs in the system. Already, evidence suggests that these and other strategies can dramatically reduce certain types of error.

Most hospitals have systems to track staffing and acuity issues. Some have separate forms which are utilized. Others ask staff to use their incident forms. The new CHW event form includes an opportunity to identify staffing issues as contributing to the occurrence. It is anticipated that this system should be instituted in all CHW facilities by the end of FY 01.

We have also begun to track staffing concerns identified as a part in our investigations of potentially compensable events. Information from both data sets—claims and event reporting—will be reported to management and Boards as they establish priorities and assess how to allocate resources.

If your organization does not have such a process, we encourage you to express your concerns to management. We would be happy to discuss best practices as they've been developed and tracked by other CHW hospitals.

Appendix B: Pathways for Disclosure

No Disclosure
- No information that medical error occurred

Continue investigation
- At such time it appears that medical error more likely than not harmed patient, disclosure.

Event Occurs

Inadequate facts to conclude medical error more likely than not caused or contributed to patient harm.

Evaluation of facts by attending physician, Nurse Manager and Risk Manager to determine if medical error more likely than not caused or contributed to patient harm.

Physician only error Physician will not participate and Nurse Manager and Risk Manager are comfortable.

Hospital Only Error Physician will participate in discussion.

Hospital & Physician Error Involved physician(s) will participate in discussion.

Nurse Manager/Risk Manager identifies appropriate disclosures.

Identified Person(s) discloses and secures appropriate support for patient.

Hospital & Physician Error Involved physician disagrees with determination that medical error caused or contributed to patient harm and/or disagrees with disclosure.

Hospital Only Error Attending physician will not participate in disclosure and Nurse Manager or Risk Manager not comfortable.

Physician Only Error Attending physician believes no error occurred and hence no disclosure is necessary.

Nurse Manager and Risk Manager refer to Hospital Administrator and medical staff process for evaluation and disposition.

Nurse Manager/Risk Manager consults with Hospital Administrator.

Hospital Administrator consults with Department Chair.

Department Chair disagrees with disclosures.

Department Chair agrees with disclosure and identifies physician participating.

Hospital Administrator/Department Chair consults with Chief of Staff.

Chief of Staff agrees with disclosure.

Chief of staff agrees with disclosure identifies physician participant.

Chief of Staff and Hospital Administrator consult with Regional Risk Manager and Medical Officer.

Regional Chief Medical Officer disagrees with disclosure.

Regional Chief Medical Officer agrees with disclosure and identifies physician participant.

Hospital Administrator and Chief of Staff consult with Chief Medical Officer, VP Risk Services, VP Ethics and Justice Education.

Consensus of group is not to disclose.

Consensus of group is to disclose and Chief Medical officer identifies physician participant.

Appendix C: Catholic Healthcare West Disclosure Policy, July 1, 2002

Disclosure of Unanticipated Adverse Outcomes to Patients/Families

PURPOSE

This policy and procedure provides guidance and direction regarding communication of outcomes of treatment, including unanticipated outcomes. It furthers Catholic Healthcare West's (CHW) Mission and Values, supports CHW's Philosophy of Mistake Management and integrates with CHW's Patient Safety Standard.

POLICY

It is Catholic Healthcare West's policy to support the right of patients to be active participants in decisions about their healthcare. Patients will be provided with sufficient information necessary to make an informed decision about treatment. In addition, patients and/or their family will be informed about the outcomes of treatment, including outcomes of treatment that differ significantly from anticipated outcomes. CHW hospitals will assure that any unanticipated adverse outcome is promptly communicated to the patient or the patient's family. This policy and procedure meets the requirements of CHW's Patient Safety Standard, reflects the CHW Philosophy of Mistake Management, and is endorsed by CHW Leadership.

DEFINITIONS

Disclosure—communication, to patients or patients' families, of information regarding the results of a diagnostic test, medical treatment or surgical intervention.

Unanticipated Adverse Outcome—an adverse result that differs significantly from the anticipated result of a treatment or procedure.

PROCEDURE

Reporting

It is the responsibility of all employees to report any unanticipated outcome immediately to their immediate supervisor and the facility Risk Manager. This information will be received, and any subsequent evaluation of the facts of the event will be conducted, in a non-punitive manner. However, failure to report such events may subject the individual to progressive discipline as outlined in Human Resources policy.

The individual identifying the event will take the following steps:

1. Assure that all necessary action is taken to mitigate the extent of the harm to the patient that may be caused by the adverse event.

2. Immediately notify the patient's treating Physician, the Nurse Manager/Department Manager and the Risk Manager.

3. Complete an unusual occurrence report (incident report) per hospital policy.

4. Participate in any investigation initiated to determine the cause of the event to determine actions that may prevent future like occurrences (as appropriate).

The Risk Manager, with the cooperation of the Department Manager, will conduct such investigation as is indicated by the hospital's relevant policies. All reports of adverse outcomes will be documented by the Risk Manager and evaluated for further action, including disclosure of the outcome to the patient and/or the patient's family as appropriate.

Disclosure

Once it has been determined that an unanticipated adverse outcome has occurred, disclosure is necessary. The Risk Manager and Nurse Manager/Department Manager, in consultation with the treating Physician (others may be consulted as well, e.g. CHW Risk Services Area Claims Manager, Chief of Staff, Department Chief), will determine the most appropriate time and manner for disclosure.

The Risk Manager, Nurse Manager/Department Manager, and treating Physician or their designees should participate in the disclosure process. It is CHW's philosophy that the treating physician has ultimate responsibility for disclosure of unanticipated adverse outcomes, that the treating Physician should be encouraged to accept this responsibility, and that hospital leadership should provide necessary support to enable the treating Physician to perform this responsibility. In cases where the adverse outcome is associated with non-physician staff, the duty to disclose will rest with responsible hospital leadership, with the most thorough knowledge of the event. However, the treating Physician will be made aware of the disclosure prior to the disclosure.

If there is disagreement or uncertainty on either the means or need for disclosure, the Hospital President will make the final determination, and if the unanticipated adverse event involves a member of the medical staff, the Hospital Chief of Staff will be consulted to assist in the disclosure determination. However, the Hospital President has the ultimate responsibility for the disclosure determination. The Hospital President may seek assistance in making the final determination from CHW's Disclosure Resource Team, consisting of the Vice President of Risk Services, Chief Medical Officer, CHW General Counsel and the Vice President of Ethics and Justice Education.

Disclosure will include the following elements:

- A clear explanation of the unanticipated adverse outcome to the patient and, when appropriate the family; Disclosure will be limited to a factual explanation of the circumstances; speculative comments will be avoided.

- A clear explanation of the investigation that will take place to learn as much as possible about the event, and plans to discuss the matter further with the patient or family as more facts become known.

- An explanation of the impact of the unforeseen occurrence on the patient's treatment, and steps taken to correct or mitigate any injury.

- Information regarding resources available to support and comfort the patient and/or family.

- Expressions of empathy to include as appropriate an expression of sympathy for the patient's inconvenience, distress or discomfort.

- An apology as appropriate for the circumstances.

The disclosure process will not include acceptance of liability, placement of fault, statements of causation or other actions that may be inappropriate given the status of the investigation.

Documentation

Documentation of disclosure of unanticipated adverse outcomes shall be done by the Risk Manager or other appropriate individual participating in the disclosure, and shall be treated as part of the unusual event/occurrence reporting process. This documentation should contain a brief statement that the disclosure has occurred and shall include the following elements:

- A full description of the facts of the event, without conjecture as to the cause or attribution of fault. Care will be taken to ensure that opinion is not documented.

- A note outlining the substance of the disclosure discussions with the patient, family member or surrogate about the event, including dates, times, and a list of who was present.

- The identity of any interpreter whose services may have been used.

- In cases where a decision is made to withhold some or all of the information about the event, the reason(s) for this decision.

- Any follow-up discussions with the patient, family member or surrogate should be similarly noted.

An unusual occurrence report will be completed and maintained by the hospital's Risk Manager, in accordance with appropriate hospital policies.

Documentation within the medical record should be limited to the medical facts of the case and a brief note stating simply that disclosure occurred.

CHAPTER 7

"Missing the Mark": Medical Error, Forgiveness, and Justice

NANCY BERLINGER

The title of the Institute of Medicine's report on medical error, *To Err Is Human: Building a Safer Health System* (Kohn, Corrigan, and Donaldson 2000), is derived from Alexander Pope's "Essay on Criticism" (1711): "To err is human; to forgive, divine" (l. 525). Given how familiar this proverb is in its entirety, it is striking that the IOM report itself contains no reference to forgiveness, divine or otherwise, in its treatment of medical error, even as its title hints at a fundamental relationship between error and forgiveness. In this chapter, I provide an overview of the close links between the concepts of error and forgiveness in the religious and related cultural traditions that have helped to shape and continue to inform Western thinking and Western medical culture. I argue that a systems approach to medical error must incorporate the recognition that errors leading to injury or death—medical harm—happen *to patients*, affecting their lives, their families, and their livelihoods, and that paying attention to the role of forgiveness in medical harm, while avoiding a principlist understanding of forgiveness, may help clinicians and administrators to focus on the needs of the patient who has been harmed. I conclude by recommending practices wherein forgiveness is understood as the outcome of concrete efforts to ensure justice for injured patients.

Forgiveness in Theo-Ethical Context

The root word *het'* appears 595 times in the Hebrew Bible, more than four times more often than its nearest synonym.[1] Although this word is usually translated into English as "sin," its oldest meaning, a meaning that has parallels in other ancient Near Eastern cultures, is to "miss the mark," like an archer who takes aims at a target and "misses" it, or a traveler who "misses" the correct turn.[2] *Het'* is also used to describe breaches of social ethics, as when someone "misses" an opportunity to assist another. It also has a theological dimension when one "misses" with respect to one's relationship with God, or in the performance of religious rites.

What is interesting about *het'* is that it truly means "missing the mark"—that is, error, not "sin"—requiring close attention to context to determine if a given error was intentional, unconscious, or avoidable, a matter of judgment, skill, experience, or character. As such, the word and its associated images may make a hermeneutical contribution to the study of medical error as a situation in which "missing the mark" may be framed as technical error by medical culture, as risk management by hospital administrators, as moral error, injustice, perhaps even sin, by patients, as spiritual and psychological devastation by the individual clinicians involved. By appreciating the many ways in which "missing the mark" may be interpreted, one may be better able to comprehend how the expectations of stakeholders concerning the resolution of cases of medical error may differ and conflict.

Within the Jewish and Christian traditions, forgiveness works roughly like this: God forgives the error itself, while the injured party forgives the individual who has made the error. Thus, forgiveness has both a divine and a human component and encompasses two relationships, one between a human being and God, the other between human beings. Furthermore, forgiveness is a response to two discrete actions or series of actions: an acknowledgment of the error by the person who has made it, a practice often called "confession" (*viddui* in Hebrew) that is inclusive of disclosure and accountability; and an effort by this person to make amends for the harm he or she has done, a practice often called "repentance" or "atonement" within religious contexts.[3] In these traditions, therefore, forgiveness is understood as the outcome of a relational ethical process, rather than as a first principle.

Jewish traditions concerning forgiveness emphasize human agency to a somewhat greater extent than do Christian traditions, in which divine agency, often represented by clergy, may be more prominent. For example, the Hebrew word for "atonement," *kapparah*, specifically refers to the reconciliation of the person who has committed an error with the person he or she has injured.[4] The error is forgiven only when the injured person has been sufficiently appeased, a process that may involve concrete restitution; indeed, the word *kapparah* comes from a legal term for compensation.[5] During the Ten Days of Repentance between *Rosh Hashanah* and *Yom Kippur* (*kapparah* and *Kippur* share the same root), all Jews are responsible for acknowledging their errors of the past year, making restitution, and reconciling with those whom they have wronged.[6] The Jewish tradition's understanding of atonement as the reconciliation of *persons* thus requires the injured party, as human agent of forgiveness, to play an active role in the repentance of the person responsible for his injury. If taken literally, this expectation may be oppressive to the injured party, who may wish neither to engage directly with this person, nor to be held to her timeframe for atonement.

In recent years, the Kabbalist concept of *tikkun olam*, or "repairing the world" through acts that promote justice—in particular, social justice—has come to be associated with the Ten Days of Repentance, extending the idea of atonement beyond individual error and individual forgiveness.[7] Finally, it is worth noting that the Hebrew word for "repentance," *teshuvah*, literally means "return."[8] Recalling that one of the images associated with error as "missing the mark" is taking the wrong road, we may be able to discern an underlying metaphor for repentance after error: turning around and retracing one's missteps so as to determine where one went astray.

In *A Philosophical Disease*, Carl Elliott makes an observation concerning the continuing influence of his cultural background upon the way he makes decisions in everyday life: "I refer to no systematic moral theories or doctrines in making moral judgments, but I have no illusions that these judgments are independent of the fact that I grew up as a Presbyterian in South Carolina" (Elliott 1999, 148). Dena S. Davis argues that one of the goals of the *religious* ethicist working in a clinical setting is to "describe how real people actually believe and act" when faced with ethical dilemmas, adding that these beliefs and actions may or may not be consistent with religious doctrine: knowing what Presbyterians are supposed to believe may be an insufficient guide to understanding how growing up as a Presbyterian in the postwar American South influenced a specific individual's norms and values (Davis 1999, 10, 13). Yet knowledge of religious practices embedded in the real lives of real people may offer insight into an individual's moral formation. The extensive use of the Lord's Prayer in Christian worship, public and private, makes it a useful window through which to glimpse how individual perspectives on error and forgiveness may be grounded in formative religious influences and internalized norms.

The best-known version of this prayer comes from the Gospel according to Matthew, and includes the phrase "forgive us our debts, as we also have forgiven our debtors" (Matthew 6:12, New Revised Standard Version). The shorter, probably older version of this prayer found in Luke's Gospel makes even clearer the extent to which these early Christian texts are grounded in the Jewish understanding of how forgiveness works: "forgive us our sins, for we ourselves forgive everyone indebted to us" (Luke 11:4, NRSV).[9] God forgives the error, but people must first forgive one another. The prayer's "debt" metaphors and their epistemological implications for patients injured through medical error will be discussed at a later point.

Christian paradigms of error and forgiveness may stress personal salvation—the repair of one's relationship with God—over the concrete making of amends to the injured party—the repair of one's relationship with another human being. These tendencies can lead to a truncation, even a perversion, of the process of forgiveness that Dietrich Bonhoeffer memorably described as "cheap grace . . . cut-rate forgiveness . . . grace as doctrine, as principle, as system" (Bonhoeffer [1937] 2001, 43).[10] In this "system," disclosure, accountability, and repentance—all of the traditional, specific responsibilities of the person who has harmed another—are eliminated, as forgiveness is elevated to a "general truth" (43).

Christian feminist ethicists such as Pamela Cooper-White and Marie M. Fortune have made use of Bonhoeffer's work—written as an indictment of the readiness of many German churches to accommodate the rise of Nazism in the 1930s—to criticize the tendency of pastors (and other counselors) to forgive those who have not acknowledged, taken responsibility for, or made amends for the suffering that they have caused, particularly in situations of sexual abuse. Such a pastor may then encourage the injured person to offer forgiveness despite the absence of confession or repentance on the part of the person who caused the injury (Cooper-White 1995, 253–62; Fortune and Poling 1995, 451–63).

Fortune and Cooper-White argue that, in this scenario, an injured person may believe, whether as the result of internalized norms or the influence of a pastor, family member, or even the person who has harmed her, that she *has* to forgive, no matter what the circumstances, in order to demonstrate that she is a good person or a faithful believer. In urging well-intentioned counselors to abandon the cheap grace of what Cooper-White calls "an ethic of instant forgiveness," these feminist critics assert that "[f]orgiveness will always be premature, pseudo-, or at best partial . . . until [the injured person has] uncover[ed] enough of the factual story to know what really happened to her"; that "forgiveness is not a right," but is contingent upon justice; and that "the deepest form of justice involves the calling to account, subsequent repentance, and amendment of life" of the person who has harmed another (Cooper-White 1995, 253, 255–56). Forgiveness, therefore, is a response not to the harm itself, but to evidence of change after harm.

Bonhoeffer's "cheap grace" formulation is useful to contemporary discourse on medical error in another respect: its rejection of forgiveness understood as a "principle" or a "system."[11] When forgiveness is elevated to a first principle, instead of understood as the outcome of a process that requires something of the party whose actions have led to harm, it may obscure, or be misunderstood as a surrogate for, the ethical principle of justice. And when discourse on medical error misuses the language of "systems" to dodge the issue of individual responsibility, or when information about a patient's health, including injury resulting from error, is withheld from that patient, the ethical principle of respect for persons is undermined. In either case, what is ignored is what Bonhoeffer calls the "concrete place"—here, the reality of human suffering resulting from harm—and its attendant responsibilities (Bonhoeffer [1949] 1995, 87).[12]

A principlist approach to forgiveness is evident in many contemporary, secular projects, including A Campaign for Forgiveness Research, an initiative of the John Marks Templeton Foundation that promotes the scientific study of forgiveness, and developmental psychologist Robert Enright's Wisconsin-based

International Forgiveness Institute.[13] The goal of A Campaign for Forgiveness Research is to support sixty research projects on "the power of forgiveness and reconciliation" in four categories: forgiveness among individuals, among families, and among nations; and the biology and human evolution of forgiveness.[14] While none of the projects funded to date focuses on forgiveness after medical harm, information published online by several projects focusing on "forgiveness among individuals" suggests that responsibility for repairing damaged interpersonal relationships lies with the person who extends or withholds forgiveness.

Thus, the Heartland Forgiveness Project at the University of Kansas describes "persons who are stuck in unforgiving, unproductive patterns of interacting with themselves, other people, or situations" as those who may benefit from "forgiveness interventions."[15] The Stanford Forgiveness Project asserts that "[a]ll major religious traditions and wisdoms extol the value of forgiveness" and describes its focus as "training forgiveness to ameliorate the anger and distress involved in feeling hurt"—adding that "the need for forgiveness emerges from a body of work demonstrating harmful effects of unmanaged anger and hostility on health." The Stanford Project offers a "unique and practical definition of forgiveness," which "consists primarily of taking less personal offense, reducing anger and the blaming of the offender, and developing increased understanding of situations that often lead to feeling hurt and angry."[16] While clinical research by Enright and others strongly suggests that the ability to forgive is a marker of psychological health and may be indispensable to the healing of relationships, identifying forgiveness as a norm or virtue characteristic of a physically, emotionally, and morally healthy person, without closely examining the roles that disclosure, accountability, and repentance play in allowing one person to forgive another, potentially conflates someone who has been injured through medical harm or other trauma with someone who has a tendency to "feel hurt" and "take offense" (Freedman and Enright 1996; Kaminer et al. 2001). As the sole agent of forgiveness in this scenario, the injured person must both be good *and* be God, responsible for saving herself and other people from her own unhealthy, "unproductive" anger.

Forgiveness Rituals in Western Medical Culture

Forgiveness as ritual and system is deeply embedded in medical education and culture. Charles L. Bosk's *Forgive and Remember: Managing Medical Failure* (1979), a classic study of how surgeons handle error and other types of medical failure, provides a detailed description of forgiveness norms and practices—as well as a title that directly suggests a relationship between error and forgiveness. The following excerpt is from the section titled "Forgiveness and Punishment":

Superordinates tend to be tolerant and forgiving of technical error and intolerant and unforgiving of moral error [which Bosk defines in this context as "failure to follow the code of conduct on which professional action rests"]. . . .

Forgiveness itself operates as a deterrence to further technical error. First, it obligates the subordinate who is forgiven to the superordinate who shows him [sic] mercy. To repay this obligation, the subordinate becomes more vigilant in the immediate future. Following a technical error, it is quite common for a subordinate to spend extra time with each patient . . . to make sure results are satisfactory. . . . Second, when a subordinate sees his technical errors are forgiven, he recognizes that he has no incentive to hide them. He is less likely, therefore, to compound his problems by attempting to treat problems that are over his head for fear of superordinate reprisal. Forgiveness encourages "help-seeking" behavior and removes the stigma from uncertainty.

Forgiveness also serves to reintegrate offenders into the group. We see this most directly in the "hair-shirt" ritual that is part of the Mortality and Morbidity Conference [M & M]. The self-criticism, confession, and forgiveness that are all part of this ceremony allow the offender to reenter the group. The "hair-shirt" ritual promotes group solidarity. In tightly knit communal groups such ceremonies are a regular part of group life. . . . "Hair-shirt" rituals are a form of public exorcism. Through them, whatever demons that led to incorrect practice are driven from the group. . . .

Forgiveness binds the confessor to the group and exacts a pledge from him to live up to standards in the future. Since in time all make errors in techniques, all are obliged in time to go before the group and humble themselves. Through this practice of confession and forgiveness, the group exacts the allegiance of all its members to its standards. . . . [T]he group can afford to be merciful in the face of technical error since its members openly confess them. (Bosk 1979, 177–79)

Bosk's richly descriptive account of the "hair-shirt" ritual that is such a prominent feature of the mortality and morbidity conference allows theologically and anthropologically attuned readers to identify vestiges of ancient Jewish and Christian practices concerning forgiveness.[17] Both Jewish and Christian communities have long incorporated ritualized public confession into their religious practices.[18] The "hair-shirt" that functions here as a metaphor for "self-criticism" was (and is) a real garment, woven of animal hair and worn as an act of penance during religious rites and as an ascetic practice.[19] "Exorcism" may have been a feature of early Christian rituals associated both with the reinstatement of penitents within the community, and with the preparation of catechumens for baptism (Dujarier 1979, 52; Hatchett 1980, 448–49).[20] We can even see, in the sequencing of ritual actions—confession through the "hair-shirt" ritual, forgiveness by the superordinate, and then repentance through vigilance and spending extra time with patients—a parallel with the reordering of Christian penitential rites in the late medieval period, as the practice of private confession, followed by absolution and then by the performance of penitential acts assigned by one's parish priest, superseded public rituals of forgiveness (Hatchett 1980, 449–50). Viewed through the lens of Western religious tradition, then, the morbidity and mortality conference "hair-shirt" ritual and related penitential practices are neither modern nor wholly secular, whether or not contemporary participants recognize the ancient religious and cultural roots of their "ceremony."

What is perhaps most striking in Bosk's account, from the perspectives of theology and of cultural anthropology alike, is the role of the "superordinate"—the erring physician's superior—who combines religious and secular roles, functioning as deity, high priest, judge, pastor, peer group representative, and injured party, forgiving both the error itself and the physician who makes the error. According to a taxonomy devised by British moral philosopher J. L. Austin, who catalogued the ways rituals can fail to fulfill their cultural, religious, or psychological functions through "infelicitous performances," this conflation of roles constitutes a "ritual misapplication": a legitimate ceremony that fails because of the involvement of inappropriate persons (Grimes 1996, 285, 288). The "hair-shirt" ritual, *qua* ritual, fails because it excludes the patient, whose roles as injured party and as human agent of forgiveness are usurped by the erring physician's superordinate. The patient has no role, no voice, and no representation within this closed ritual, and cannot rely upon it for justice, or for the possibility of being able to forgive and to heal.

This is *not* to say that injured patients should be included in M & M conferences. Rather, it is to say that the ritual of confession, repentance, and forgiveness, enacted within a culturally appropriate context and with reference to the needs and expectations of the injured party, may be as important to patients as it is already understood to be among physicians, and should be available to them.

The "hair-shirt" ritual may be infelicitous in another way. In recent interviews and correspondence conducted with physicians, nurses, and chaplains on the topic of forgiveness after medical error, *self-forgiveness* has emerged as a constant theme. All stressed that some form of self-forgiveness—their phrase—was essential in restoring confidence and morale after incidents of medical harm, even as one physician acknowledged that while self-forgiveness is "something we all have to face when we make an error that harms someone . . . [i]t is hard to get physicians to think in these terms."[21] None described any existing institutional process, such as the "hair-shirt" ritual of M & M, as capable, in and of itself, of helping clinicians who have made errors to forgive themselves. Instead, the single most important factor in the clinicians' ability to forgive themselves appeared to be the ability to have private, unguarded conversations with colleagues (what one physician called a "cadre of friends") or chaplains (described as a "safe space")—conversations in which they could discuss incidents of medical error and their own roles in and emotions concerning these incidents.[22]

One physician questioned the appropriateness of the term "self-forgiveness," and the theological premise underlying it: that one could be the agent of one's own salvation. Taken literally, self-forgiveness would be another example of cheap grace, in which the other—the injured party, God—is pushed out of the frame, while the person who has made the error is forgiven without any assurance that the relational actions traditionally described as confession and repentance have first taken place. This physician suggested an alternative definition for so-called self-forgiveness—"freedom from guilt and self-hatred"—while arguing that forgiveness itself must be understood to be relational: "there must be a self-transcending aspect to forgiveness—or it does not occur."[23]

Among my interview subjects, the need for self-forgiveness was held in tension with the belief that there was not "much of a possibility" of being forgiven directly by a patient or a patient's family following an incident of medical harm.[24] There is in these words a poignant echo of Christopher Marlowe's version of the Faust legend: in his despair, Dr. Faustus believes—incorrectly—that his "offense can never be pardoned" (*Dr. Faustus*, 1604, Scene 14). Lest the contemporary reader imagine spiritual despair to be a quaintly "religious" notion or literary conceit, here are some of the words that the clinicians interviewed used to describe their responses to their own errors: "devastated"; "heartsick . . . demoralized, worthless."[25]

These clinicians also reported that even peripheral involvement in an error—referring a patient for a procedure, then learning that the patient was injured while being moved, or knowing a patient by sight, then learning that this patient has committed suicide—can result in feelings of "devastation" and "failure" among many staff members.[26] The word "devastating" also came up with respect to legal liability, both in terms of what being sued can do to one's career, and in terms of "the folk wisdom" among physicians concerning the percentage of patients who do sue.[27] Given this snapshot of the psychological and spiritual dimensions of how medical harm is experienced by clinicians, it is not surprising to learn that, according to a director of pastoral care who also serves as a medical school instructor and chaplain, "theological concepts can be useful even if you don't use [theological] language" when counseling clinicians following incidents of medical error.[28]

Other conversations, with clinicians and scholars from non-Western religious traditions, have proven to be an essential corrective to any notion that forgiveness is universally understood as a principle, norm, or religious or secular practice.[29] Recalling Arthur Kleinman's "category fallacy"—the "imposition of a classification scheme onto members of societies for whom it holds no validity"—is instructive (Kleinman 1995, 13). It would not be appropriate to talk about the "Buddhist" or "Hindu" understanding of forgiveness, for example—not because these traditions are "unforgiving," but because forgiveness as a metaphor for a relationship between autonomous persons may not be appropriate in traditions in which there may be no concept of the self independent from other persons or one's past lives. Similarly, in traditions in which suffering is understood to be inevitable, compassion (literally, "suffering with"), not forgiveness, is the predominant metaphor for right relationship between persons. At a time when one in five physicians practicing in the United States today was born and raised in Asia, it is ever more important to be aware of the extent to which apparently "universal" norms and rituals concerning error and forgiveness are grounded in Western culture, Western religions, and Western ideas about the self.[30]

While there is virtually no literature on the role of pastoral care in dealing with medical harm and promoting patient safety, my preliminary research suggests that professional chaplains in some hospitals—notably, palliative care and psychiatric hospitals—are regularly involved in counseling individual physicians and other staff members, and in playing what one chaplain on a psychiatric unit describes as a "prominent role" following critical incidents.[31] These chaplains, whose profession has been transformed in the past generation due to the Clinical Pastoral Education (CPE) movement, which trains clergy and laypersons for ministries in health care, view working with clinical staff, as well as with patients and families, as a "recognized part of [their] ministry."[32] A student chaplain, who had previously worked as a nurse for over thirty years, said she could imagine creating a "ritual of forgiveness" on her palliative care unit to help clinicians come to terms with their own errors: "I could picture me doing it—I don't think it's far-fetched at all."[33] Perhaps not surprisingly, clinicians and chaplains at these specialized hospitals work closely with one another in general, developing relatively nonhierarchical peer relationships that can be relied upon in times of crisis. They may also develop closer relationships with patients, whose average stays in these hospitals may be much longer than the three-day average in an acute-care facility, a situation that may promote an ethos of disclosure and accountability in cases of medical error. More empirical research on this topic is needed, particularly among pastoral care and clinical staff in acute-care hospitals.

What is true for the "hair-shirt" ritual of M & M is also true for these alternative rituals that are developing elsewhere within hospital culture: even if a clinician is officially forgiven by her superior through an established ritual, or comes to forgive herself following peer discussions and pastoral counseling, *the injured patient is not a member of these "congregations."* As such, these rituals, in and of themselves, do not provide the patient with an opportunity to forgive if he chooses to do so, because they do not ensure that the patient has received justice following medical harm.

From the Patient's Point of View: A Theory of Forgiveness after Medical Harm

This brings us to an epistemological problem. "Forgiveness" is a Janus word, in that it holds contradictory meanings—to engage and to detach—that are often conflated or insufficiently distinguished in discourse. In the Jewish and Christian traditions, the deepest meaning of forgiveness is *detachment*. Thus, in the Lord's Prayer, the "debt" language, which has many antecedents in the Hebrew Bible, means God forgives sin by releasing the believer from the error that is holding him captive, and that one human being forgives another by detaching from that person, and the harm that person has caused, as a source of pain, anger, and injustice. The underlying metaphor is the cancellation of a financial debt that can never be repaid; the metaphor itself is grounded in a culture in which debt-servitude was common. Forgiveness as "cheap grace," as principle rather than outcome, ignores this deep meaning, forcing engagement or acquiescence on the injured party, and even forcing this human into a divine, salvific role, instead of allowing detachment to take place over time—in what the Christian Bible refers to as *kairos*, the appropriate time, as opposed to *chronos*, chronological time—once justice has been secured.[34]

This does *not* mean that injured patients—or clinicians who have made errors, for that matter—should simply be encouraged to "detach" from incidents of medical harm, and from their feelings concerning these incidents. Detachment, as I have noted, takes its own time, and, in cases of injury or other trauma, may be conditional upon disclosure, accountability, and the making of amends. Even in mundane interpersonal situations, forgiveness-as-detachment can be problematic: after we have succeeded in detaching ourselves from a painful situation, we may still hesitate to *say* "I forgive you" if we believe that, by doing so, we are excusing bad behavior rather than affirming changed behavior.

Because forgiveness—as a word, a metaphor, a virtue, a process, a ritual, a principle, a system—is so vulnerable to the category fallacy and other misinterpretations, some scholars have proposed "reconciliation" as an alternative name for the outcome of the justice-making project. Writing about forgiveness after personal trauma, Pamela Cooper-White notes that reconciliation literally means *re-concilium*, regathering, the restoration of community, and calls for an understanding of forgiveness as a communal ethic of truth-telling, accountability, and care, resulting in justice (Cooper-White 1995, 261–62). Writing about forgiveness after political trauma, Donald W. Shriver suggests that reconciliation is "the end of a process that forgiveness begins," with forgiveness understood as "an act that joins moral truth, forbearance, empathy, and commitment to repair a fractured human relation," and with repentance understood to be the "twin" of forgiveness in the project of restoring "civil relationship between strangers" (Shriver 1995, 6, 8–9).[35] If we consider patients and clinicians to be members of the same community, we may prefer Cooper-White's definition of reconciliation; if we consider them to be strangers, we may prefer Shriver's definition. We may also reject both of these definitions: philosopher Susan Dwyer argues for a definition of political reconciliation that is "conceptually independent of [personal] forgiveness" and "might be psychologically possible where forgiveness is not" (Dwyer 1999, 23). None of these definitions is necessarily concerned with the reconciliation of *persons* that we have observed in traditional religious paradigms; nor are these definitions specifically concerned with individual forgiveness. Rather, they are closer to the recovered Jewish tradition of *tikkun olam*, with its underlying image of the repair of a shattered world.

And what might the justice-making project encompass in cases of medical error? Here are some preliminary suggestions, building on a Western theological framework and with reference to pastoral concerns:

The practices traditionally described as *confession* would include:

- promptly acknowledging error and disclosing to the patient a cogent and complete narrative of what happened;

- being personally accountable even in cases of systems error, bearing in mind that some patients may comprehend error in all cases as an individual rather than a collective or systemic failure;

- providing opportunities for clinicians to process incidents and receive counseling in a "safe," i.e., nonpunitive or demoralizing, environment;

- nurturing as a communal principle that withholding the truth violates patient autonomy and has a corrupting effect upon care providers;[36]

- avoiding the scapegoating of subordinates; and

- avoiding the abuse of the unequal distribution of power between a physician and an injured patient, which may be further skewed by gender, race, income, age, culture, disability, or other factors. Relevant abuses of authority would include making a patient complicit in error by labeling her "noncompliant"; conflating known incidents of error with "complications" in general; and taking advantage of a patient's religious beliefs, e.g., "It was God's will," to hide or excuse error.[37]

With respect to the legal and financial ramifications of "confession," i.e., full disclosure, Steve S. Kraman and Ginny Hamm, the authors of the oft-cited multiyear study of the full disclosure policy of the Veteran Affairs Medical Center in Lexington, Kentucky, in effect since 1987, observe that "[t]his practice continues to be followed because administration and staff believe that it is the right thing to do and because it has resulted in unanticipated financial benefits to the medical center," and conclude that "an honest and forthright risk management policy that puts the patient's interests first may be relatively inexpensive" (Kraman and Hamm 1999, 964).

The practices traditionally described as *repentance* would include:

- apologizing and expressing remorse to injured patients—and allowing oneself to feel remorseful after harming a patient;

- not forcing the patient to interact with the person responsible for her injury if the patient does not wish to do so;

- appreciating the difference between appropriate feelings of guilt and destructive feelings of shame;[38]

- offering injured patients and family members immediate access to pastoral care or other counseling services should they desire them;

- covering the cost of treating injuries resulting from error, and meeting other concrete needs resulting from loss of income due to injury or death resulting from error;

- recognizing that asking for "forgiveness" may be oppressive to an injured patient; and

- working to create conditions that may allow that patient, at some point in *her* future, to detach from this incident as a continuing source of pain, anger, and injustice. Kraman and Hamm, for example, observe that the Lexington facility's practice of "offer[ing] timely, comprehensive help in filing claims . . . diminishes the anger and desire for revenge that often motivates patients' litigation." (Kraman and Hamm 1999, 966)[39]

The practices designed to promote *forgiveness* or *reconciliation* would include:

- inviting patients to be part of the hospital's quality improvement process, to allow them, *if they wish*, to take an active role in working with clinicians and administrators to create a patient-centered culture of safety by sharing their experiences of medical harm and their perspectives on hospital culture. This is *not* to suggest that injured patients are responsible for participating in quality improvement efforts to prevent other patients from being harmed, or to solve systemic problems;

- using Clinical Pastoral Education and clinical ethics education opportunities to help chaplains, local pastors, counselors, patient advocates, clinical ethicists, and clinicians explore the psychological and spiritual aspects of medical error; develop their capacity to "see the world from the victim's point of view"; learn how to frame human forgiveness as detachment predicated upon justice; recognize non-Western paradigms of reconciliation; and work toward making justice for injured patients;[40]

- offering a ritual or other forum for hospital staff to explore their emotions and responsibilities concerning medical error; and, finally,

- identifying and challenging any aspects of institutional culture that deny the fallibility, and therefore the humanity, of clinical staff, or that work against truth-telling, accountability, compassion, and justice in dealing with medical error and promoting patient safety.

Acknowledgment

I wish to thank Virginia A. Sharpe, Albert Wu, my colleagues at the Hastings Center, audience members of the Hastings Center Bioethics Colloquia, doctoral students and faculty of the clinical ethics program at Saint Louis University, Professor Larry L. Rasmussen and Jennifer Harvey of Union Theological Seminary, and Kristin Bryant, whose comments have contributed to the development of this chapter.

Notes

1. Werblowsky and Wigoder 1997, s.v. "sin"; Freedman 1992, s.v. "sin, sinners."
2. Ibid.
3. Werblowsky and Wigoder 1997, s.v. "atonement." Technically, the actions of confession and repentance lead to the *state* of atonement, although in colloquial terms one may "atone" for one's errors through these actions.
4. Ibid., s.v. "atonement."
5. Ibid.
6. Werblowsky and Wigoder 1997, s.v. *"Aseret Yemei Teshuvah,"* "atonement," *"Yom Kippur."* It is important to note that rituals of penance—prayer, fasting, charitable giving— undertaken during the Ten Days of Repentance will atone only for sins against God, while "atonement for a wrong against a fellow human involves the seeking of forgiveness" from, "and appropriate restitution" to, that person (s.v. "atonement").
7. Werblowsky and Wigoder 1997, s.v. *"tiqqun 'olam."* The phrase *tikkun olam* has been adopted by Jewish congregations and organizations in the U.S. to describe their faith-based social justice projects, and as a framework for discussing the relationship between traditional rituals and contemporary ethical obligations. I am grateful to Charles L. Bosk for drawing my attention to the recovered tradition of *tikkun olam* with respect to the observance of *Yom Kippur* in particular.
8. Werblowsky and Wigoder 1997, s.v. "repentance."
9. On the dating of the material included in the Lord's Prayer, see Cross 1997, s.v. "'Q'." In biblical studies, "Q" represents the "hypothetical sources of those passages in the Synoptic Gospels where Matthew and Luke show a close similarity to each other but not to Mark." The hypothesis holds that the "Q" material in Luke is closer to the original than is the comparable material in Matthew.
10. For a comprehensive theological overview of the themes of forgiveness and repentance in Bonhoeffer's writings, see Jones 1994, 149–69.

11. Bonhoeffer's theo-ethical critique of principlism extends beyond the issue of forgiveness, and would doubtless have included a critique of the notion that biomedical ethics can be reduced to four principles. In his *Ethics*, Bonhoeffer rejects any principlist understanding of the nature of God: "[I]t is not written that God became an idea, a principle, a programme, a universally valid proposition or a law, but that God became [hu]man [in the form of Jesus Christ]. . . . He affirms reality." What follows from this theology is "an ethic which is entirely concrete . . . beyond formalism and casuistry" (Bonhoeffer [1949] 1995, 86–87).

12. See also Bonhoeffer, "After Ten Years": "[I]t is much easier to see a thing through from the point of view of abstract principle than from that of concrete responsibility" (Bonhoeffer [1951] 1997, 7). As Bonhoeffer sees it, the "ease" of using principles alone to assess ethical dilemmas is not an argument in their favor.

13. In addition to sponsoring A Campaign for Forgiveness Research, the Templeton Foundation's Program to Encourage the Scientific Study of Forgiveness has commissioned an annotated bibliography of social science research on forgiveness (available on the foundation's website, www.templeton.org) and has published several collections of essays and symposia papers. Information on the International Forgiveness Institute, founded and directed by Robert Enright, is available from the institute's website: www.forgiveness-institute.org (accessed 8 December 2001).

14. The website of A Campaign for Forgiveness Research (http://forgiving.org) includes descriptions of the twenty-nine projects fully or partially funded as of 1999. The funding category "forgiveness among individuals" includes six subcategories: the relationship between forgiveness and health; models and theories of forgiveness; developing forgiveness; forgiving after sexual, alcohol, or drug abuse; forgiving after trauma, grief, loss, or violence; and forgiveness in place of revenge (accessed 8 December 2001).

15. Heartland Forgiveness Project website, www.ukans.edu/~forgive/ (accessed 8 December 2001).

16. Stanford Forgiveness Project website, www.stanford.edu/~alexsox/forgiveness _article.htm (accessed 8 December 2001).

17. See Bosk 1979, 127–46, for additional description and analysis of this ritual.

18. For example, on *Yom Kippur* in Jewish congregations, and on Ash Wednesday in Roman Catholic and some other Christian congregations.

19. Cross 1997, s.v. "hair-shirt." J. F. Powers includes a fictional account of the use of (real) hair-shirts by mid-twentieth-century American priests and seminarians in his novel *Wheat That Springeth Green* (2000, 41–56).

20. Dujarier identifies the ordinary laying on of hands as "probably a gesture of exorcism" and cites Tertullian's descriptions of formal exorcisms that were part of the baptismal rite itself. Hatchett suggests that the laying on of hands, a practice described in the Hebrew Bible, was "possibly" part of the ritual of reinstatement for penitents.

21. Albert Dreisbach, M.D., Assistant Professor, Department of Internal Medicine, Tulane University School of Medicine, New Orleans, Louisiana; personal communication.

22. Lyla Correoso, M.D., attending physician, Calvary Hospital, Bronx, New York; personal communication. Staff chaplain, personal communication.

23. Dreisbach, personal communication.

24. Ibid.

25. Correoso, personal communication. Student chaplain, personal communication.

26. Ibid.

27. Dreisbach, personal communication. Curtis Hart, M.Div., Director of Pastoral Care, New York–Presbyterian Hospital; personal communication.

28. Hart, personal communication.

29. These conversations, with visiting international scholars at The Hastings Center, focused on Hindu and Buddhist traditions in particular.

30. The "one in five" statistic was quoted by Bryan Liang, at the July 2001 meeting of the *Promoting Patient Safety* project team at the Hastings Center.

31. Staff chaplain, personal communication.

32. Student chaplain, personal communication.

33. Staff chaplain, personal communication.

34. The eschatological dimension of *kairos* is discussed in Cooper-White 1995, 262.

35. Shriver's "civil relationship between strangers" is derived from Jean Hampton's discussion of biblical metaphors of forgiveness: "These ways of speaking suggest that when the wrongdoer is forgiven, it is presumed that he has committed an immoral action, but the forgiver nonetheless 'forgets' what the wrongdoer has done to him; not literally, but in the sense that he will not let the wrongdoing continue to intrude on his dealings with the wrongdoer in order that they can reestablish some kind of relationship—at the very least, the 'civil' relationship that prevails between strangers in a human community" (Hampton 1988, 37).

36. Observations made by Hart, personal communication.

37. Anne Fadiman describes an immigrant family's stigmatization as "noncompliant" with respect to their epileptic daughter's complicated medication regimen. A review of the child's case following a catastrophic seizure concluded that this event was triggered by an infection that may have resulted from an immunosuppressant drug that was administered by the parents as directed; the reviewing physician concluded, "[T]he family didn't do this to the kid. We did" (Fadiman 1997, 255).

In a recent article, physicians Timothy E. Quill, Robert M. Arnold, and Frederic Platt conflate "responding to medical complications or errors" as a single "representative clinical scenario" for the purpose of offering "sample responses" for their peers, although elsewhere in the article the authors do distinguish between complications and errors. Their sample response for "medical complications or errors"—"This is so hard for you—just when our hopes were so high, for her to have this complication, I wish it had been otherwise"—could be misused in cases of error, by misleading the patient or family into believing that "this complication" is of unknown origin, or even the fault of the patient (Quill, Arnold, and Platt 2001, 554).

Sandra M. Gilbert, whose husband died as the result of medical error, recounts a story from her lawyer, about one of his other clients, a benefactor of a Catholic hospital who had been repeatedly assured by his wife's doctor that it was "God's will" that his wife was comatose after routine surgery and later died. The husband sued to find out what happened in the operating room, and learned that "'everyone knew all along'" that the patient's coma and death had resulted from error (Gilbert 1997, 218–19).

38. A distinction made by Hart, personal communication.

39. By contrast, not addressing patients' questions and needs may increase their anger. A director of pastoral care reports that patients who "sense that something's gone wrong . . . start to ask questions, and if they're put off, they become angry. The longer they're put off, the more their anger increases" (personal communication).

40. The phrase "see the world from the victim's point of view" is taken from the title of physician David Hilfiker's keynote speech to the American Society of Bioethics and Humanities (ASBH) at its annual meeting in 1999. Hilfiker suggests that a goal of ethicists in the field of health care "should be to develop in those who care for others an empathy with the outsider, with the excluded, with the victim. . . . [I]f doctors and nurses and therapists and others cannot—to some extent—see the world from the victim's point of view, they'll have a difficult time developing an ethical framework in which to work" (Hilfiker 2001, 255).

Hilfiker's own ability to "see the world from the victim's point of view," honed through living and working in community with homeless men suffering from AIDS and other illnesses, is similar to Bonhoeffer's "view from below," which he identifies as "the perspective of those who suffer," and which he was able to comprehend through his role in the anti-Nazi resistance movement (Bonhoeffer [1951] 1997, 17).

CHAPTER 8

Is There an Obligation to Disclose Near-Misses in Medical Care?

ALBERT W. WU

Introduction

In its report *To Err Is Human*, the Institute of Medicine concluded that improvements in quality of care and patient safety depend on voluntary reporting systems (Kohn, Corrigan, and Donaldson 2000). These systems were viewed as particularly useful for identifying errors that occur too infrequently to be detected by individual health care organizations examining their own data, and patterns of errors that reflect systemic issues. Some of these errors are "near-misses" that do not cause harm to the patient. Reporting near-misses offers several advantages for achieving improvements in quality and patient safety: they have not resulted in patient harm and are thus less painful for workers to report; they are much more common than adverse events; and recovery strategies ("good catches") can be captured and incorporated into improvement efforts (Vincent et al. 2000; Leape 1999; Wu, Pronovost, and Morlock 2002; Callum et al. 2001). It should be noted that in this context, reports are made to an institution or other body, rather than to the patient or family.

There is professional and social consensus that physicians and health care organizations have an obligation to disclose errors and other incidents that cause significant harm to the patient and/or family, particularly those that are likely to be remediable, mitigable, or compensable (Wu et al. 1997; JCAHO 2002, RI 1.2.2). An ethical and practical question is: Is there also an obligation to disclose near-misses to patients? In the following discussion, I examine ethical arguments for and against disclosing near-misses to patients. I also provide practical suggestions for when and how to discuss these incidents with patients.

Definitions

A health care incident can be defined as "an event or circumstance which could have, or did lead to unintended and/or unnecessary harm to a person, and/or a complaint, loss or damage" (Australian Safety and Quality Council 2000). This definition is closely related to the Institute of Medicine's definition of an error, which is "the failure of a planned action to be completed as intended or the use of a wrong plan to achieve an aim" (Kohn, Corrigan, and Donaldson 2000, 156; Reason 1990). I have also used "an act or an omission with potentially negative consequences for the patient that would have been judged wrong by skilled and knowledgeable peers at the time it occurred" (Wu et al. 1997).

A "near-miss," also referred to as a "close call" by some and a "near hit" by some wags, can be defined as "an incident that did not cause harm" (Australian Safety and Quality Council) or "a medical error that resulted in no harm." Carol Bayley has distinguished between a near-miss and a harmless hit, defined as an error in which the departure from plan is executed, but with no appreciable effect on the patient (Bayley, this volume). Examples of near-misses might include a prescription that is written in error but noticed and corrected before being taken to the pharmacy, or a medication that is dispensed in error but is not administered to the patient. Examples of harmless hits might include a radiograph that is performed on the wrong patient but with no discernable consequence beyond delivery of a small amount of unnecessary X-rays, or a minor overdose of a medication that is administered to the patient with no ill consequences. Although the epidemiology of near-misses is not well-defined, it has been estimated that near-misses are much more frequent than errors that affect the patient (Bates et al. 1995; Bates 1996). In one study of transfusion medicine, near-misses were five times more frequent than completed errors (Callum et al. 2001).

Policy and Evidence

In general, policy statements of professional societies and regulatory bodies either do not mention near-misses, or exclude them from the obligation to disclose. The AMA Code of Medical Ethics section E8.12 states: "Patients have a right to know their past and present medical status and to be free of any mistaken beliefs concerning their conditions. Situations occasionally occur in which a patient suffers significant medical complications that may have resulted from the physician's mistake or judgment. In these situations, the physician is ethically required to inform the patient of all the facts necessary to ensure understanding of what has occurred" (AMA 1999). The 2001 Joint Commission on the Accreditation of Healthcare Organizations (JCAHO) Standard RI 1.2.2 states: "Patients and, when appropriate, their families are informed about the outcomes of care, including unanticipated outcomes" (JCAHO 2001c). The intent of this standard is that the responsible, licensed, independent practitioner or his or her designee clearly explains the outcome of any treatments or procedures to the patient and, when appropriate, the family, whenever those outcomes differ significantly from the anticipated outcomes. The Johns Hopkins Hospital Interdisciplinary Clinical Practice Manual states: "All health care professionals and trainees have an obligation to report medical errors as a means to improve patient care delivery and to help promote safety and quality in patient care"; the manual also states: "It is the right of the patient to receive information about clinically relevant medical errors" (Johns Hopkins Medical Institutions 2001). None of these statements addresses the subject of near-misses.

One exception is the disclosure policy of the Sunnybrook and Women's Hospital (Toronto) Administrative manual's section on "Disclosure of Adverse Medical Events and Unanticipated Outcomes of Care," which states: "Non-significant medical events are minor incidents that do not have a negative impact on patient outcomes, now or in the foreseeable future. No extra procedures affecting the patient are required to prevent negative patient outcomes. These events are not significant from the patient's perspective and disclosure to the patient and/or substitute decision maker or family is discretionary" (Sunnybrook 2001).

What Do Patients Expect?

There have been few studies of patients' expectations about disclosure of near-misses. Results from a survey by Witman, Park, and Hardin (1996) of 149 patients from an academic general internal medicine outpatient clinic suggested that virtually all (98 percent) desired some acknowledgment of even minor errors. In a study by Sweet and Bernat (1997), 95 percent of physicians surveyed reported that they would disclose a minor error, but some questioned their ability to do so in a real-life situation. As the severity of the injury increased, patients expected more substantial explanations. In a related study, Hingorani, Wong, and Vafidis (1999) found that fewer physicians than patients felt that the patient should be informed of an adverse event (60 percent versus 92 percent).

Considerations

The following discussion will outline arguments for and against disclosure of near-misses and harmless hits. Arguments are presented first based on consequences (a consequentialist approach), then based on a physician's duties (a deontological approach). In each case the potential effects of disclosure on patients and on physicians are considered separately. Although harms and benefits from disclosure might accrue to a health care organization or system as a whole, these will not be discussed here.

Most earlier discussions of error disclosure have focused on clear-cut individual errors. However, there is now consensus that most errors are caused by a combination of individual and system-related factors. While individuals are fallible, most near-miss incidents are caused by a combination of momentary and long-standing conditions that may involve specific tasks being performed, team functioning, the work environment, and organizational factors (Vincent et al. 2000). Failures are frequently required in several systems simultaneously in order for an incident to happen. This implies the possibility of shared responsibility among multiple individuals as well as the institution itself as a corporate entity. It may sometimes be appropriate for disclosure to be made by one or more nonphysician members of the health care team, including nurses and pharmacists, or a risk manager or other institutional representative. Recent regulations and statutes reflect this, setting forth the requirement that both individual physicians and organizations are responsible for informing patients and families. For example, under the new Pennsylvania Medical Care Availability and Reduction of Error Act (MCARE Act), signed into law on March 20, 2002, institutions are now obligated to report to the patient an "event, occurrence, or situation involving the clinical care of a patient in a medical facility that results in death or compromises patient safety and results in unanticipated injury" (State of Pennsylvania 2002, article 13). Nonetheless, the attending physician is still legally responsible for the care of the hospitalized patients. In addition, an individual patient is likely to expect information from his or her personal physician, rather than from less familiar members of the staff. This would apply even if the physician were explaining to the patient a series of events that occurred in various places within the institution. Therefore, most of the following discussion will center on the case of a straightforward, individual error made by a physician. However, in some cases, particularly those where system factors rather than individual factors are the primary cause of an incident, it may be most practical or desirable for others to discharge this obligation.

It should also be noted that particularly for patients who are seriously ill, family members may serve as surrogate decision makers. This has been recognized by the JCAHO in the standard cited above, which dictates that "[p]atients and, when appropriate, their families are informed about the outcomes of care, including unanticipated outcomes" (JCAHO 2001c). Family members or other designated decision makers might act as a proxy for the patient and be the recipients of disclosure about an incident. Discussion about ethical implications of disclosure should also take into account potential benefits and harms to family proxies, and possible responsibilities of the physician to them.

Potential Benefits of Disclosure to the Patient

The patient could benefit in some ways from knowing that a near-miss had occurred. In cases where it is evident to the patient that something has gone awry, disclosure can provide an explanation and help to relieve worry. It could prompt the patient to be more vigilant, thereby decreasing the potential for future harm to the patient, or it might encourage the patient to take more responsibility for his or her own care. If the patient's expectations are unrealistically high, disclosure could lead to more realistic expectations about the fallibility of physicians and the medical system. In some cases, it might inform a decision to switch physicians. In other cases, disclosure of a near-miss could promote trust in the physician because of this display of honesty and could strengthen the patient-doctor relationship.

Potential Harms of Disclosure to the Patient

Despite the absence of physical harm, learning of a near-miss may cause shock, anxiety, or disappointment. For some, it could reduce faith or confidence in the ability of the individual physician, or of medicine in general, to provide help. This may cause the patient to refuse beneficial treatments or advice, effectively reducing access to care. Disclosure of a series of near-misses could be confusing or demoralizing, particularly for a patient who is seriously ill or who has limited capacity. For example, it is possible to envision a patient in an intensive care unit being informed of multiple near-misses a day. This would be stressful and distressing even for a family member acting as proxy for the patient. The patient or family member might be overwhelmed with information and feel paralyzed.

Potential Benefits to the Physician

If a physician discloses a near-miss, patients may appreciate the physician's honesty, and the disclosure could actually strengthen the patient-doctor relationship. Disclosing a near-miss may also help physicians to acknowledge their own fallibility and make plans to improve their practice in the future (Wu et al. 1991). However, it is not known the extent to which this applies to near-misses as opposed to errors with adverse consequences for the patients. Disclosure of a near-miss could provide a relatively risk-free opportunity for the physician to practice the skill of disclosure.

Potential Harms to the Physician

Perhaps the greatest harm to the physician is the time and hassle that would be required for the disclosure of all near-misses—and the resulting loss of

efficiency. Depending on the operational definition of a near-miss, a busy practitioner might be responsible for disclosing several incidents per day. If the
physician were also responsible for disclosing near-misses that occur
throughout the system (near-misses by other staff members, the pharmacy,
scheduling, laboratory services, etc.), the burden could be substantial. Disclosing all near-misses could make it difficult for the physician to do his or her
job. It seems that this would be especially true for physicians with the heaviest
clinical workload, and for those taking care of the most severely ill patients,
some of whom require upwards of 200 activities per day (Donchin et al. 1995).

Disclosure of a near-miss could potentially expose the physician to litigation.
In the absence of injury or other damages, the lack of a tort greatly diminishes
the risk of a decision against the physician. Nonetheless, a lawsuit can be considered to be a taxing and stressful adverse outcome in itself.

Fiduciary Arguments for Disclosure of Near-Misses

The fiduciary (i.e., trust-based) character of the doctor-patient relationship dictates that it is the physician's ethical duty to disclose incidents to a patient when
disclosure benefits the patient's health, respects the patient's autonomy and personhood, or enables compensation for serious harm. There is no obligation for
physicians to disclose to the patient every detail of his or her case; nor would
this be desirable or practical. Patients trust the physician to inform them about
aspects of their health and care that they want and need to know. In some cases,
but not all, the physician's fiduciary responsibilities to the patient might impel
disclosure of a near-miss; in other cases not. For example, it would be well
within the scope of the physician's responsibility to tell a patient with a penicillin allergy that she nearly received a prescription for this medication. On the
other hand, investigating a variety of near-misses that occur at various points
throughout the health care system, and informing the patient about all of them,
would extend beyond the physician's usual role. On these grounds, I would
argue that there is no routine obligation for physicians to disclose a near-miss.

Assuming that the patient's family caregivers also have a relationship with the
doctor both as such and as proxy for the patient, the physician's fiduciary obligation may extend to family as proxy. In addition, Virginia Sharpe has argued that
fiduciary obligations should extend beyond the physician and other clinicians
to hospital administrators and health-plan administrators who play an indirect
but significant role in the delivery of health care (Sharpe 2000a).

Summary of Arguments for and against Disclosure of Near-Misses

Neither harms nor benefits provide a compelling argument for or against the disclosure of near-misses in all cases. In some cases, benefits to the patient might prevail, whereas in others, harms to the patient and the physician might predominate. An obligation to disclose all near-misses seems likely to place an undue burden on some physicians, particularly those caring for the sickest patients. I conclude that a uniform rule for disclosure of near-misses would not produce a greater balance of benefits in even the majority of cases. If this is true, then disclosure should be discretionary, and practical considerations and the specifics of each situation should prevail. However, I would argue further that although disclosure of near-misses is discretionary, it is also desirable, and these incidents should be disclosed whenever it is convenient. Since there is no tangible patient harm, disclosure of a near-miss is unlikely to result in significant negative consequences for the physician. Some of these instances may provide a "teachable moment" to impart useful advice to the patient (Nutting 1986). Most should provide an opportunity for honest discussion and can benefit the relationship with the patient or family.

When to Disclose a Near-Miss

Granting the physician's option to disclose near-misses, there are practical issues concerning whether, when, and how to tell the patient. One criterion for disclosure of a near-miss is whether the patient could benefit from knowing. The concept of a "teachable moment" can be applied here, whereby disclosure of a near-miss could be used to help reinforce an important point. For example, in the case in which a patient was prescribed a medication to which she is allergic, the physician could mention this with the advice to always give this information to all health care providers, to avoid the same thing happening again. In cases where it is evident that something unusual has occurred, disclosure can provide an explanation and thus provide relief of uncertainty.

A near-miss might best be disclosed as soon as possible after it is noted. However, there is probably little disadvantage to delaying disclosure, and it could be made at a time when it is convenient or particularly relevant. For example, mention of a near-miss involving an incorrect dose of a medication could be timed to correspond to a discussion of the patient's medication regimen.

Disclosure can be difficult, even when disclosing a near-miss, in part because teaching this skill is not a routine part of undergraduate or graduate medical education. Disclosure of a medical error should be seen as an instance of "breaking bad news" (Campbell 1994). Care should be taken to be as empathic as possible with the patient's response, and not to react in a defensive manner. The physician should begin by stating simply that he or she made a mistake. The physician should describe what happened, taking care to avoid medical terminology and jargon. The nature of the mistake, the consequences (or lack thereof), and any corrective action should be described. The physician should express personal regret and apologize for the error. The physician should ask if there are any questions or concerns. Finally, any advice or a lesson to be gleaned should be stated. For example, in the case where a physician attending to a hospitalized patient intercepted an antibiotic that was intended for another patient, she might say: "That was a close one. This wasn't intended for you. Every now and then it is possible for a medication to be given to the wrong person. I am so sorry that this happened. I will certainly get to the bottom of this to see that it doesn't happen again. It's a good thing I was here. You can also pay attention to the medications you are getting, and if you have any doubts, don't be afraid to speak up."

Conclusion

A near-miss is a medical error that does not result in harm. There is consensus that physicians and health care organizations are obliged to disclose errors that cause harm. It does not seem that there are either substantial harms or benefits for patients or physicians in the majority of cases of disclosing near-misses. Therefore, since disclosure of near-misses could place a substantial burden on physicians, particularly those caring for the sickest patients, disclosure should be discretionary. However, near-misses should be disclosed when it can provide an object lesson or some other benefit. In these cases, disclosure should be timely, and may be treated as an instance of breaking bad news. Disclosure should include a statement that an error occurred, a description of what happened, an apology, and, if appropriate, a statement of what can be learned or done differently to improve safety in the future.

Acknowledgment

This chapter was funded in part by an Agency for Healthcare Research and Quality grant, no. U18HS11902-01.

CHAPTER 9

God, Science, and History:
The Cultural Origins of Medical Error

KENNETH DE VILLE

Introduction

Many Americans appear to believe that we are currently experiencing a plague of medical errors. A decade ago, the Harvard Medical Practice Study reported that 4 percent of hospital patients suffered iatrogenic injuries, two-thirds of which were due to medical error (Leape et al. 1991; Leape 1993). These and other error studies reported high rates of missed diagnoses, mistaken treatments, medication errors, and a wide range of other mistakes in patient care (Leape 1994; Bedell et al. 1991; Shimmel 1964). More recently, of course, the Institute of Medicine (IOM) report *To Err Is Human: Building a Safer Health Care System* estimated that medical error was responsible for 44,000 to 98,000 inpatient deaths a year (Kohn, Corrigan, and Donaldson 2000). The IOM study received much attention from governmental bodies, regulatory agencies, and the mainstream media. For example, the *New York Times* compared the IOM rate of error in U.S. hospitals to three jumbo jets crashing every two days. "If the airlines killed that many people annually," the writer observed, "public outrage would close them over night" (Weinstein 1998).

As a healthy and laudable consequence of these reports and observations, the public, the government, health care administrators, health regulators, the medical profession, and a plethora of multidisciplinary groups are taking a long, hard look at medical error, its origins, and its prevention. Much has been made of the statistical limitations of the IOM study, and it should be. But I want to focus on another curiosity, the seemingly prevalent notion that medicine has suddenly become more dangerous and error-prone. The relatively recent reports of widespread error and mistake in medicine have led observers in some quarters to suggest that health care workers are careless or reckless. Richer explanations, however, have demonstrated that this evident plague of error is just as likely to have arisen from faulty systems designs that conceal "error traps," or that require health care professionals to work too hard or too long or press their cognitive abilities beyond that which is safe for patients (Reason 1990; Perrow 1999; Leape et al. 1995). Systems analyses have been applied to error in other contexts—the airline industry, for example—to great benefit and will likely play an important role in preventing and mitigating human harm in the medical context.

For practical reasons, it is important to focus on the prevention of both individual and systems error in response to the current groundswell of concern regarding medical error. But despite the usefulness of a systems approach (or other approaches), there is much that is left unexplained. Such approaches, for example, do not fully explain why medical error has increased, or has seemed to increase, at a time when medical professionals have almost certainly become better educated, more skillful, and more careful than their historic counterparts. In addition, there is no definitive agreement or even working definition of what constitutes error or culpable error (Hofer, Kerr, and Hayward 2000). Charles Bosk has explained that the definition of error is, and is likely to remain, "contested." It is contested in part because a society's view of what incidents to construe as error and culpable error is highly dependant on cultural conventions and historical context (Bosk 2000). The origins of medical error are multifactoral, relating both to the individual health care practitioner and to organizational deficiencies. But medical error, like disease, is an amalgam of physiological explanation and social definition (Rosenberg 1962).

In this chapter, I argue that the apparent rise in medical error in the U.S. must be seen not merely as a product of human action or inaction, or of flawed systems, but as a product of our culture and history. I attempt to connect the way that Americans explain medical misfortune to three discrete but related changes that have occurred in American culture over the past several centuries. First, the weakening of providential views of the world has led Americans to explain misfortune as the result of actions or inactions on the part of human actors, rather than as the work of God. In Anglo-American culture, the gradual transformation of society's view of God's role on earth has gradually allowed and encouraged society to search for human agents of misfortune, thus giving the title of the IOM report, *To Err Is Human*, great poignancy. Second, the proliferation of medical technology, knowledge, and expertise over the last two centuries has profoundly affected what "errors" we see, how those "errors" are perceived, and what "errors" concern us. Specifically, new knowledge about, and approaches to, illness and injury have generated higher expectations about what is possible and desirable. Moreover, these approaches typically require greater degrees of skill, learning, and care than the procedures and explanations they replaced, thus carrying with them a greater susceptibility to human fallibility, carelessness, and ignorance. Third and finally, society's focus on error may be changing in lockstep with the historical change in the way society relates to the medical profession. A society that tends to view medical professionals more like commercial providers of ordinary goods and services and the medical encounter as a consumer exchange may focus on different errors than a society that views physicians as possessing a special status based on their calling as caregivers.

The distinction between culpable and nonculpable error may be important in a number of contexts, morally and legally. Although I do not attempt to distinguish explicitly between the two, my analysis does suggest reasons why the line defining culpability is not static and why society's view of responsibility is the result of a number of interlocking historical transformations. My primary goal in this chapter, though, is to explore the factors that induce individuals to view undesirable outcomes as medical errors.

Man Proposes and God Disposes?

When an individual or a society conceptualizes an unfortunate event as an error, he, she, or it also makes an important statement about the prevailing cosmology. Although a society's view of humankind's relationship with the cosmos is never monolithic and varies from person to person and from denomination to denomination, a number of broad, relevant trends are apparent. For example, as late as the seventeenth and eighteenth centuries, many Americans believed in some version of the doctrine of *direct* or *specific* divine providence. Providential theory reflected the belief that nothing in heaven or on earth, including physical misfortune, occurred by chance or without the connivance of the Supreme Being. God sustained the earth from moment to moment, willing every sparrow's fall (May 1983). Supernatural explanations may have helped believers accept what would have otherwise been unfathomable and perhaps unbearable physical misfortunes (Thomas 1971, 5–7, 651–63). God might punish sinners or reward the blessed on earth as well as in the afterlife. He might conversely rain misfortune on the holy as a means of testing or teaching them (Miller 1939). Such tests in sixteenth- and seventeenth-century America might include: lightning, bad crops, earthquakes, epidemics, a sick horse, or the death of a child (Miller 1953, 345–66; Tilton 1940; Clark 1965). The journals of seventeenth-century American colonists are filled with examples of individuals who felt the "special providence of God." The "righteous hand of God" spared or smote individuals with fire, drowning, Indian attacks, accidental injuries, smallpox, and birth defects (Winthrop 1908).

Physical misfortune, viewed through the mantle of divine providence, appeared as a work of God and affected the ways in which individuals could acceptably respond to adversity. Individuals who subscribed to this version of special or direct providence would be unlikely to look for temporal or human causation and blame. Rather, they would assume and look for the wise hand of God at work and would attempt to believe that God ultimately worked only to good ends. This variant of special providence, of course, was not held by all individuals or all denominations with equal and unvarying dedication. But the notion of special providence was strong among broad segments of the American population through the eighteenth century. Change was already on its way by the 1700s, but religious historian Lewis Saum has argued that providential sentiments remained strong in many parts of the country through the early 1800s (Saum 1976). For example, one inhabitant of Philadelphia who lived through the 1793 yellow fever epidemic reported that "most if not all were convinced it was a judgment sent by the immediate hand of God" (Gribbin 1972, 287–89). Cholera epidemics in the early 1800s provoked a similar analysis, with most of the population viewing the epidemics as a "rod in the hands of God." This view persisted even though many physicians and scientists had begun to search for earthly causes of the disease and infections (Rosenberg 1962, 15).

Not surprisingly, medical malpractice cases were nearly unheard of during this period, although by the mid-nineteenth century the medical profession would be faced with the country's first malpractice "crisis" (De Ville 1990, 25–64). Obviously, if God ordained the harm that befell a patient, it was fruitless to look for human causation or to assign blame, much less seek some manner of remuneration. Humble acceptance of God's will, not a lawsuit, would be the appropriate response to physical misfortune. Yet a rare 1824 medical malpractice accusation illustrates the apparent power of providential explanations for medical error even in a culture in which the process of change was already well under way.

Dr. Gerard Bancker vaccinated the four-year-old son of Michael O'Neil for smallpox. Soon after, the young boy became fatally ill, with some of his symptoms resembling those of smallpox. Before dying, the boy went blind, lost his hair and teeth, his jaw disintegrated, and he developed an ulcerous hole in his neck. O'Neil sued Bancker for malpractice, claiming that the physician, when preparing the vaccination, had mistakenly drawn material from a smallpox sore rather than a cowpox sore, thus wrongfully exposing the boy to the risk of the dread disease instead of protecting him. Moreover, many of the young boy's most horrible symptoms are classic signs of mercury-based calomel poisoning, a frequent remedy of the period. Therefore, it is possible that there are two medical errors present in this case: infection with smallpox and excessive and fatal use of calomel. Clearly the boy's father was able to view his son's death as human error and demand an accounting from human actors. But the notion of providence still appeared to carry substantial influence in the first third of the nineteenth century. The physician's lawyer, in his argument to the jury, declared that the child's disease was nothing short of miraculous. "Providence," the defense attorney declared, was responsible for boy's death. "In a word," the attorney claimed, "we expect to prove the child died of smallpox, proceeding from the visitation of God, and not from any negligence or any want of skill of the physician." The jury found in favor of the physician (*Michael O'Neil v. Gerard Bancker*, 1827).

The defense attorney's use of a divine explanation for disease, and its apparent success, suggests that the notion of direct providence commanded at least some influence as late as the 1820s. Indeed, in an 1823 article, a writer declared that providence "extends to all beings that have existed, or ever will exist; to all events that have occurred or ever will occur. . . . [T]he humble Christian will discern in them all the hand of a wise and holy God" (Christian Spectator 1823, 172–74). In the same magazine, another writer proclaimed that "without [God's] permission, no power can harm, no ill can befall us, and every afflicting stroke is meant for our good" (Christian Spectator 1836, 2).

But these sentiments were increasingly rare and limited more and more to religious leaders outside the cultural mainstream. Theologians who believed that God literally willed every sparrow's fall lost ground rapidly both in intellectual circles and among the general populace. Many of the sociological and theological debates of the 1820s and 1830s centered on the relationship between God and earthly occurrences and frequently focused on the apparent contradiction between free will and God's providential control. Some writers explicitly attacked the notion of direct providence for this reason, contending that it devalued the responsibility and accountability of the individual. Critics, anxious to usher in reforms to address social ills, assailed strict belief in the immediate power of providence because such a position encouraged inertia in regard to the status quo and encouraged acceptance of otherwise remediable social problems. American intellectuals and theologians were influenced by European philosophers such as John Stuart Mill and Auguste Comte. According to historian Charles Cashdollar, these writers' conception of God's relation to man "forced man away from a pietistic or providential to a naturalistic view of social problems, from prayer to human action" (Cashdollar 1976). Therefore, misfortunes that had once been viewed as divinely ordained burdens could now be justifiably viewed as remediable ills that demanded human solutions.

The gradual but clear move away from providence as a central feature of day-to-day life varied from person to person, from region to region, and from denomination to denomination, but as the nineteenth century progressed fewer Americans viewed social and physical ills as the will and work of God. Such views never disappeared entirely, but the predominant part of society had begun to believe that God worked in the world through natural law and influenced events largely by creating the context for the unfolding of His will from a distance (Cashdollar 1978; De Ville 1990, 119–37). Secular interpretations of specific physical misfortunes frequently started with scientists, physicians, and intellectuals, then were embraced by broader segments of society. Where Americans once saw yellow fever and cholera as moral retribution, they now began to view such diseases and others in scientific terms. For example, by the time of the widespread cholera epidemics of the 1860s, the majority of Americans had abandoned the notion of divine intervention and recognized and accepted that the disease was spread through contaminated water (Rosenberg 1962, 193–96). During this period, a vast number of movements eager to address human suffering with human intervention flourished, including movements for the abolition of slavery, prevention of cruelty to animals, child protection, and prison reform (Walters 1978). And significantly, contemporary with the social and theological debates over the nature of providence, physicians reported a massive and unprecedented attack of malpractice prosecutions ostensibly aimed at compensating patients for medical error (De Ville 1990, 25–64).

Religious attitudes have continued to evolve, of course. Scientific and medical explanations of various natural and physiological phenomena accelerated further the decline in the perception and acceptance of different varieties of misfortune as divine will. Medical researchers in the nineteenth and twentieth centuries explored and explained the functions and malfunctions of the body in patho-physiological terms. Statistical and scientific analyses of diseases, treatments, and cures began to engender the hope of a scientifically predictable medicine. These changes, both scientifically and theologically, loosened the grip of providence on the American mind. Slowly and gradually, providence and fatalism were replaced by a secularized, optimistic view of the merits and promise of material and social progress (Marty 1970, 188–98). But such confidence brought greater demands and expectations. When these expectations were not met, individuals increasingly blamed others for their physical and other misfortunes. The decline in the importance of providence in the public mind may have paved the way for a variety of reform movements, but it may have also encouraged the search for, and identification of, human error and the proliferation of lawsuits by removing the possibility of divine intent and highlighting human culpability. This process, beginning at least in the eighteenth century, continues to the present. While the notion of providence still plays a role in the lives of many individuals, its nature has been altered and its potency profoundly diluted.

The Paradox of Technological, Scientific, and Medical Progress

Broader cultural recognition of human error inside medicine, and without, has been facilitated by the gradual but unmistakable transition from divine to human explanation for physical misfortune. Indeed, without such a shift in a society's cosmological mind-set, it would have been impossible to search on a broad scale for either human causation or human culpability. But another factor has played a central role in the cultural tendency to view physical misfortune as medical error. Specifically, technological innovation and scientific advancement in the medical world has multiplied many times over the types of incidents and results that might be characterized as medical mistake or error. Moreover, in many instances technological advancement has increased the likelihood of those mistakes and errors occurring. Because advances in medical technology and knowledge both improve care and create a larger space for error and blame, the role of technology is paradoxical.

Mark Grady has produced one of the more cogent articulations of this phenomenon (Grady 1988). According to Grady, medical innovation and technological advancement capture what was previously "natural risk" and transform it into "medical risk." Before the development and perfection of a given medical technique or explanation, individuals and society at large tend to accept physical misfortune as part of the known and expected sequelae of an injury or illness. In such a state, human error cannot exist. As Kurt Baier has explained, in order to identify human error, "we must know how to intervene suitably in the natural course of events so as to prevent such harm or avoid bringing it about" (Baier 1987). Stated another way, when the injury or condition is insufficiently understood and no effective treatment appears to exist, judgments, decisions, and actions that retrospectively prove incorrect or harmful are ordinarily not considered mistakes or errors—much less culpable errors. These "state of the art" errors are typically not recognized as such, because the physician or health provider could not have decided or acted in a more advantageous way given the current state of the art and existing knowledge. This situation and perception changes once the public and the profession see a new medical technique or explanation as effective, even if it is not. Under these circumstances, a failure in treatment related to the technique or its denial may now be viewed as a harm or a mistake. The availability of the technique means that the patient may be denied a potential benefit, and the patient may view the absence of the expected benefit as a mistake or error—and a potentially culpable one.

For much of medical history, there were relatively few medical explanations or procedures that were sufficiently developed to generate predictable results and benefits, thereby engendering professional and public confidence. But as medical theory and practice boasted advances in a progressively greater number of areas, lay and professional expectations increased and their view of error was transformed. At the same time, technical and intellectual demands on practitioners increased, and success or failure appeared to rest on human performance and knowledge rather than on the vagaries of a poorly understood medical problem or God's will (De Ville 1998).

Analysis of the specific medical advances through the nineteenth and twentieth centuries illustrates how medical progress both helps patients and increases error. At the end of the eighteenth century the standard of care for severe fractures and dislocations was amputation. Although amputations resulted in horrible disfigurement and very frequently in death, the procedure generated very few claims of incompetence or malpractice (Elwell 1860, 54–58). Social and professional expectations were low for severe orthopedic injuries; amputations and/or death were the norm. By the late 1830s, however, in nothing less than a revolution in orthopedic treatment, the medical profession had developed a range of new techniques that allowed physicians to save rather than amputate badly fractured limbs. By 1850, amputation was no longer the standard of care (De Ville 1990, 94–108; Walker 1848). Medical literature began to refer to the treatment of such fractures as a relatively mechanical procedure in which physicians and patients could expect predictable and nearly perfect cures. Fracture treatment of course, then and now, is neither mechanical nor predictable. The new treatment protocols required more skill, knowledge, and care than did amputations. Physicians were faced with a broad range of new concerns and complications that continued through the convalescent period. Finally, although physicians had improved patient care by saving rather than amputating limbs, patients usually were either left with permanent injuries (shortened or deformed limbs or frozen joints) or suffered from complications during their usually long recovery periods (Hamilton 1886; Ohio Medical Society 1856). Because medicine now *appeared* to offer a treatment for severe orthopedic injuries, both physicians and the lay public frequently viewed these side effects of what was in fact *successful* fracture treatment as "medical error," rather than viewing them as a less severe "natural" consequence or risk of suffering a compound fracture. Only after the physical misfortune has been transformed to "medical risk" from "natural risk" can it be attributed to human agency. Less than perfect results following orthopedic injuries constituted the most common type of malpractice suits from the mid-nineteenth century through the late 1930s (Sandor 1957).

Medical advancements affect the evolution and recognition of medical error in two other respects as well. As Grady has explained, new medical procedures more often than not require greater skill, learning, and care than the remedies and explanations they replace. They therefore place greater demands on medical practitioners and expand the opportunity for incompetence, ignorance, or lapses of attention (Grady 1988). Thus, surgeons who eschewed amputation and instead saved limbs were more likely to make mistakes. When these expected results were not achieved, it was easier to point to lapses in the skill, care, and knowledge that are often required in progressively greater quantities as medical science advances. Primitive medical procedures promised little and required relatively low levels of vigilance, knowledge, and skill (Grady 1988). So not only did they promise little, they were easier to complete successfully. Finally, advancements in medical knowledge and technology can create the preconditions for another form of error springing from a physician's failure to keep current on evolving practices.

The foregoing discussion of the evolution of fracture treatment in the nineteenth century exemplifies the contention that human error is more likely to surface as a recognized cause of misfortune when medical science most appears to promise results. The medical profession's experience with fracture treatment and the identification of medical error illustrate a cycle that has recurred in the guise of other medical procedures and treatments in the twentieth century. Specific improvements in medical treatment have continued to incite cycles of heightened expectations, greater clinical demands, unforeseen complications and opportunities for error, and resultant disappointments when expectations are frustrated.

Consider the path of body cavity surgery. Before the 1880s, operative surgery was limited. When a patient died of peritonitis or an intestinal blockage, the death was not viewed as medical error. Instead, the death was viewed as the result of a poorly understood medical condition for which no effective treatment had been developed. But by the first third of the twentieth century, the prevalence of surgical procedures had become somewhat more common. Results remained uneven though, as surgical success was limited by factors such as surgical shock, infection, inadequate training, and primitive instruments (Rothstein 1972, 251–59). Still, when these very frequent surgical failures occurred, they were typically not conceptualized as errors and generated few malpractice suits. Surgeons, although they frequently did not accomplish the desired goal and undoubtedly harmed many or most patients, could not have decided or acted in a more advantageous way given the then-current state of the art and existing knowledge. Thus, they were neither deemed the cause of the patient's harm, nor held responsible.

It was not until the late 1920s and the advent of sulfa drugs, the refinement of aseptic practices, transfusions to assuage surgical shock, better training, and more appropriate instruments that surgeons were able to claim regular, numerous, and noteworthy successes (English 1980, 57–68). It was only then that "[s]urgical intervention could be represented as the inevitable, scientific solution to disease" (Howell 1995, 57). Surgical progress had transformed the "natural risk" of an appendectomy into the "medical risks" associated with surgery. And, given the nature of the medical innovation, these medical risks were more likely to come to fruition. Like the new orthopedic treatments of the mid-nineteenth century, surgical remedies were typically more complex and exacting than previous treatment modalities, which were sometimes in fact nonexistent. Surgeons in the post-1930s world had to monitor and manage shock, bleeding, and vital signs while they were performing complex and new medical procedures. Surgeons were thereby exposed to exponentially higher opportunities for error, lapses in skill, knowledge, or care, in intrinsically dangerous procedures that were now expected to generate beneficial results for patients. Thus, surgical error became a possibility and a reality.

The appearance of widespread surgical malpractice suits, one sign of the public recognition of culpable medical error, may be evidence of this shift in public perception. Body cavity surgery was performed for nearly four decades without generating large numbers of medical malpractice suits. Even in the face of failures, surgery did not incite suits until the treatment modality (like fracture treatment before it) reached a threshold of lay and professional expectation and confidence. After that time, however, legal claims against surgeons increased dramatically and overtook orthopedics as the most common source of malpractice suits by the 1940s (Sandor 1957) and, according to one report, accounted for 57 percent of the total claims between 1950 and 1971 (USDHEW 1973).

Obstetrical care appears to have run a similar historical course. Obstetrics was the source of relatively few medical malpractice claims—a particular type of error claim—until the 1970s, accounting for only 2 percent of suits as late as 1972 (Guinther 1978). This was the case even in light of the dangers of childbirth, with maternal and fetal risk remaining considerably high through the mid-twentieth century. After that time, however, obstetrical care improved rapidly and dramatically. In the next two decades, new drugs, medical techniques, and technologies provided obstetricians with "an armament which is unsurpassed in the history of medical practice" (Chamberlain and Turnbull 1989, vi). These advancements have undeniably improved patient care and delivery results, but have complicated treatment decisions, placed greater demands on physicians, and increased the potential for the perception of "error" when a mother or child is injured. Not coincidentally, obstetrical medical malpractice claims increased dramatically during the same period of dramatic medical advancement, amounting to nearly 10 percent of claims by 1985 (Rostow, Osterweis, and Bulger 1989). A similar path seems to have been followed by any number of other modern medical practices. Recent decades have brought profound advances in sophisticated pharmacological therapies. The application of drug regimes provides great benefit, but they are also complex and potentially harmful. Again, the perception of error in the application of pharmaceutical remedies has accompanied an exciting period of advancement in a medical modality.

Late-twentieth-century advances in diagnostic technologies have played a similar but even more striking role in contributing to the increase in perception of medical error. These technologies have improved care but may have influenced the perception and identification of error in a number of ways. First, they have engendered the expectation that illnesses can be foreseen and thwarted by early intervention. Some of this enthusiasm is well-founded, some exaggerated. Patients and sometimes even physicians are not fully aware of the limitations of diagnostic technologies, leading to surprise and disappointment when they do not perform as intended, and paving the way for claims of error (Black and Welch 1993; Anbar 1984; Council on Scientific

Affairs 1993). Advances in diagnostic technologies have also created the context for the recognition of an entirely new type of error—that of misinterpretation and the failure to diagnose an illness correctly. Second, some diagnostic technologies carry with them their own danger of iatrogenic injury that may be construed as "error" even when such risks are known and disclosed. Third, diagnostic technologies might increase the perception and discovery of error by providing a record of previously unseen and unrecorded information. Such records provide evidence that error has occurred and were not always available before the advent of the diagnostic technology. This was clearly true of the introduction of the x-ray in the late nineteenth century. The x-ray helped physicians avoid misdiagnoses, but it also increased the expectations of laypersons and the profession, carried risks of its own (e.g., risk of burns from early equipment or risks associated with use of contrast mediums), and was susceptible to mis- and ambiguous interpretations. The x-ray also displayed the physician's work visually for third parties and made it easier to identify physician error. These features allowed the x-ray to play a role in an entirely new class of error and mistake (De Ville 1990, 221–23). To take a more recent example, electronic fetal monitors (EFM) were initially viewed as an improvement in care and as protection against obstetrical error and medical malpractice. This technology, though, has proved a mixed blessing for both patient and physician, increasing the rate of cesarean section, and increasing the likelihood that an anomaly will be interpreted as medical error and will generate a medical malpractice suit.

Other diagnostic technologies that have come into use in the last half-century may have had a similar impact on society's ability and propensity to identify and perceive error. Similar observations might be drawn regarding the use of ultrasound, bronchoscopy, endoscopy, magnetic resonance imaging, and computed tomography. They might also be drawn regarding other diagnostic practices refined in the late twentieth century, including laboratory tests, genetic screening procedures, and the medical record itself. All of these may serve as sources of medical error and may, at the same time, provide evidence of error that was not discernible before their introduction. The heightened and sometimes inflated expectations inspired by these diagnostic technologies are analogous to those raised by fracture treatment in the mid-nineteenth century, surgery in the 1930s, and obstetrics in the mid-twentieth century. And as with these other advances, a dramatic increase in medical malpractice suits has followed a period of dynamic improvement in a particular medical modality, in this case diagnostic technologies. Currently, the fastest-growing malpractice allegation is the failure to diagnose an existing illness or injury, a result not surprising given the vast array of diagnostic technologies that have entered conventional medical practice in the latter third of the twentieth century (McCormick 1996).

The errors that seem to arise out of the dynamic of medical advancement do not necessarily remain static. After a technological innovation or improvement becomes a conventional practice, clinicians may not realize the range of new error traps associated with the procedure. Over time and with experience, collectively the profession responds to discovered error traps in new technologies with precautions, safeguards, and additional training. Some precautions may involve simple routines such as instituting sponge counts in operative theaters. As safeguards are introduced to deal with newly discovered dangers, successes increase and iatrogenic injuries and errors typically decline. Consider the case of anesthesia-related patient injuries, low-frequency but high-cost events. After an increase in anesthesia-related medical malpractice cases in the 1970s, the American Society of Anesthesiologists established a set of detailed standards for patient care during surgery. These reforms included refined training programs, higher monitoring standards, documentation requirements, and mechanical safeguards such as pulse oximeters, electrocardiograms, and alarms on the anesthesia system itself (Cheney et al. 1989; Eichhorn et al. 1986). These reforms, aimed at decreasing both error and medical malpractice claims, were credited with decreasing the rate of anesthesia-related malpractice claims in the 1990s. However, while safeguards are frequently successful in addressing newly discovered error dangers, they, like other technological improvements, frequently serve as yet another fertile source of potential mistakes. First, safeguards can sometimes increase the perception that the procedure can be conducted in a near-error-free environment. And second, as Charles Bosk has observed, a central lesson from the study of normal accidents is that "safety systems folded into a complex organization are just as likely to provide incorrect cues, become routinized, and malfunction as any other component of the system" (Bosk 1979, 45; Richards and Walter 1991).

The advent and spread of minimally invasive surgical procedures may provide another example of this process of innovation, resulting error, and professional reaction. When laparoscopic cholecystectomy was introduced in the late 1980s, it "revolutionized" the treatment of gallstone disease. In many ways it was "safer" than traditional "open" procedures and decreased pain, as well as inpatient and recovery time. It was adopted rapidly by physicians and embraced by patients. But while open procedures had extremely low complication rates, the initial introduction of the laparoscopic version of the procedure was accompanied by an increased risk of adverse events on any given patient—most frequently, injuries to the common bile duct, intestine, bowel, and liver (Legorreta et al. 1993; Steiner et al. 1994). Given these complications that occurred at a rate significantly higher than under the open procedure, it is not surprising that medical malpractice suits related to cholecystectomies increased 500 percent, by some estimates, after the introduction of the laparoscopic technique (Kern 1992, 1994). The error and suit generating complications were unknown to the profession at the time of the initial proliferation of the technique. After several years of use, however, the profession can warn patients of procedure-specific complications and can moderate expectations. More importantly, surgeons have instituted specific precautions to decrease the likelihood of adverse events and have discovered that laparoscopic complication rates can be decreased further by better training, experience, and credentialing. As in other procedures, experience and informed consent have made expectations more accurate, and better training and pre- and postoperative safeguards have helped control the complication rates of the procedure. As a result, the complication rates associated with the laparoscopic procedure have dropped nearly to the level of the previously used open technique. Related lawsuits have decreased as well (Soper et al. 1992). Like fracture treatment, surgery, obstetrics, diagnostics, and a host of other medical and treatment innovations, laparoscopic techniques proceeded through a similar cycle of introduction, proliferation, inflated expectations, and errors and lawsuits when expectations were not met and unforeseen complications led to injury or less than perfect results.

During the period in which the medical profession, health care institutions, and the public must adjust their expectations regarding a new technology, discover error traps and complications, and institute safeguards, the new technology is a substantial source of error and, usually, increased lawsuits. If the process goes through a sequence similar to that experienced with anesthesia or laparoscopic surgery, then error (and suits) will gradually decrease until they reach a point of relative equilibrium. I say "relative equilibrium" because it is likely that in many instances the number of errors and suits generated by the technological or procedural innovation will be higher than before the improvement was introduced. This paradoxical effect occurs in part because the new mode of practice generates higher professional and lay culture expectations, requires a greater degree of care, skill, and learning, and thus provides more opportunity for oversight and accident. Thus, even after adjustments, medical improvement is likely to lead to an overall increase in the number of medical mistakes and errors (as well as to new classes and varieties of error) identified both professionally and among the lay public.

What Kind of Error?

Finally, historical transformations in the way that society views the medical profession itself may have contributed to the late-twentieth-century focus on a particular type of medical error. In short, I tentatively suggest that a change in the public view of the medical profession and the source of its duties may have led to a concomitant shift in the kind of concern paid to various forms of medical error: a transformation from a search for normative error to the search for technical, result-based error.

A classic theory in the history of jurisprudence suggests that legal relationships and responsibilities in modernizing societies tend to evolve from "status-determined" duties to "contractual or commercially determined" duties (Maine 1884, 164–65). Under the "status" model, rights, duties, and liabilities are derived more from a person's role, calling, position, or status in society, than from explicit, conscious agreements made by the persons involved in the relationship (Graveson 1941, 261–67; Gilmore 1974). Although the existence of a "contract" frequently signals the existence of a medical relationship, the duties and responsibilities of the physician have typically been drawn from the nature of the calling of the physician and the special features of the physician-patient relationship.

Society, policy, law, and physicians especially, have long resisted the notion and importance of contractual relationships with patients because it conflicted with the image of the physician as a public servant with a distinct social status. Worthington Hooker, an influential mid-nineteenth-century physician who wrote on medical ethics and etiquette, contended: "The relation of a physician to his employers is not shut up within the narrow limits of mere pecuniary considerations. There is a sacredness in it, which should forbid its being subjected to the changes incident to the common relations of trade and commerce among men" (Hooker 1849, 410). Thus, even though the doctor-patient relationship may in some instances have been initiated by a contract to treat, the duties emanated not from the contract but from the physician's status or calling. As John Ordronaux, another mid-century physician commentator on medical law and professional propriety, explained: "[T]he very nature of the relation between patron and client raised it [the doctor-patient relationship] above all taint of a mercenary character" (Ordronaux 1869, 73). Professional responsibility had its origins in "the character publicly assumed by him who undertakes to render such services." The duties that physicians owed patients could never be enumerated in or bound by contract. This notion was enshrined in the law in a number of ways, but explicitly in the developing medical malpractice precedents of the nineteenth century—which relegated such actions to tort law instead of contract. A trial judge explained to a medical malpractice jury: "[T]he action is not for a breach of contract, it is not for the defendant's not doing what he agreed to do, but for doing what he did agree to do in a careless, unskillful and negligent manner" (Ordronaux 1869, 96).

The consequence of this cultural view is that when the bulk of duties of the medical relationship are defined by the status of the professional, not by a contractual or commercial arrangement, there is a predominant focus on what have been referred to as "role responsibilities" rather than "task responsibilities." Thus, one might expect that the errors that are most important under this "status-based" relationship are those errors that arise from their status as caregivers—the kind of "normative" or moral errors described by Charles Bosk (1979). At least within the medical profession, Bosk has shown that the focus has predominantly been on "Did we do what we were supposed to do?" rather than "Did it work?" Accordingly, technical/performance error is granted less attention and concern (Bosk 2001).

To the degree that society shared the medical profession's view of itself, society would respond similarly to errors and mistakes; a focus on normative errors and role responsibilities might, in fact, limit a comprehensive search for task-related errors. The general population, especially patients, undoubtedly tended to focus more attention and concern on technical error, task responsibilities, and "Did it work?" than did the medical profession. But the general population too, to a considerable degree, internalized the notion that medicine is a calling and not a business and that physicians' responsibilities were defined by their membership as medical professionals more than by contract and commercial concerns (Sulmasy 1993). Given this perspective, might even the public's search for technical/performance errors have been blunted somewhat, leading them to accept the profession's focus on normative errors and internal judgments on appropriate performance?

In any event, in the last half of the twentieth century, it is reasonable to suggest that American society's view of the medical profession has gradually but consistently moved toward a more commercial conception of the medical profession—a shift from "status" to "contract," if you will. A growing segment of the population and even the profession itself has again begun to view physicians in a more commercial light. Patients have attacked paternalistic features of the relationship and have argued in favor of a greater role for the patient in the decision-making process. Patients are increasingly characterized as "consumers" of health care. Scholars have argued that there is no internal ethos in medicine to distinguish it from other human exchanges. Given these transformations, which have still not fully matured, the notion of the physician as a special actor with special duties has been substantially undermined. This transformation, which devalues the physician's special role, may allow and lead the public to alter likewise the focus of their attention on physicians' responsibilities and on error. When professional relationships are viewed by society as contractually defined, one might expect the locus of attention and concern to shift to technical/performance errors, rather than merely internal normative errors—as indeed it did in the late twentieth century.

Conclusions

The rise in the perception and identification of medical error and the attendant rise of medical malpractice suits in the last thirty years cannot be attributed solely to human action or inaction. This historically based framework begins to explain the paradox of why medical error appears to be increasing in the face of what appears to be unceasing medical progress. These observations seem to have ambivalent and unsettling implications for the discussion regarding the appropriate response to the current "apparent" wave of medical error. This discussion does underscore the dangers in adopting and embracing technological innovations and treatment protocols before assessing systematically the novel opportunities for error that these advancements are likely to create (Thacker 1989; Reiser 1994; McKinlay 1981). Such evaluations might uncover the value, limits, and dangers associated with medical advancements and might moderate some of the new opportunity for error that will inevitably come with clinical improvements.

But this thesis, if correct, also seems to suggest that events currently identified as errors will likely be replaced by new ones as innovative technologies bring new expectations, new demands, and new opportunities for inadvertence and mistake. This dynamic also has implications for the utility of ascribing culpable responsibility to individuals (i.e., blaming) for the increased levels of identifiable error. While only humans can make errors (either individually or through the design of systems), the history of the development of medical technology suggests that the demands on individuals working in the medical environment have been increasing apace with medical progress. At the same time, this historical dynamic has increased the types of misfortune that are likely to be viewed as error. This chapter does not attempt to define clearly what might constitute medical "error" or "mistake." Even less does it attempt to distinguish a blameworthy or culpable mistake from one that is not. But it does provide a description of how and why mistakes appear in the public perception and suggests a reason why the contemporary medical environment seems plagued by both medical error and medical malpractice. To say that medical error is historically constructed is only to contend that what is considered error or culpable error changes over time given particular background conditions, primarily a society's overall view of the role of providence in the day-to-day affairs of humankind and the development and refinement of medical practice and scientific explanation. What is preventable and/or culpable error changes over time and will continue to change. When medical knowledge in a particular area is spare or a trusted treatment unknown, actions, decisions, and judgments that retrospectively prove mistaken or incorrect are typically not viewed as mistakes by the profession or by society. The physicians involved could not have acted or decided differently given the then-existing state of the art. However, advances in medical science and practice will eventually transform these so-called "flawed state of the art" incidents into culpable errors that at least appear to be predictable and preventable given the current state of knowledge and medical practice. Given this phenomenon, it is not unexpected that advanced American medicine is an error-rich environment. It is also not surprising that reformers will never be fully successful in defining or eliminating error or its causes, given that it is, and will remain, a moving target.

CHAPTER 10

Reputation, Malpractice Liability, and Medical Error

WILLIAM M. SAGE

The purest treasure mortal times afford is spotless reputation.
—*William Shakespeare*

Reputation is not of enough value to sacrifice character for it.
—*Miss Clark, U.S. charity worker, quoted in* Petticoat Surgeon

Introduction

For over a century, opposition to malpractice litigation has been a litmus test for membership in the medical profession. Doctors hate malpractice suits. They hate them passionately and continuously. Being sued becomes a recurring nightmare for many physicians, and occasionally an obsession. Eliminating malpractice suits takes precedence over every other political objective—whether public-interested or self-serving—for the American Medical Association and state medical societies. No contradictory belief, however well-reasoned, empirically based, or sincerely held, succeeds in crowding out antipathy toward malpractice from physicians' minds. Not the large number of patients who die unnecessarily each year from medical errors; not the desirability of allowing patients to sue HMOs for improper care.

Why does malpractice stimulate the medical profession's "common bile duct"? For every straightforward explanation, there is an equally persuasive counterargument. Medical malpractice awards can be staggering, but they are almost entirely paid by liability insurers. Defending a lawsuit consumes large amounts of physicians' time and energy, but lawsuits are still the exception rather than the rule. The cost of malpractice insurance is considerable, but physicians are far from impoverished by it. Periodic "crises" of insurance availability and affordability produce stress and uncertainty, but these episodes punctuate much longer periods of stability and prosperity.

Yet none of these mitigating factors succeeds in taking the edge off doctors' suffering. The answer to this paradox may best be captured by a single word: "reputation." The dictionary definition of reputation reads: "overall quality or character as seen or judged by people in general; recognition by other people of some characteristic or ability; a place in public esteem or regard: good name." A thesaurus offers the following synonyms: eminence, face, fame, honor, image, legacy, memory, popularity, standing, celebrity, character, distinction, name, place, position, prestige, prominence, rank, renown, repute, self-respect, station, status. As this suggests, reputation is a complicated concept. At bottom, however, a malpractice suit is a genuinely felt professional insult—an assault on both physicians' self-esteem and their esteem by others.

Reputation interacts with law in interesting ways. Since ancient times, society has used both formal and informal means to police itself (Hunter 1994). Recently, legal scholars have begun to analyze in detail the importance of social norms to law (McAdams 1997). Adherence to both law and norms typically, but not always, heightens reputation. Violations of law and social codes tend to lower reputation. Reputation also protects against legal (and norm-based) sanctions, usually because prosecutors, judges, and juries exercise their discretion in that manner. At some point, however, perceptions of trust betrayed may lead to harsher-than-usual treatment of violators whose offenses belie their reputations. While members of the nobility of the Middle Ages were often immune from criminal charges (so-called "fur-collar crime"), aristocrats in eighteenth-century France met a very different fate (Hanawalt 1998, 53–69).

Reputation is frequently referenced by courts in malpractice suits and other health care litigation. In an early case involving chiropractors, *Foster v. Thornton* (1936), the Florida Supreme Court invoked reputation to establish a legal standard for proving malpractice. According to the court: "In cases arising from charges of malpractice, the sum of money involved regardless of its size, is a mere gesture in comparison with the professional character and reputation of the defendant. He should not, therefore, be condemned on evidence that does not point conclusively to his negligence." However, the importance of reputation was assumed rather than elucidated. For example, the court did not specify whether the physician's self-esteem was its primary concern, or the commercial harm to the physician's livelihood that might follow a finding of liability.

More recent cases have cited both aspects of reputation, and have connected the latter to structural features of physician practice. In *Raine v. Drasin* (1981), the Kentucky Supreme Court allowed physicians to recover damages for malicious prosecution where most of the harm was emotional. The court noted that the defendants "[testified] to their embarrassment, humiliation, mortification and mental anguish at having been publicly accused of malpractice. . . . [One doctor testified] that he suffered an acute anxiety reaction." In *Elbaor v. Smith* (1992), by contrast, three Texas Supreme Court justices focused on economic effects when strongly dissenting from the majority's decision that a physician who had entered into a contingent settlement agreement with the plaintiff was precluded from participating in the trial of the remaining defendants. The dissenters argued that the physician's "reputation in the community . . . has hereby been declared legally worthless, and any effect a jury verdict attributing significant negligence to him may have on hospital privileges, the cost and availability of malpractice insurance, and [his] patients is completely ignored."

In this chapter, I explore the relationship among reputation, malpractice liability, and medical error. The exercise has public policy relevance beyond offering an intellectual anodyne to physicians. Concern for reputation is cited by some as the principal reason why physicians scrupulously avoid injuring patients. Others attribute "defensive medicine" and similar socially undesirable phenomena to the specific affront to reputation that malpractice litigation poses. Changes in the structure and financing of health care, such as the trend toward delivering services through larger professional and nonprofessional organizations, may alter these tendencies. I suggest that factoring reputation into the design of legal and extralegal systems for policing medical quality and patient safety is less straightforward than economic analysis of incentives might predict, and more dependent on hard-to-quantify factors such as history, culture, and human impulse.

Reputation and the Health Care System

> One can survive anything these days, except death, and live down anything
> except a good reputation.
> —*Oscar Wilde*

Recent advances in patient safety pose a central question about the role of reputation. Since the publication of the Institute of Medicine's (IOM) landmark report *To Err Is Human*, reductions in medical errors have been predicated on replacement of punitive, individually oriented quality control processes such as professional discipline and malpractice litigation with cooperative, systems-based peer review and consultation (Kohn, Corrigan, and Donaldson 2000). Left ambiguous in both the critique of the old paradigm and the design of the new paradigm is the degree to which behavior is assumed to be the result of rational self-interest, and the mix of monetary and nonmonetary motivators involved.

Reputation is important to this analysis. Reputation is generally held to be a powerful driver of human behavior, but is open to a variety of interpretations regarding the source and direction of that power. Historically, reputation, perhaps even more than wealth, was what each generation passed to the next. As such, it constituted an inherited trust as much as an individual achievement. It was also inextricably linked to the myriad personal and family characteristics that define the self. Practical considerations connected to reputation, such as commercial or social advantage, were layered on top of this core value.

The evolution of the health care system in recent years alters reputation's potential influence on medical services and therefore on patient safety. Because "tort reform" has been an *idée fixe* of the medical psyche for so long, however, there is a tendency when debating malpractice liability to disregard the modernization of health care in ways that would be absurd in a discussion of virtually any other health policy issue. Does it not seem odd that the principal malpractice legislation being debated in Congress in 2004 is basically the same as that adopted in California in 1975? The fact that health care delivery is far more sophisticated, institutionalized, and competitive is largely ignored, as is the fact that the aggregate increase in malpractice premiums during those three decades is a ballpark equivalent to the aggregate increase in overall health care spending.

Although battle lines between physicians and lawyers over malpractice hardened by the late nineteenth century, technical progress since that time has created a modern medical science that would strike historical observers as nothing short of miraculous. The need for specialization, coordination, and capital financing, coupled with the breakdown of guild barriers to explicit management of professional services, converted American medicine into a corporate endeavor. Equally dramatic changes have occurred on the demand side. Urbanization and population mobility, along with medical specialization, reduced the continuity of therapeutic relationships. Medical paternalism receded as bioethicists focused attention on patient autonomy, and a consumerist mentality began to take hold. The tragedy of America's uninsured and the persistence of racial disparities notwithstanding, mainstream health care was universalized beyond the wealthiest enclaves, with the medical profession's acknowledgment of diverse perspectives being accompanied by a retreat from noblesse oblige into technical perfection.

These changes raise several questions about the role of reputation in the contemporary health care system. Is reputation still primarily a matter of professional pride, dependent on the judgments of peers? Or is it principally a commercial construct, with its value determined by buyers' goodwill in the marketplace? What about ways the two might connect, such as the importance of peer esteem in developing and maintaining referral networks or the subtext of professional jealousy, personal animosity, or economic rivalry in decisions to grant or to withhold affiliations with hospitals or managed care organizations? For patients who are the ultimate consumers, health care is unusual among goods and services because the process of receiving it is inseparable from the product received (Arrow 1963). Does this imply that gossip that breaks reputation can be in itself destructive of quality as well as competitively harmful to physicians? Does reputation operate differently for health care organizations (hospitals, HMOs) than for individual professionals?

How does tort law interact with reputation? Should reputation and malpractice liability be regarded as complements, both necessary to channel physicians' efforts in the direction of better patient care? If this is the case, one would expect the public's insistence on legal accountability to rise as physicians' reputations for competence improve. Or should they be regarded as substitutes, so that physicians whose reputations are on the line can be considered sufficiently cautious as to obviate the need for tort litigation? In this case, one would expect legal remedies to have greater currency in situations where considerations of reputation hold less sway over physicians. Finally, does concern over reputation promote appropriate care, or does it predispose to waste, as has been claimed regarding malpractice liability and fee-for-service payment (Kessler and McClellan 2002)?

Reputation and the Physician

> It will do you no good if I get over this. A doctor's reputation is made by the number of eminent men who die under his care.
> —*George Bernard Shaw, age ninety-four, said to his doctor*

The sociology literature views professions as personal vocations set in collegial and cultural context—in Roscoe Pound's words, "the pursuit of a learned art, as a common calling, in the nature of a public service" (Pound 1953, 5). Therefore, a first foray into the relationship between reputation and the quality of medical care should focus on the personal and professional reputations of the individuals who enter the healing professions.

Reputation and Conservatism

> The relatives of a suicide hold it against him that out of consideration for their reputation he did not remain alive. —*Friedrich Nietzsche*

A starting point for understanding how reputation affects the public policy of medical malpractice is the conservative force that concern for reputation exerts on social actors. Reputation distills down to one's position in a web of social relationships. Once reputation is attained, one alters these relationships at one's peril—dislodging even a single strand of the web risks a nasty fall. Furthermore, reputation is sufficiently ethereal as to exist largely in the perceptions of its possessor. Therefore, reluctance to change one's worldly circumstances for fear of the reputational impact is compounded by cognitive biases that tend to overestimate the fragility and the determinism of those circumstances.

Why is reputation so lastingly important to physicians? Perhaps it inheres in the notion of profession, in the supposed continuity of identity and purpose that leads every physician at least occasionally to measure him- or herself against Cushing, Osler, Harvey, Galen, or Hippocrates. The conservatism of medical reputation increases physicians' attachment to the status quo. Because modern medical training is long and intense, and the position of those who complete it relatively secure, entrepreneurship regarding reputation occupies an early and brief period in most physicians' careers. After that point, change that potentially compromises relative standing is viewed more as a threat to reputation than an opportunity for improvement. Small-area variation studies show that medical communities adhere closely to modal practices, though those practices differ markedly from place to place (Wennberg 1999). Efforts to measure physicians' practice against objective standards are resisted. In this climate, it is unsurprising that a malpractice suit alleging serious divergence from prevailing standards strikes most physicians as terribly disruptive.

Reputations also help maintain stability in the face of adversity. Even in the corporate context, reputations insulate firms from the immediate effects of controversy (Schultz, Hatch, and Larsen 2000, 79). Historically, challenges to established reputations were conducted through "ordeals." Allegations of malpractice likely strike some physicians as ordeals, but with notable differences from the historical model. The classic ordeal was a test before God, not man. Accordingly, physicians confer little legitimacy on the lawyers, judges, and juries who conduct malpractice litigation, especially since the impulses that determine legal outcomes are human and therefore profane rather than scientific and pure. Moreover, classic ordeals were limited to cases where doubts had been raised about an individual's trustworthiness, and were used to resolve that doubt and therefore to promote and maintain reputations (Nock 1993, 75–82). By contrast, physicians recognize that closure is not achievable from litigation, that even a decision in their favor is at best a temporary salve when the threat of additional claims is ever-present.

Reputation and Community

> How happy the lot of the mathematician! He is judged solely by his peers and the standard is so high that no colleague or rival can ever win a reputation he does not deserve. No cashier writes a letter to the press complaining about the incomprehensibility of Modern Mathematics and comparing it unfavorably with the good old days when mathematicians were content to paper irregularly shaped rooms and fill bathtubs without closing the waste pipe.
>
> —W. H. Auden

Defining the boundaries within which the norm of reputation operates raises another set of issues. Because reputation is constructed informally, individual reputations seldom permeate large societies. Rather, reputations are typically formed within communities constituted according to local geography, employment, interests, or other common characteristics. Within which community do physicians feel the greatest concern about exposure? A century ago, the answer would often have been a small group of well-to-do neighbors who were simultaneously paying patients, social peers, and opinion leaders. By the middle of the twentieth century, however, urbanization, specialization, scientific progress, and health insurance had greatly reduced most physicians' dependence on reputation among local gentry for their livelihoods and prospects of advancement. Instead, reputation within one's professional peer group became paramount, both for general self-esteem and for bread-and-butter reasons such as hospital privileges and patient referrals.

Communities use different methods to disseminate the information required to police reputation. Before modern journalism, the most rudimentary was word-of-mouth (Hunter 1994, 96–119). In many communities, gossip has both a negative and a positive influence. Gossip can shred reputations undeservedly, but it can also help define and preserve values by publicly embarrassing those who violate accepted norms. Whether constructed by locality or by practice institution (e.g., hospitals), physician communities are sufficiently close-knit that allegations or findings of malpractice liability can generate rumors that influence reputation, even where the fact of litigation is not formally connected to eligibility for specific professional benefits.

Medicine, like other professions, has a long tradition of self-policing errors and closing ranks against external accountability. Notwithstanding the fact that the legal standard of care is supposed to reflect professional custom, a malpractice claim represents a clear challenge from outside the fold. Accordingly, physicians often assert that being sued is a random event, and therefore no reflection on the ability of the individual involved. It is somewhat mysterious that physicians care about the reputational effects of malpractice suits if their peer group considers tort law illegitimate. Nonetheless, physicians take allegations of malpractice to heart. Even proxy indicators of prior involvement with litigation, such as purchasing liability coverage from state joint underwriting associations or other insurers of last resort, carry a significant degree of stigma. One explanation is that professional self-confidence is fragile whenever success depends largely on experience and judgment, which is the case for medicine despite its veneer of scientific precision. Another explanation is that a lawsuit criticizes the peer review process itself, and therefore challenges every physician's belief that he or she can distinguish good from bad practitioners.

A different explanation is that secondary communities have emerged in response to intensified government regulation and market competition. For example, health insurers may use malpractice history to determine eligibility for managed care networks. In *Potvin v. Metropolitan Life Insurance* (2000), an obstetrician was denied renewal of his preferred provider status because he had incurred more malpractice claims and payments than the health insurer considered desirable. Unlike hospital privileges decisions, these determinations are not made by self-governing medical staffs (i.e., professional peers), but by commercial contracting partners. Furthermore, nonprofessional audiences, such as insurers, are heterogeneous compared with physician groups, heightening uncertainty over how particular information will be reflected in reputation. The American Medical Association's recent experience evidences the difficulties of juggling internal and external reputation. Scandals such as Sunbeam (placing endorsements on household appliances) and Axicom (selling physicians' contact information) can be seen as resulting from the AMA's failure to accurately predict the blend of public and professional norms that will be applied to its behavior (Marconi 2001, 174–78).

The degree to which formal information exchange extends the reputational reach of liability experience is also relevant. When mobility is limited or when information is widely disseminated, harms to reputation carry great weight because one can neither live them down nor escape them (Nock 1993). This helps explain physicians' continued resistance to the National Practitioner Data Bank, which collects information on disciplinary actions and malpractice liability in order to prevent substandard practitioners from relocating from one state to another with impunity. To physicians, the Data Bank greatly magnifies the reputational effects of litigation by sharing that information across communities. Moreover, the Data Bank and similar state-based compilations regarding physicians' practice histories resemble to a degree consumer credit reports, raising the related point that reputations in mobile societies depend on impersonal data rather than personal references (Leary and Hudson 1985).

The Data Bank's threat to physicians' reputations has been noted by the courts in malpractice litigation. In *Sedlitsky v. Pareso* (1993), a Pennsylvania appeals court considered a physician's objection to the trial judge having given the jury a common instruction that effects on professional reputation were irrelevant to their conclusions about negligence in the specific case being tried. The physician argued, unsuccessfully, that "under the new [Data Bank] law . . . [the jury instruction] falsely trivializes the importance of the case to the defendant physician." In *Burgos v. Giannakakos* (1998), the court disqualified the law firm for a physician malpractice defendant from representing defendants in unrelated litigation in which the physician was serving as an expert for the plaintiffs because the physician would have confided his "inner most professional secrets" to the lawyer. The court opined that the "most serious" consequence of a malpractice suit for physicians was "the fact that any adverse result . . . will be reported to the National Clearing House . . . thus affecting the physician's very career and livelihood."

Reputation and Reality

> Character is like a tree and reputation like its shadow. The shadow is what we think of it; the tree is the real thing.   —Abraham Lincoln

Reputation is a social shorthand for qualities that are not easily measured. Reputation therefore reflects perception, not reality. The information base that determines reputation is contentious. Particularly when dealing with strangers, various proxies for reputation come into play. Interestingly, the accoutrements of "professionalism" exemplify these factors: formal education, government endorsement, membership in learned societies, acceptance of ethical codes. For example, educational degrees convey not only learning but also morality and etiquette—"portable reputations" (Nock 1993, 68–69). Another scholar notes: "A diploma could act as a kind of letter of introduction. What did a diploma certify? Certainly literacy, but also manners" (Kett 1977, 155).

Physicians' distaste for malpractice litigation is in part a statement that claims history is an unfair basis on which to judge reputation. As previously noted, most physicians feel that allegations of malpractice, and even findings of liability, are either random or motivated by greed on the part of patients and their lawyers. In fact, studies have shown that jury awards do not correlate strongly with actual negligence, or even iatrogenic injury (Brennan, Sox, and Burstin 1996). The mismatch between findings of liability and actual negligence after objective medical record review suggests that single allegations of malpractice are poor indicators of quality (Danzon 2000). Nonetheless, like the gossip that informs reputations in other contexts, lawsuits are appealing proxies for physician competence because of their narrative quality. Human beings have well-established cognitive biases. The greater salience of malpractice suits compared to physician "report cards" or other aggregate, statistical information is a striking example of a larger problem in health policy: the urge to focus on the personal anecdote and the identified life, even when it contradicts the data (Hyman 1998).

Physicians must also grapple with the uncomfortable fact that, despite their belief in the scientific foundation of modern medicine, relatively little of medical practice is scientifically proven. Given that fact, on what should physicians' reputations depend? Peer review? Hard data on outcomes? Patient satisfaction? A related problem is that different communities may have different realities. Physicians may seek to be judged "on the merits" by their peers rather than by the lay public. However, it is far from clear that reputation in professional communities is based on true competence, as opposed to collegiality and other niceties. And who is to say that reputation among patients is irrelevant, that only technical and not interpersonal skills determine medical quality (Sage 2002)? For example, studies correlating malpractice litigation with failures of physician-patient communication, lack of respect, or similar indignities imply that basing reputation on accusations of malpractice may be a reasonable indicator of professional qualities that matter to patients even if they are poor indicators of legal fault (Vincent, Young, and Phillips 1994; Hickson et al. 2002).

Reputation and Expectations

> The greatest dangers have their allurements, if the want of success is likely to be attended with a degree of glory. Middling dangers are horrid, when the loss of reputation is the inevitable consequence of ill success.
> —*Philip Dormer Stanhope, 4th Earl Chesterfield*

Because reputation is a matter of perception, the effect of particular events on reputation depends as much on relative factors—how those events comport with expectations—as on their absolute characteristics. Failure when failure is expected is a disappointment but no shame, while triumphing over extreme adversity—even if the result of good fortune rather than skill—can establish lifelong reputations. On the other hand, as politicians have found, when you lose and are in the favorite's position can mean banishment, as much because people hate to be reminded that their initial impressions were flawed as because actual ability proved to be limited.

The law of evidence reflects these considerations in its disregard of reputation as proof of negligence. The court commented in *Hinson v. Clairemont Community Hospital* (1990) regarding the defendant's performance in medical school and subsequent exclusion from two residency programs: "A doctor's reputation for skill and ability will not exonerate him. . . . Nor can the fact that a doctor is reputed to be negligent or unskillful be allowed as proof to establish negligence or unskillful treatment in a particular case." In reaching its decision to exclude such evidence, the *Hinson* court drew on legal authority from a full century earlier. In *Holtman v. Hoy* (1886), the Illinois Supreme Court wrote: "The veriest quack in the country, by his peculiar methods, not infrequently becomes very famous for the time being in his own locality, so much so that every person in the neighborhood might safely testify to his good reputation. It is true that one's reputation, thus acquired, is generally of short duration. His patrons sooner or later must pay the penalty of their credulity by becoming the victims of his ignorance, and with that his good name vanishes. Yet, according to the principle contended for, the quack, in such case, when called to account for his professional ignorance, might successfully entrench himself behind his prior good reputation."

This is one respect in which medicine is a victim of its own success. Considered in historical perspective, advances in medical technology have been the primary impetus for rising malpractice litigation (De Ville 1998; De Ville, this volume). This effect has been mediated by several factors, such as easier proof that treatment delay caused injury, rising costs of medical care necessitated by iatrogenic injury, greater financial resources among defendants, and more readily available scientific evidence that care was negligent. Most importantly for reputation, medical progress increases patients' and jurors' expectations and therefore intensifies the disappointment that follows failure. And the spectacular failures that traditionally induced tolerance or forgiveness become rarer as medicine improves: explicitly "experimental" treatments are presumed effective, "heroic" efforts are converted into daily achievements, and "medical miracles" become routine.

Reputation is therefore a lightning rod for litigation: it both attracts and dissipates it. A sterling reputation provides immunity from attack by creating a presumption of skill and diligence, but also magnifies the shock of a bad outcome because it is so unexpected. An implication of this observation is that testing reputation through malpractice litigation may have more to do with well-placed faith, confidence, and trust than with technical ability. Indeed, evidence of potential disloyalty, such as acceptance of financial incentives to limit treatment in managed care, tends to carry great weight in malpractice cases (and for that reason probably should be admitted in court only occasionally). Tort standards do not accord well with this notion, because the formal legal duty is one of care rather than loyalty.

Reputation and Elitism

> Henri IV's [unattractive] feet and armpits enjoyed an international reputation. . . . It was precisely because great men tried to seem more than human, that the rest of the world welcomed any reminder that, in part at least, they were still merely animal.
>
> —*Aldous Huxley*

One can see from the preceding discussion that medical elitism is a mixed blessing. On one hand, patients often draw comfort from believing that physicians who care for them are superhuman and infallible. On the other hand, the public has a natural tendency both to vent their disappointment when performance does not meet expectations, and to take special pleasure in seeing the mighty humbled. Correspondingly, malpractice litigation goes through cycles of greater or lesser deference to physicians. In general, it is difficult to persuade juries that physicians are negligent, and nearly impossible to extract punitive as opposed to compensatory damages even if liability is clear (Studdert and Brennan 2000). This is particularly true in smaller communities where individual reputations are personally known—some plaintiffs' lawyers complain that juries in these locations apply quasi–criminal law standards of proof to civil suits for medical negligence. However, unlike earlier historical periods when juries were drawn exclusively from the privileged classes—such as Norman juries in England that routinely nullified laws to exonerate well-reputed Norman defendants—jury pools today if anything tend in the other direction. Urban jurors, for example, may be less sympathetic to physician defendants, arguably reflecting both higher expectations of prosperous city doctors and resentment of the racial and class divides that often separate juries from professional defendants.

One set of questions these observations raise is whether and how physicians' risk of litigation might be correlated with social status. Certainly, physicians who practice sophisticated specialties such as orthopedic surgery or neurosurgery have greater malpractice exposure than family practitioners, seemingly in proportion to their respective degrees of social prominence. But confounding factors make any statistically valid comparison difficult. Higher-prestige fields in American medicine tend to be those that apply lifesaving technologies to very sick patients, which also increases the likelihood and worsens the severity of complications. These specialties tend to de-emphasize communications skills and limit the duration and scope of personal involvement with patients, which itself increases litigiousness. They are also practiced more in urban areas, and more in behalf of wealthier patients, both of which predispose to lawsuits. Finally, medical prestige is closely linked to earnings, which influences litigation as much through "deep pocket" effects as through anti-elitist feeling. Comparisons between the United States and other countries in which physicians have lower social status, such as Russia, reveal even greater differences in malpractice litigation but suffer from correspondingly more complex cultural confounders.

Still, it is possible that physicians could protect themselves against litigation by moderating their reputations in certain respects to appear less godlike and more human. New ethical standards for the medical profession emphasize honest disclosure of errors, and studies suggest that prompt apology can improve patient satisfaction and avoid lawsuits (Cohen 2000). The goal of these communication strategies would be to maintain physicians' reputations for technical proficiency, but simultaneously to enhance their reputations for trustworthiness by demonstrating openness. Indeed, the title of the IOM's exposé of medical error, *To Err Is Human*, subtly attempts to convey this point both to the medical profession and to the public.

Reputation and Finances

> A good reputation is more valuable than money.
> —*Publilius Syrus*

A principal lesson of the preceding analysis is that feelings and beliefs apart from rational economic incentives are very important to understanding the effect of reputation on malpractice litigation involving individual physicians. As prelude to the next section, in which we consider *corporate* reputation in an increasingly industrialized health care system, however, it is worth recapitulating the purely commercial considerations affecting physicians who face potential damage to reputation.

A quirk of malpractice insurance markets, explainable in part actuarially and in part politically, is that physician liability policies are not "experience-rated." Instead, premiums vary according to specialty, exhibiting as described above a general tendency toward higher prices in more highly compensated areas of medical practice. Because malpractice law operates at the state rather than the federal level, of course, state-to-state premiums may vary widely within specialties, especially during periodic insurance crises. In addition, the acuity of the current malpractice insurance crisis compared to its predecessors can be explained in part by constraints that have evolved on physicians' ability to pass through liability insurance costs to payers and patients. Unlike the generous third-party payment that prevailed in 1970 and even in 1985 (Danzon, Pauly, and Kington 1990), aggressive price negotiation by health insurers and restrictive Medicare and Medicaid reimbursement mean that recent, rapid increases in liability insurance costs have been borne primarily by physicians. Combining these facts, one realizes that liability insurance does impose real economic costs on physicians, although not in direct relation to their individual tendencies to attract or avoid lawsuits.

Malpractice litigation also places other financial burdens on physicians, costs that insurance does not cover: the time, inconvenience, and opportunity cost of having to prepare a defense, and several more mediated by loss of reputation. As noted, these include word-of-mouth among patients, referrals from other physicians, admitting and practice privileges at hospitals, and affiliations with managed care organizations. Courts have long been sensitive to the "uninsurability" of physicians' reputations. In *Clark v. Gibbons* (1967), Justice Tobriner's dissenting opinion observed that "[a]lthough the vast majority of medical practitioners are protected financially by liability insurance covering such accidents, and although doctors and hospitals can readily transfer the cost of this insurance protection to their patients through higher medical fees, no technique yet devised can protect a doctor from the devastating impact which an adjudication of malpractice can have upon his professional standing." From the perspective of liability insurance markets, of course, reputation acts as essential coinsurance, allowing insurers to issue policies with first-dollar coverage at community rather than experience rates without exposing themselves to moral hazard.

Because of the economic importance of reputation, judicial opinions in several cases have addressed the question of whether defense counsel may argue that the jury should consider the impact on the physician's reputation of holding him or her liable for malpractice (Habeeb 1960). Most courts have decided that effect on reputation is not a proper consideration in malpractice litigation. In *Zaretsky v. Jacobson* (1961), for example, the appeals court reversed a jury verdict in favor of the defendants because the trial judge had instructed the jury that "even should they conclude that the physicians had been negligent, . . . they were entitled to weigh against that the effect that their findings and verdict would have upon the professional character and reputation of the defendants." Among other things, these rulings suggest that many courts give primacy to the compensatory function of tort law (to which reputational effects are irrelevant) over its goals of encouraging safety and providing justice (to which reputational effects are indispensable).

Reputation and the Law

> No splints yet invented will heal a lawyer's broken reputation.
> —*Paul O'Neil, on attorney Edward Bennett Williams*

Thus far, I have speculated on how malpractice liability, or the fear of it, might influence physicians' reputations. I have said less about the specific role of reputation in legal proceedings. One reason is that, although some experts continue to support "shaming" as a pragmatic approach to misconduct, the evolution of formal legal sanctions can be seen as a principled alternative to penalties aimed at diminishing reputation (Kahan 1996; Whitman 1998). In this section, I consider law explicitly and conclude somewhat surprisingly that law has interacted with reputation primarily through its protection of information, not its rules of substantive conduct.

Reputation and Privacy

> At every word, a reputation dies.
> —*Alexander Pope*

It would be a mistake to equate reputation with achievement, ability, or character. Reputation is chiefly determined by judgments based on intimate information gathered, evaluated, and shared in private. Secrecy is therefore central to the formation and maintenance of reputation. For this reason, one talks about reputation as being "protected" or "safeguarded" as much as "established." One way in which courts hearing malpractice cases have addressed this issue is by protecting conversations between physicians and their lawyers from discovery by injured patients. In *Brown v. Foley* (1963), the court invoked the "work product" doctrine and denied the plaintiff access to information from a meeting at which a committee of physicians who belonged to the medical society that sponsored the defendant's malpractice insurance discussed the case with the defendant and his attorney. The court justified its holding in part by "the desire to obviate an individual's fear that his communication . . . if made public, would . . . so embarrass him that he would forego [*sic*] legal counsel rather than suffer the consequent humiliation."

The stridency with which the medical profession has lobbied for heightened "peer review" protection in the aftermath of the IOM's report can be interpreted in this light. Drawing analogies to aviation safety, the IOM observed that the threat of legal discovery and disclosure, with attendant reputational risk, discourages voluntary reporting of "near-misses" and chills collaborative analysis and feedback by professional peers (Kohn, Corrigan, and Donaldson 2000; Liang 1999). However, one can also sense in the powerful support these proposals have received from the medical profession a desire to shield reputations by limiting information to certain communities with which physicians are comfortable, regardless of the ultimate impact on patient safety.

There is a tension between privacy and reputation, however. Nock writes: "Privacy . . . makes it difficult to form reliable opinions of one another. Legitimately shielded from others' regular scrutiny, we are thereby more immune to the routine monitoring that once formed the basis of our individual reputations" (Nock 1993, 1). Sacrificing relevant information to privacy considerations invites other forms of surveillance, as well as intricate attempts at evasion. For example, the architectural response to the Calvinist obsession with the connection between openness and unblemished reputation placed large-windowed, curtainless front rooms facing the street in Dutch cities, while discreetly hiding L-shaped chambers, where life was really lived, behind one's neighbor's "front" (White and Boucke 2001).

One surprising implication of this analysis is that, under the proper conditions, transparency and accountability can serve as guardians of reputation, mainly by inducing the recipient of malicious gossip to discount its truthfulness. However, few individuals in modern society are required to meet this standard, and cover-ups are common even among public officeholders for whom it is supposedly the norm. Transparency is more commonly applied to the finances of corporations, a context in which revelations of its failure can bring dire consequences, as has been recently and vividly demonstrated by the bursting of the stock market bubble. Physicians have yet to adopt a disclosure-based regime for preserving reputation, although the financial incentives concocted by managed care have provoked some movement in this direction (Sage 1999; Hall et al. 2001). By and large, physicians expose to their colleagues and their patients only those facts about themselves that they desire to be known. Medical error, or even a patient sufficiently dissatisfied to take legal action, is something to be held in strictest confidence. Furthermore, as much for modern-day medical malpractice as for Victorian indiscretions, it is the accusation and not the resolution of the claim that generates headlines and saps reputation. Many physicians therefore resist the idea of disclosing unanticipated bad outcomes of care to patients, whether or not they amount to malpractice as a legal matter. This is the case despite the AMA's adoption of error disclosure as an ethical obligation of the medical profession.

Reputation and Defamation

> Libel actions, when we look at them in perspective, are an ornament of a civilized society. They have replaced, after all, at least in most cases, a resort to weapons in defense of a reputation.
>
> —Henry Grunwald, *editor of* Time *magazine*

It is the violation of privacy that directly connects reputation with law. Reputation is no stranger to the courtroom. Legal actions for intentional torts of defamation such as libel and slander are the traditional contexts in which reputation receives a judicial hearing (Soloski and Bezanson 1992; Waddams 2000). Significantly, truth is not always a defense under these legal principles, which exist as much to protect private information aired by the defendant with malice toward the plaintiff as to punish deliberate falsehoods. Because physicians tend to regard malpractice suits as baseless, the public nature of suit and the community gossip it often triggers lead physicians to feel defamed. Physicians consequently go to considerable lengths to preserve their reputations if they are sued, such as insisting on vindication through trial rather than settling out of court, or pressuring hospitals to offer payment in exchange for having the physician dropped from the complaint. As Syverud observes: "The filing of a malpractice suit, and its attendant publicity, may seriously damage a doctor or lawyer's professional reputation and self-image. Settlement of the suit, even for a nominal amount, may do little to repair that damage, whereas a judgment for the defendant may help a great deal" (Syverud 1990, 1174). Physicians on occasion have sued their liability carriers for both loss of reputation and increased premiums if nuisance claims are settled rather than fought. As was the case in *Shuster v. South Broward Hospital District Physicians' Professional Liability Insurance Trust* (1990), provisions in insurance contracts that allow carriers to settle as each "deems expedient" generally preclude these arguments, although a number of insurers (usually physician-owned companies) have adopted "consent-to-settle" clauses giving physicians a veto over proposed settlements. An innovative approach that succeeded for the physician plaintiff in *Arana v. Koerner* (1987) was to sue insurance defense counsel for legal malpractice on the grounds that they "knew or had reason to know that their settlement . . . without [their client's] consent or knowledge was highly likely to result in injury to [his] reputation."

Physicians' perception of litigation as defamatory is heightened by the fact that the source of the accusation is a patient to whom the physician feels intimately connected and whose legal claim therefore seems at best ingratitude and at worst betrayal. At common law, formal suits for defamation were unusual against family members, but were typically reserved for strangers who gained and abused access to intimate matters. The publicity of a tort suit for malpractice therefore represents a double affront from a patient because it breaches the decorum of the relationship as well as airing private facts. Similarly, well-intentioned regulatory regimes that require mandatory reporting of malpractice judgments and settlements so that they can be made available to licensing and credentialing bodies (e.g., the National Practitioner Data Bank) or to the public (e.g., websites operated by state licensing boards) accentuate the reputational threat of tort litigation and worsen physicians' resistance to it.

As one would expect, actual defamation suits by doctors against their patients are rare, though not unheard of. The court in *Morrman v. Khan* (2002) summarized the case as follows: "[As a result of] the defendant's response to a hospital survey in which he made derogatory comments about the medical care he received . . . plaintiff alleges that . . . he has suffered damage to his reputation and brought a single-count complaint, sounding in libel." Because the defendant's motive in making the allegedly defamatory statements was a factual question, the plaintiff succeeded in getting his case to the jury. That the physician in *Morrman* pursued the traditional form of defense to reputation, a libel suit, may reflect the increasingly impersonal nature of modern health care—an emergency department physician engaging in a brief technical interaction with a patient, never to be repeated, with each party regarding the other as a stranger. However, the decision (if it survives on appeal) is in tension with efforts to promote informed consumerism and to instill a customer-service ethos in hospitals and other corporate health care organizations. It would also seem to discourage patients from bringing grievances directly to health care providers so that they could form the basis for internal quality improvement efforts, rather than airing them publicly in the form of malpractice litigation.

Physicians who have had malpractice suits against them dropped or dismissed also may bring suit for malicious prosecution or abuse of process against plaintiffs' lawyers and even patients themselves. Harm to reputation is the main injury alleged in these cases, such as *Carruth v. Stoike* (1978): "As a direct and proximate result of the [lawyers] bringing the . . . action against [the physician], [he] has been injured in his good name and reputation and . . . has been caused grievous mental and emotional suffering and distress." These claims rarely succeed (Yardley 1984; Sokol 1985). Many jurisdictions limit malicious prosecution claims to "special injuries" beyond the pecuniary and nonpecuniary costs of being a defendant, and have been unreceptive to arguments, usually made during malpractice insurance crises, that "the fact that [malpractice] actions are particularly harmful to the reputations and livelihoods of physicians calls for a modification of the rule" (*Berlin v. Nathan*, 1978). As the Michigan Supreme Court pointed out in *Friedman v. Dozorc* (1981), one risk of expanding the availability of suits against lawyers without full legislative evaluation of costs and benefits is that "[a] legal malpractice crisis may arise as serious as the medical malpractice crisis."

Legal action for reputational injury also demonstrates the importance of the news media to the formation of medical reputations. The tension between unfounded affronts to reputation and the public's legitimate right to hear facts that might lead it to question professional practices has a long history. Over a century ago, the libel case brought by Dr. Mary Amanda Dixon Jones against the *Brooklyn Daily Eagle* showcased the courtroom as a forum for evaluating professional conduct and standards, established the power of the media to create harm to reputation, and led physician societies to recognize the importance of maintaining a united front against the media, lawyers, and patients (Morantz-Sanchez 1999, 199). More recently, a physician who claimed her reputation had been damaged by the media-generated investigation of *Boston Globe* reporter Betsy Lehman's death from a medication error at Dana-Farber Cancer Institute was awarded $4.2 million by a Massachusetts jury (Dembner 2002). Half that amount was assessed against the *Globe* for libel (although its desire to protect confidential sources precluded the newspaper from contesting liability), and half against the hospital for violations of privacy (but not defamation).

Without the possibility of legal recourse for malicious misstatement, modern publishing enables self-styled victims of malpractice to engage in reputational vigilantism well beyond gossip, such as writing a book or supplying information for an article as both cathartic and revenge. In *Gannett Co. v. Kanaga* (2000), the Delaware Supreme Court, despite a vigorous dissenting opinion, upheld a jury award of compensatory and punitive damages in a libel case brought by an obstetrician who claimed damage to reputation and professional standing because a local newspaper had responded to an aggrieved patient by printing a story titled "Patient feels betrayed—Says proposed hysterectomy wasn't needed." An irony of the jury finding was that the obstetrician's high earnings before the story was published (a net income of $441,149—64 percent above the national average in 1991), plausibly the result of performing unnecessary surgery, served in court only to increase her damages. Another interesting aspect of the case is that the patient had sought a second opinion and had received successful treatment without surgery, rendering an actual malpractice claim unavailable to her for lack of provable injury.

Defamation lawsuits, especially those involving the media, are often better as metaphor than as practical defense. The process of going to court can be more destructive than restorative of physicians' reputation, in effect adding injury to insult. The courtroom is a bully pulpit for reinforcing negative publicity, both to influence the jury and to pressure settlement. Moreover, a claim of libel against the press is difficult to win because of free speech concerns. A loss on First Amendment grounds may even be perceived by the public as confirming the truth of the challenged assertions.

All in all, the emphasis physicians place on vindicating reputation turns an action for malpractice on its head, with the injury to the physician's dignity rather than the patient's physical injury often driving the litigation. That there is a de facto defamation suit buried in the defense of many malpractice suits constitutes a significant obstacle to offering a plaintiff fair compensation. It also highlights the incompatibility of tort litigation with what is really at stake in many malpractice suits. Money damages end up being inadequate both for the physical injury of the patient and for the reputational injury of the physician, because restoring to each what each believes was wrongfully taken is impossible (Soloski and Bezanson 1992, 162).

Reputation and the Courtroom

> I rather like my reputation, actually, that of a spoiled genius from the Welsh gutter, a drunk, a womanizer; it's rather an attractive image.
> —*Richard Burton*

Stepping into the courtroom carries its own risks to reputation. Litigation used to be theater. A trial was often a town's chief entertainment, a blood sport that captured its attention and fed its appetite for gossip. Historically, physicians experienced the connection between litigation and reputation mainly in this context, and not just as defendants in malpractice actions. Each time a physician was sworn as an expert witness, whether to opine on cause of death in a possible homicide or to assess mental competency in a testamentary dispute, he put his professional reputation on the line (Mohr 1993).

This was a precarious position for a capable if inarticulate physician, because damaging a well-known doctor's reputation in open court enlarged the professional reputation of the lawyer who accomplished the feat. Antipathy between medical and legal professions in the United States reflects to a substantial degree the number of physicians who wilted under aggressive cross-examination by lawyers with far greater natural affinities for the stage. Physicians, trained to be cautious and scientific, came to regard the hyperbolic oral advocacy of lawyers as unscrupulous, while attorneys' standing in their own communities depended on a separate set of ethical considerations and was rarely jeopardized by courtroom rhetoric. Consequently, lawyers may have dismissed doctors' grumblings as poor sportsmanship by a bested adversary without fully appreciating the impact that the courtroom experience might have on a doctor's career.

Modern litigation, by contrast, is a war of attrition—a grimy group tug-of-war rather than a dramatic, decisive duel between two nimble adversaries. Extensive depositions and documentary discovery, costly expert reports, maneuvering over procedural advantages, fingerpointing among multiple defendants and their liability insurers, overcrowded court dockets, and reluctance by both sides to risk the caprices of a jury trial have sapped malpractice disputes of much of their immediacy and impact. In this environment, the intensity of physicians' concern for their reputations when sued may reflect received wisdom more than reality. Not only have the pace and tone of litigation changed, but a run-of-the-mill malpractice case (not involving a major celebrity) is unlikely to captivate the public in communities that are bigger, less unified, more mobile, busier, and blessed or cursed with a wider variety of apprehensions and amusements. At the same time, of course, physicians' fantasies about being publicly vindicated (and the accuser correspondingly humiliated) are rarely fulfilled. Moreover, the anticlimax of resolving a negligence claim by settlement after years of strategic positioning detracts from the traditional goals of tort liability. Compensation for injured patients is often too remote and speculative to be meaningful, while delay and uncertainty attenuate any signal to providers regarding the need for quality improvement.

Nonetheless, physicians still react strongly to the reputational threat of courtroom proceedings. For example, a Maryland appeals court confronted the question of whether a malpractice defendant's attempt to discourage other physicians from testifying against him constituted grounds for professional discipline in *Commission on Medical Discipline v. McDonnell* (1983). The defendant, a professor of orthopedic surgery at Johns Hopkins who "[a]pparently . . . enjoys an enviable reputation" and was "incensed" about the potentially damaging testimony of the plaintiff's experts, had used his academic connections to have intimidating phone calls made to prospective witnesses by senior physicians who had been their mentors in medical training. The court concluded that this "attempt to protect and preserve his professional reputation [was] conduct 'in his practice as a physician'" and therefore was appropriate grounds for discipline by the state medical board.

Reputation and the Corporation

> In business a reputation for keeping absolutely to the letter and spirit of an
> agreement, even when it is unfavorable, is the most precious of assets, although
> it is not entered in the balance sheet.
>
> —*Lord Chandos*

Not only individual physicians but corporate entities can suffer reputational harm related to medical error and malpractice litigation. Widely publicized tragedies in high-profile hospitals, such as Boston's Dana-Farber Cancer Institute or Memorial Sloan-Kettering Medical Center in New York, place their reputations for quality in jeopardy (Chassin et al. 1998). When settlements in malpractice litigation exceed the damages available under state law, as occurred in the Ben Kolb case in Florida, one can surmise that preserving reputation rather than legal exposure was the principal motivator for the defendant hospital to be generous at the negotiating table (Boodman 1996).

Reputation and Management

> Two-year-olds are not "terrible," but their reputation is.
>
> —*Bernice Weissbourd*

The economic importance of reputation is most clearly demonstrated in the corporate context (Dowling 2001). Reputation is often said to survive the death of the person it relates to. While the transcendent quality of individual reputations takes on quasi-religious significance, immortality in the corporate realm serves a much more practical purpose as a store of goodwill, a motivator of employees, and a determinant of business value. In health care, Arrow postulated that nonmarket social institutions, such as physicians' ethical codes and nonprofit hospitals, serve to maintain trust in medical care despite the lack of information that plagues the typical patient (Arrow 1963). As corporate organizations grow in importance in the health care system, reputation that enables trust is easier to see as an objective of market participants than as a phenomenon external to markets. Many health care services are "credence goods": goods bought on faith (Fombrun 1996, 7). Furthermore, reputation for quality (including honesty) is an important source of product differentiation, and therefore brand equity (Fombrun 1996, 4). It has taken time for business reputation to evolve from a personal model of contacts and connections to a measurable, manageable asset. In the early twentieth century, reputation for business purposes largely depended on admission to a fraternity or club, preferably at the national level, and the display of membership in that organization (Nock 1993, 47–48). Modern corporate images, by contrast, are strategically designed, carefully cultivated, and diligently defended. Furthermore, a core function of some corporate entities, such as investment banks, bonding organizations, and accrediting bodies, is to associate their reputations with their clients' products, thereby certifying quality or value to those doing business with their clients (Gilson and Kraakman 1984; Mann 1999). Organizations may also invoke gains in commercial reputation as justifying broad programs of corporate social responsibility (Peters 1999). However, empirical studies do not always support the notion that reputational "ill will" from events such as toxic releases or other corporate environmental damage is financially harmful to firms (Jones and Rubin 2001).

Reputation plays an important motivating role within organizations. As Schultz and colleagues observe, "reputation not only accrues to better-performing companies, but also enables their performance" (Schultz, Hatch, and Larsen 2000, 79). A good reputation attracts corporate partners, sponsors, and employees in addition to customers, and reassures government regulators. In repeated transactions, reputation serves to enforce contracts without recourse to law (Milgrom and Roberts 1992, 259–69). The premium paid by acquirers for goodwill also provides incentive for each successive owner to invest money and effort to preserve a firm's established reputation (Tadelis 2002).

Corporate reputation depends on corporate leadership. Marconi notes that "[c]orporate reputations, like individuals' reputations, can be managed both assertively and defensively" (Marconi 2001, 99). In some health care organizations whose complacent belief in their own superiority was shattered by deadly, avoidable medical errors—such as the hospitals mentioned above—senior management stepped up in defense of reputation, restored morale, and brought about significant, coordinated change by instilling a new sense of mission. In other settings, however, managers have misguidedly denied errors and bred employee confusion and patient distrust, or have placed their short-term exit strategies ahead of the organization's long-term interests.

Reputation and Marketing

> You need not rest your reputation on the dinners you give.
> —*Henry David Thoreau*

Corporations engage in a more organized process of measuring and molding reputation than do individuals, approaching issues of mass or targeted communication proactively rather than reactively (Gray 1986). Research is the key to effective marketing (Marconi 2001). Media interest, market trends, and political agendas are among the factors that can be evaluated in assessing present reputation and planning image improvements. This presents a greater risk of manipulation with respect to facts that might reflect poorly on the organization, but it also implies greater sensitivity and responsiveness to consumer preferences. In many instances, for example, companies have to actively solicit reputation information from stakeholders. Marketing experts also exhort companies to exercise swift damage control when things go bad: monitoring potential problems, taking prompt corrective action, and publicizing the response (albeit with "spin").

Health care organizations, whether hospitals, physician group practices, or managed care companies, take great pains to portray the care they provide as "cutting-edge" in safety and effectiveness. Litigation, especially accusations of physical harm such as malpractice, can rapidly undo years of costly corporate image-making. Courtroom proceedings are typically protracted and therefore less controllable than other sources of reputational damage. Cases may be tried in the press if it serves the plaintiff's interest. The adversary process also rewards extreme positions and tends toward escalation, both of which run counter to principles of strategic communication with customers, regulators, and the public.

Reputation and Responsibility

> Although the employer may perhaps lawfully destroy its own reputation, its employees should be and are barred from destroying their employer's reputation by misappropriating their employer's informational property.
> —Judge Lawrence Pierce, upholding the conviction of a former
> Wall Street Journal reporter for insider trading

Ultimately, one must ask whether corporate organization in health care improves accountability in the event of medical error and therefore enhances incentives for safety improvement. Arrow viewed corporations optimistically, noting that their greater financial resources, internal checks and balances, bottom-line orientation, and institutional stability all improve their capacity to self-regulate their conduct and that of their employees (Arrow 1972). Yet others consider large corporations to be powerful but depersonalized—faceless bureaucracies that can only be held to account by aggressive litigation.

Corporate reputation deserves consideration where malpractice liability is concerned for two reasons. First, the rise of the modern hospital and the more recent growth of managed care, with its spillover effect on physician organization, signal that twenty-first-century health care will be dominated by corporations rather than solo professionals. Second, the patient safety movement has demonstrated that systematic and organizational flaws are the source of most medical errors, rather than individual "bad apple" physicians that traditional peer review has failed to cull from practice. Accordingly, legislatures and courts continue to expand the malpractice exposure of institutional health care providers, both for their own negligence and for the negligence of their employed or affiliated physicians.

This liability risk also connects institutional reputation in health care to the component reputations of individual physicians who work within a corporate organization. Institutions may be held legally responsible for failing to evaluate the qualifications of those with whom they affiliate, with reputation again serving as an imperfect proxy for more specific measures. "Negligent selection" has a long history of being used to justify direct recovery by plaintiffs for the acts of third parties with respect to whom the defendant was not legally responsible on a theory of vicarious liability. In an early case, *Atlantic Coast Line Railroad Co. v. Whitney* (1911), the court affirmed "the wisdom of adhering to the general reputation, rather than isolated incidences, to bring home to the principal guilty knowledge of incompetence. . . . [T]he railroad company is not responsible for the negligent work of its surgeon if not negligent in selecting or retaining him, [but] . . . [h]is general reputation may be so bad that the law will impute knowledge."

For these and other reasons, proposals to unify legal accountability for error in a single corporate entity such as a hospital or health plan—termed "enterprise liability"—continue to attract support from the policy and scholarly communities, notwithstanding the political backlash that occurred during the debate over the Clinton administration's health reform plan (Kohn, Corrigan, and Donaldson 2000; Sage 1997). Incorporating reputation into the analysis of enterprise liability may significantly strengthen the concept. Specifically, displacing liability risk from individual physicians onto medical institutions may substitute a relatively clear, consistent set of corporate reputational concerns for the murky and variable considerations that drive physicians facing threats to personal reputation. Ideally, this heightened predictability might facilitate the replacement of fault-based liability with an administrative system that would offer faster, cheaper, surer compensation for avoidable error (Corrigan, Greiner, and Erickson 2002).

However, two questions persist. First, will corporate medical organizations defending their reputations be more or less forthcoming than individual physicians about the occurrence of error? Second, when public responsibility rests most visibly on the physicians or other health professionals proximately connected to a particular adverse outcome, will institutions shield the individual reputations of those involved as part of a coordinated plan of acknowledgment and corrective action, or will they attempt to deflect responsibility onto them and discard them? Neither answer is clear. The reputational interests of corporations are less convoluted than those of individuals, and their smaller number makes them easier to monitor both as a market and as a regulatory proposition. On the other hand, corporate concentrations of wealth and power can increase both the temptation and the ability to conceal misdeeds.

Conclusion

> Hope is the only universal liar who never loses his reputation for veracity.
> —*Robert Green Ingersoll*

Society looks to medical malpractice law to achieve four goals: compensating victims, improving safety, surfacing explanations for tragedy, and providing corrective justice. The incentives for plaintiffs to trigger this process, and the responses by defendants, are significantly influenced by concern over a lawsuit's effect on reputation, regardless of its monetary implications. Although reputation's effect on medical practice is complex, it seems safe to draw three conclusions. First, self-regulatory models that rely on professional peer review and informal sanctions to surface, analyze, and prevent error are inadequate substitutes for public surveillance and accountability given the hazy yet intransigent quality of individual physician reputation. Second, no-fault alternatives to malpractice litigation that require physicians to confess error in order to obtain fair compensation for patients, such as the state funds that operate in Sweden and New Zealand, will be difficult to implement in the United States without solving the problem of the American medical profession's defensiveness regarding reputation. Third, the predominantly economic interest of corporate entities in goodwill, coupled with the emphasis that modern management science places on effective communication to protect corporate reputation, signals that the "corporatization" of health care delivery, despite its other uncertainties, may bring greater clarity to reputation as a competitive and social benefit.

Acknowledgment

The author thanks Nancy Cooney for research assistance. This work was supported in part by a grant from The Pew Charitable Trusts' Project on Medical Liability in Pennsylvania. All epigraphs that appear in this chapter were taken from Andrews et al. 1996 and Simpson 1988.

CHAPTER 11

Ethical Misfits: Mediation and Medical Malpractice Litigation

EDWARD A. DAUER

Introduction: The Hypothesis

Reducing injuries from medical error is a central focus of current health care policy and research. A traditional presumption of the law of civil liability, or torts, is that charging a negligent person with the monetary consequences of his or her lack of due care will cause others similarly situated to exercise greater care in the future. This proposition, known to legal scholars as the "deterrence" function of torts, would suggest that a sound system of civil liability can make a positive contribution to the quest for patient safety.

Quite to the contrary, fault-based tort law has recently been subjected to serious criticism (Gosfield et al. 1992; Hiatt et al. 1990; Kessler and McClellan 1997). The empirical facts of the deterrence function are in doubt (Weiler 1991; Sloan et al. 1993; Conrad et al. 1998), and the law's unintended but demonstrable inhibitions of other patient safety initiatives have been sharply critiqued (Liang, this volume). The once-robust swagger of torts in the councils of safety has been changed to that of a still-important but somewhat clumsy and warily regarded guest. Medical malpractice liability law is in disrepute.

In addition to the increasing skepticism about the substantive aspects of the law of torts, there is reason to believe that the quest for improvements in patient safety may also be affected, again adversely, by the *process* through which malpractice law is applied and imposed. To give a convenient name to a complex device, we may refer to this as the "conventional system" for managing claims alleging iatrogenic injury. It includes litigation and litigation's appurtenant procedures of pretrial discovery (e.g., depositions) and motion practice. It also includes the more frequent process of insurance claims management and attorney-managed settlement negotiation, all of which is profoundly shaped by the imminence or potential of a courtroom trial, however rare actual trials may be. Based on both theoretical and empirical considerations, I wish to hypothesize that this conventional system, occurring in the aftermath of a medical mishap, is problematic; and that a form of mediation applied to appropriate cases in lieu of the conventional system may be able to advance the cause of patient safety more effectively than litigation can.

Mediation is a form of alternative dispute resolution, which is generally known as "ADR." Its applications in diverse areas of legal and organizational conflict are well-understood. ADR's risks, when it is properly applied, are low and its benefits well-demonstrated. It would seem, therefore, that in an environment in which tort law is under siege and patient safety is of prime importance, those who are in a position to employ alternatives such as mediation would be doing so eagerly. The fact is, they are hardly doing so at all.

This reluctance to explore the mediation alternative, largely on the part of the liability insurance industry and the defense bar (less so on the part of the plaintiffs' bar), requires an explanation. One possibility is that the hypothesis is wrong—that despite all we know about mediation in every other setting where it has been successfully applied, for some reason it has either fewer benefits or greater risks in medical malpractice than I have supposed. While I am not unalterably opposed to accepting that explanation, for the moment I reject it as both facile and implausible. There are other possibilities. For one, the legal system itself has features that tend to inhibit everything other than the conventional process—which is to say, that the future of mediation may require amendments to more than just the claims-management process itself. For another, we have learned through focus group research that there are sources of resistance deeply embedded in the litigation process that are artifacts rather than intended features of its structure. There is as well a belief system about litigation that is more resonant than empirical—resonant, that is, with the simplistic but widely observed value of vindication, and with a common and possibly adaptive instinct that harm causing anger justifies revenge.

These factors, however, seem not to explain all of the reluctance there is. That is of course a judgment call, but it inspires a thought that, if correct, could have an even broader importance. That thought is that the operators of the conventional medical malpractice liability system live in a world suffused with ethical values that they find comfortable; and that mediation, in the form I will describe, confronts those values with implicit but contrary values of its own. For a person steeped in the world of conventional torts, moving into the ethical framework of mediation is an unpleasant challenge. That, together with the other explanations—the legal and the organizational—may account for the reluctance to supplement the conventional system with interest-based mediation.

There is a practical importance to exploring this possibility. If an objective is worthy and the causes of resistance to it are known, it becomes that much easier to pursue the objective. There may be a wider value as well, which I explore again near the conclusion of the present discussion. Examining this small hypothesis calls for an explicit description of what the ethical values of medical malpractice law are, adding another dimension perhaps to the policy discussion about how much tort law we want or need in the practice of American health care.

I begin with a reprise of how and why mediation is thought to be beneficial in the cause of patient safety. I then report what is known about its actual, rather than expected, employment. I briefly discuss the two candidates already mentioned, for explaining the gap between the theory and the practice. Then comes the core of the analysis—explicating the ethics of malpractice litigation, the ethics of malpractice mediation, and the misfit between them. Finally, I conclude with some additional implications that may follow if the hypothesis turns out to be true.

Litigation, Mediation, and Patient Safety

The case in favor of mediation is based positively on mediation's characteristics, and negatively on those of the conventional process, which for this purpose I will use interchangeably with the word litigation.

Litigation is enormously inefficient as a device for compensating injured patients. It is not at all unusual for the contending sides together to spend over $2.50 in legal and processing costs to deliver $1.00 to the injured plaintiff (Weiler, Hiatt, and Newhouse 1993). If tort law is social insurance, it is insurance with an administrative overhead no private market would ever allow.

More to the point, litigation often fails to meet the needs of the parties who engage in it. The outcome of a lawsuit can only be money. Courts cannot heal wounds, physical or psychological; they cannot order that corrective actions be taken in the future; they cannot force apologies or expressions of regret and concern; they cannot make right what has been made wrong. They can only award or not award money. For a variety of reasons, the settlement negotiations and claims-management activities that go on "in the shadow" of the formal law tend to share this narrow remedial capability. Comprehensive data are lacking, but anecdotal evidence and such empirical inquiries as there are bear it out. Conventional settlements occur along the single axis of more money or less.

It is now beyond serious doubt that money is not what motivates most medical malpractice plaintiffs. Some patients, but a minority, describe "financial consequences" as the dominant effect of their injury. Lost wages are often covered by disability insurance, and excess health costs by comprehensive health insurance. Many more report that their dominant response after their injury was anger, or betrayal—the latter as often caused by the provider's defensive silence as by the fact of the medical mishap. The motivations for bringing claims and lawsuits are likewise partly, but only partly, economic. Of equal sway are the drives for "justice" or "accountability," and, most telling, simply to have an explanation of what happened, or to assure that such a thing must never happen to anyone else (Hickson et al. 1992, 1994; Huycke and Huycke 1994; May and Stengel 1990; Berlinger, this volume; Gilbert, this volume). These objectives can be powerful motivators. A money judgment or a money settlement is often a pale surrogate. The patient-now-plaintiff's energies are steered by the conventional process into a debate about fault and damages, rather than being channeled and employed as a force for correction. Mediation offers a very different set of possibilities, including that of explicitly corrective outcomes.

The traditional apology for tort law, that the threat of liability deters future carelessness and thereby fosters future safety, has also been put in doubt. On the margin at least, the most recent evidence shows no statistically significant benefit from more or more certain liability. For one thing, the presumption that liability imposed on one provider will cause others to be more careful assumes that the others believe their care or carelessness is related to the risk of being held liable. With some good reason, many physicians do not believe that. They see the incidence of liability as being correlated with medical outcomes, not with the exercise of care. There is little to be learned by correlating claims and liability with factors over which physicians believe they have no control. "Risk management" thus becomes largely an effort to avoid liability, rather than an effort to avoid error. Deterrence does not justify the conventional system any more than compensation does.

There is also reason to believe that the *process* of conventional claims management may in fact have the opposite of the hypothesized deterrent effect. It has been suspected for some years that the stress physicians experience while being subject to malpractice claims may result in a degradation of their performance (Charles 1985; Passineau 1998). Partial isolation from peers and patients (self-imposed or otherwise), excessive rumination, self-doubt, anger, and hostility contribute to altered mental states and concomitant effects on judgment and performance. One major liability insurer that has examined its own claims records found evidence strongly suggestive of these effects (Passineau 2000). Specifically, physicians against whom a malpractice claim had been made exhibited a sharply elevated risk of incurring a second "loss" (insurance argot for payment on a claim) during the year after the first claim was brought. In the first two quarters after the filing of the first claim, the odds ratio is as high as three-to-one. The fact that the loss experience declines to normal levels after eighteen to twenty-four months suggests, though it does not prove, that the effect is attributable to the pendency of the first claim rather than to any unusual propensity toward error.

The data are now being carefully examined, and other claims repositories are being surveyed to see if the effect is replicated elsewhere. If the findings hold up, they will be powerful reinforcement of the idea that litigation is decidedly "antitherapeutic" for those who are involved in it (Wexler and Winick 1996).

Again, mediation is structured in a way that may ameliorate these effects. It is nonadversarial, not bent on proving "fault" or imposing blame, and intentionally focused on each party's need for restorative resolution.

There is finally, on this negative side of the case for mediation, a growing body of information about what error reduction initiatives actually require. As my colleagues and I have discussed elsewhere, major features of the conventional malpractice system are inconsistent with what we now know is necessary for effective error prevention (Dauer and Marcus 1997). To iterate just a few of those comparisons: While error prevention requires analyses of the systems within which individuals work and err, tort law focuses on individuals alone; while error prevention requires a mishap to be regarded as a window through which the more frequent process upsets can be glimpsed, tort law attaches blame to and focuses on rare and singular events; while error prevention requires that physicians become active participants in the search for quality improvement, the public and punitive attributes of tort law dissuade useful involvement; and while error prevention requires comprehensive information about errors and their causes, the risk of additional tort liability tends to cause cover-ups and reduce the incentives, if not the willingness, to examine error's root causes.

The positive side of the case for mediation is that it is confidential, fosters communication and understanding, and allows for almost infinitely flexible outcomes—attributes that, not coincidentally, can obviate the very disadvantages of the conventional process.

The confidentiality of mediation is assured by statutory legal privileges in nearly every state. It can thus be a safe harbor in which candid introspection and examination of the injurious event may take place, and where corrective possibilities can be considered without being taken as incriminating evidence of an earlier lack of due care. The confidentiality also avoids the publicity and seemingly punitive aspects of litigation, allowing a post-event opportunity for reflection that is more resonant with the requisites of error prevention than litigation is.

When mediation is employed in an "interest-based" mode, its objectives include the restoration of communication between the disputing parties. Mediators work to bring each side to an understanding of the needs and limitations of the other. The net effect may be "dealing the patient back in" to medical care, with the beneficial consequences that is widely supposed to have.

The remedial flexibility, contrasted with the frequently single-axis outputs of the conventional process, allows for explicitly corrective resolutions. In one experiment with mediation of claims against doctors brought by patients to a board of medical examiners (and thus a setting admittedly somewhat different from that of civil liability), the vast majority of all the mediated cases were resolved; the majority were resolved without the payment of money; and a larger majority were resolved with agreements by the medical care provider to take corrective action—changing office procedures, for example, or undergoing additional medical education, or implementing other changes for the future that respond to the patient's drive to see that "it never happens again" (Dauer and Marcus 1997).

The case for mediation, and for its potential to be more consonant with the goals of patient safety than the conventional system alone is, seems to be a sound one. Why, then, do so few of the right people seem to care?

The Gap between What Might Be and What Is

Accurate data about how widely mediation is actually employed are hard to come by. Most of the empirical studies to date deal with mandatory, court-annexed mediation programs, simply because they are easier to study. Mediation as it is applied in these programs, however, is very different from the form of voluntary mediation being examined here, thus making mere counts of "mediation" unuseful. Moreover, the very confidentiality of the process plays a role in keeping good information away from public view, though a relatively small number of programs have published their results. There is, in addition, undoubtedly more mediation going on than is commonly counted. Hospital risk managers and patient ombudsmen, for example, employ mediation-like techniques without calling them by that name. And some insurers that do have early-intervention, interest-based mediation programs regard both their programs and their results as proprietary and therefore confidential. In short, we do not know how much mediation goes on in medical malpractice.

In 1998 the Physician Insurers Association of America (PIAA), an association of physician-owned liability carriers, surveyed its member companies in an effort to learn how mediation was being used (Bartholomew 1999). The results of the survey are illuminating on several counts. Of the thirty-three responding companies, thirty reported having used mediation to resolve malpractice claims at least once, though in many cases they did so under court order rather than voluntarily. Nearly half of the companies, however, reported using mediation in less than 2 percent of their claims. And the overwhelming majority reported that mediation was most often used for claims with clear liability and limited damage potential.

Understanding the significance of this last point requires a brief digression. The word "mediation" has an array of different meanings. The very flexibility of the process allows for a wide variety of forms. So far no taxonomy has emerged to distinguish one from another. They are all called "mediation." But some are significantly different from others. The two polar cases may be called the "settlement conference" mode, and the "interest-based" mode. Insurers almost always mean by the word "mediation" the former. The mode that has been under examination in my work is the latter. The differences between them are substantial.

In the settlement conference mode, mediation is employed only after an insurer has determined that some amount of money will be paid to the claimant, and the only remaining question is how much. The mediator acts as a go-between, attempting to find some amount of money that is between the upset points of the competing interests. The defense side is usually represented by the insurance company and a lawyer, and only sometimes by the physician. The plaintiff is represented by a lawyer, and only sometimes by the plaintiff. As often as not, in this settlement conference mode, the parties are separated while the mediator shuttles between them, seeking just enough compromise from each to allow for a deal. This is bargaining in the shadow of the law, and it is about money.

In the interest-based mode, the mediator seeks to create a functional channel for communication between the parties directly. There is no presumption going in that any money will be paid. The search is for a solution that will respond to the parties' *interests* (needs, concerns, and limitations) rather than to their adversarial *positions* (the demand for money and the refusal to pay any). The goal of interest-based mediation is a positive-sum rather than a zero-sum outcome, and the technique includes bringing each side to listen to and come to grips with the perceptions and motivations of the other.

In a series of focus groups conducted among insurers, doctors, patients, and lawyers, my colleagues and I found that the settlement conference mode is what most insurers understand mediation to be (Dauer, Marcus, and Payne 2000). What is most interesting in the PIAA data is the finding that confirms this—of the thirty companies that used mediation, only six had *ever* had a nonmonetary result. (The proportion of nonmonetary results among the mediated cases for those six companies does not appear in the collected data.)

The PIAA survey did, however, establish that when mediation was employed, it enjoyed significant success measured in terms of settlement rates and in sharply reduced expense, in addition to the finding that the physicians who experienced even just the settlement conference mode found it far more satisfying than did those whose cases were managed in the conventional system.

Nonetheless, the usage rate is well below what should be expected. Why is that so?

Explaining the Gap

The very existence of litigation creates risks for any who would depart from it. Some lawyers believe the mediation privilege may be porous—"apologies" uttered by a contrite physician could, if the mediation does not result in a resolution, be used as evidence in a later trial in court. Apparatus related to the fault-based system has the same inhibiting effect. The National Practitioner Data Bank (NPDB), for example, and its analogues in the several states require a report of every case in which an insurer makes a payment on behalf of a physician, once a written malpractice claim has been made. There is no floor or threshold, and as yet no effective way to distinguish in the NPDB reports passed on to employing hospitals and health plans, which payments were connected to error and which were made to buy peace. A truly *early*-intervention mediation program could avoid NPDB reporting by responding to instances of medical mishap before the patient made a written demand, but defense lawyers and many insurers refer to such a practice as "trolling for plaintiffs." While a program recently mounted by one farsighted insurer has given the lie to this fear, defensive instincts die hard.[1]

Beyond these factors, we learned from our focus group studies that the traditional litigation process remains firmly in place in part because of artifacts and myths, as well as because of its undoubted real advantages. I have described these factors more fully elsewhere (Dauer, Marcus, and Payne 2000). Just one example may make the point here. Litigation, again, produces outcomes measured in dollars. The operators of the system are organized around dollars. Plaintiffs' lawyers, necessary to any litigation, generally take malpractice cases on a contingency fee. The system must, therefore, produce dollar outcomes if these essential people are to be involved. Insurance companies are organized to manage cash flows. Premiums are paid in dollars; claims are assessed in dollars; claims management is created as an investment of small numbers of dollars to protect larger numbers. Litigation, that is to say, requires these operators in order to work well, and the apparatus of operators built up around it requires that the system stay pretty much as it is. That is not to say that lawyers behave purely out of self-interest to preserve an ineffective system. Most do not, in the same way that physicians are also paid in dollars but gauge their behaviors along professional lines. Each participant sees itself, rightly, as doing the job within the system it is obligated to do. It is the whole that tends to preserve itself.

One particular anecdote may illustrate the point. We know that many patients and families injured by what they suspect was a medical error are moved to learn "what happened." During the focus group studies, we learned of one major insurer that imposed on its insured physicians two rules. First, if a patient appears to be asserting a complaint about a medical error, the physician would be asked (or told) not to speak with the patient until the insurance company has provided the doctor with legal counsel. Rule number two is that the company does not provide legal counsel until there is a formal claim. To make such a claim a patient must hire a lawyer, who must be paid in money. Thus, the motive to learn what happened inevitably becomes a dispute about money. The system, in other words, in this case is perpetuating itself.

The Residual Question

All of these factors, and perhaps others like them, operate to make any movement toward mediation seem riskier or more jarring than it actually could be, in a world dominated by the fault-based tort system we presently have. Having pondered the question of why mediation is used so infrequently, however, and having experienced both focus group conversations and personal involvement with a fair sample of the insurance and legal defense sectors, it is my judgment, and admittedly only that, that there is probably more going on. The tone and timbre of many conversations, for example, suggest an additional source of reluctance lying underneath what the speaker was saying.

In particular, I suspect there may be a clash of inconsistent moral values between those who live daily in the world of conventional tort law, and the unspoken but undeniable moral pretensions of mediation. The litigation industry, that is, may be resisting the inroads of mediation because it senses, perhaps correctly, an ethical misfit. What an interesting possibility that is, if it is true. To examine whether such a misfit is among the causes of the curious phenomenon—the resistance or reluctance to supplement litigation with interest-based mediation—requires first asking whether there is in fact any such difference in the ethical frameworks of the two. We therefore look at the ethics of medical malpractice litigation, and the ethics of interest-based mediation in turn.

The Ethics of Torts

Before getting into the details of this, I wish to make clear exactly what I am trying to say. Tort law, as it is applied to malpractice cases, has both a substance (the fault-based rules of negligence) and a process (the adversary process that goes on in and around a court). Both substance and process have a content, and each has a job to do.

For anyone who is professionally mature, the rules of the game they play every day cannot be sensed as being arbitrary. The rules must, somehow, be "right" in the sense of being proper, or useful, or appropriate. Legal rules, both substance and procedure, purport to be based on values. Hence the values underlying the rules must also be "right," in this same sense. People who must spend their professional lives as operators of the system but whose personal values are out of sync with the values necessarily implied by the rules of the game they play, will tend to experience a dissonance that eventually drives them either to feel cynical about their profession or to leave it. I am therefore suggesting that if we can locate the values implicit in the rules of torts, we will have described some of the values held by those who operate the tort system day after day. When those values address matters of right and wrong and morality and the way in which people do or should behave toward each other, they may properly be called ethical values. The values of tort law are in that sense ethical values, and the operators of the system—defense lawyers and insurers, principally, and many plaintiffs' lawyers as well—may be said to subscribe to them, or at least to live comfortably among them.

To gain a sense of what these values are, we can begin by noting three fundamental moral antinomies that occur in negligence law, and particularly in medical malpractice. First, two equally injured patients are treated in completely different ways by the law of torts, if one was injured through a physician's negligence while the other was injured through an unavoidable event or adverse outcome. In ordinary moral discourse, the two patients are equally deserving of having society act to compensate them, or to restore them from their loss. Their conditions and their intrinsic moral claims on society for assistance are identical. But the tort system treats them differently.

Second, two equally negligent physicians will be treated in very different ways if the act of one happened to result in injury to a patient, while the identical act of the other for whatever reason did not. If catnapping while administering anesthesia is negligent and wrongful, it is a behavior that is negligent and wrongful whether harm results or not. Yet as between two equally culpable physicians, one will be punished by the tort system and one will not be, depending on the differential occurrences of other things over which, *ex hypothesis*, neither of the catnapping anesthesiologists had any control.

The third problem tort law must face is even more difficult, and may be the central problem any reasonable explanation of torts must face. Tort law imposes wildly disproportionate penalties on those who commit small errors. Absent-mindedly using a tongue depressor twice on two different people is stupid if not just careless, but it is not, in ordinary life, morally reprehensible. Likewise for accidentally misreading a dosage, or confusing two similar-looking vials. Yet in each of these cases the consequence can be catastrophic; and if that catastrophe happens, the question put to the tort system is simply which of two people should bear it—the innocently injured patient, or the negligent but morally innocent provider. If the tortfeasor was negligent even in the limited sense just described, that person must bear the economic equivalent of all of the resulting harm, however enormous and disproportionate it may be compared with the moral magnitude of the careless act. (Comparative negligence and similar doctrines do not play any significant role in medical malpractice and can be disregarded for purposes of this analysis.)

How are these moral dilemmas to be resolved? We have already dismissed both deterrence and compensation as validating explanations for the essential features of tort law. Most contemporary torts scholars who are not committed to an unremitting and purely theoretical economic approach would agree.

To explore this question, I took what an empirical researcher might disdain as the ultimate convenience sample—a handful of popular anthologies of essays on the philosophical foundations of tort law (Levmore 1993; Owen 1995; Postema 2001; Rabin 1995). Two things should be said by way of explanation, or what code-pleading lawyers would call confession and avoidance. First, this is a very preliminary exploration. My goal was only to see whether the idea of an ethical misfit had enough plausibility to be a useful working hypothesis, which a more refined investigation of contemporary torts scholarship might later confirm. I mean to use the writings of torts scholars in a very tentative, suggestive way. What matters for my present purposes is not the graceful structure of philosophical disquisitions, but the rough-and-tumble reality of life in the tort-litigation system. That life is to the philosophy of torts as what happens on a used car lot is to academic economics. In both instances the concrete case is an instantiation of some part of the theoretical or social whole; and in most instances the single real case is doing the social job ascribed to the larger system. But it doesn't necessarily feel that way, exactly, on the used car lot or in the malpractice settlement conference or trial. Eventually, if the hypothesis seems worthy of further work, the description of the ethics of torts will come from a blend of philosophy and professional sociology. At this point, the convenience sample and some anecdotal experience in litigation may suffice.

It is fair to say that there is no uniformity among torts scholars about what tort law is about. As the paradigmatic common law system, built up over the years case by unique case, it may not be about anything very coherent. It might be about lots of things, all at once. As Holmes observed, the life of the common law has not been logic, but experience. Nevertheless, three main themes describe the commonly accepted modern understanding.

The first theme, and perhaps the most traditional, is that, to misquote the now-popular bumper sticker, hurt happens. In a complex society, people's activities and foibles bump into each other and do damage. The state runs a relatively civil system by which the injured can call the injurer to account, and the rules adopt the simple notions that there is no reason for the state to act unless there has been an injury; there is no reason to move the loss from the plaintiff to the defendant unless the defendant had a duty to act in a better way and failed to do so; and there is no reason to measure the damages by anything other than the harm resulting to the victim. This, perhaps the most accessible understanding of torts, has been called a "naive moral theory" acting, so to speak, wholesale (Postema 2001). Tort law is a set of ground rules for the playing field of complex social interactions. Without disregarding it as an acceptable description, as a wholesale theory it is of limited interest to the ethical texture of daily reality within the system.

A second and equally wholesale theme is the rationalizing economics first assembled by Calabresi (1970). Torts rules imposed today channel the behavior of people tomorrow in ways that may optimize the collective welfare potential of a society marked by people, accidents, and limited resources. There is a certain moral sterility about this as well. The choice about where to allocate a disproportionate loss ignores the personhood of *this* injured patient and *this* careless but not necessarily reprehensible defendant, subsuming their interests to a larger calculation of aggregate social welfare.

The third theme is actually a collection of differing ideas driven, so it seems, by the inability of either of the first two to explain in a philosophically consistent way all of the major themes actually found in tort law, including the three antinomies—and particularly the problem of disproportionality. A quick romp through them discloses the following kinds of ideas:

Restoring the reliability of social conventions. A negligent act with resulting harm upsets the reliability of the usual rules of social behavior. When the state acts through its laws to enforce a payment in consequence, the amount or disproportionality of the payment is secondary to the fact that simply by interceding and enforcing compensation some reliability has been reassured.

Freedom and equality are primary moral values. Violating another's freedom, as by injuring them, is therefore a wrongful act. The principle of equality forbids anyone from injuring another's interests just to advance their own. Doing so by prior choice (viz., the choice not to exercise due care) is therefore morally wrongful. "Wrongful" means blameworthy, and worthy of penalty.

Life, happiness, and well-being are fragile. It's a precarious world out there, and one who puts well-being at risk is (metaphorically) Satan's own agent, whose acts are worthy of revulsion if not just reproach.

Torts are social wrongs like, though lesser than, crimes. Accordingly, they justify monetary penalties, even if not incarceration.

As Aquinas taught us (or at least the neo-Thomists among us), prudence is a cardinal virtue. Therefore imprudence is a cardinal vice.

Tort compensation effects equality of risks. By acting negligently, the tortfeasor has imposed a risk of loss on the victim. The existence of the tort system *ex ante* as well as *ex post* places the same quantum of risk and loss back on the tortfeasor, thereby restoring the justice of their interaction. This is a retributive, not a corrective morality—"You did X to me, therefore I am justified in doing X to you."

Rawls's notion of equality forbids nonreciprocal risks. We are all entitled to equal security against risks of harm. Hence A's subjecting B to an excess or nonreciprocal risk justifies a redress of the balance.[2]

And finally, tort law papers over some of its most difficult moral cracks with a linguistic sleight-of-hand—"responsible for" in the sense of physical causation becomes "responsible for" in the sense of moral desert—without always attending to how slick and enormous that equation really is.

I shall return in a moment to comment on these quick summaries as a group. What is notable at this point, however, is their "retail" character—they focus blame and blameworthiness on a single individual, the tortfeasor, finding justification for disproportionate penalties in the moral character of the *person* in the context of having done the act. (*"You* were negligent, Dr. Welby.") Even recognizing the risk of reading too much of this in, that I believe is the common theme which the academic philosophy of torts injects into the everyday ethics of those who practice within the system. There is good medical practice and there is bad medical practice; it is blameworthy to practice medicine badly and expose patients to excess risk; and the legal system exists to say whether this one doctor was good or bad in this case at that moment.

To the philosophy of the law we should add the ethics of the arena, for tort law is practiced in courts and in their shadow—a venue that, like the law itself, has attributes that distinguish it from ordinary social life. To cite just a few from a universe of many:

For one party to be right, the other party must be wrong. There will be but one outcome. The defendant was either negligent or not, and responsible for the plaintiff's loss or not. There is accordingly a "right" result. The system is here to help find it.

Responsibility for the outcome of a trial is externalized. A judge or jury hears the case and makes the decision. Neither party is responsible to do so, but rather plays the role of advocating relentlessly a single point of view, with virtually no constraint on the ability to exaggerate either the rightness of one's own position or the wrongness of the other's. This is the ethic (and the ethics) of the arena—within very wide compass, finding the "right" decision demands unalloyed self-interest and partisanship.

An adversary system affords each party's champion discretionary moral capital (Fried 1976). It is acceptable for a lawyer to cross-examine a truthful witness to make him or her appear untruthful. That is what truth's crucible demands.

Information can be secreted. Factual information may be subject to disclosure, but strategic information is protected by, inter alia, privileges between lawyer and client and privileges for the attorney's work product. Ambush and surprise are therefore still allowed, and still allowed to affect the outcome. Litigation is an athletic sport.

Unequal access to the process is tolerated. Plaintiffs whose cases cannot command large verdicts cannot have their cases adjudicated. Defendants benefit from this threshold cost of access to the arena, and the legal system permits it to exist.

Admitting again the risk of overstatement, these are among the common features of everyday life in the torts world. Taking them together with the more intrinsic rationales of the law itself, what picture do they paint of the ethics of that daily world? This is to ask, again, how would lawyers or insurance claims agents who regularly operate in that world justify what they see and what they do? What personal set of ethical ideas allows them to be comfortable in that very special place?

I make no claim that these selective and qualitative descriptions of both tort law and tort practice are a complete description of the whole. It would be understatement to confess selection bias in the sources and interpretation bias in the analysis. Again, the claim here is not the strong one that this is what tort law is about. It is rather the weaker claim, that it is a reasonable hypothesis that this is what tort law—and the ethics of tort law—are about. Taken with that recognition, I believe it is plausible to say that the ethical texture of tort law, and particularly of medical malpractice, immerses its operatives in—and therefore imbues them with—an ethical matrix that includes the following propositions:

- Responsibility for the personal consequences of the outcome of the conflict is externalized. There is an umpire whose responsibility is to manage the process justly, and a neutral agent sworn to reach a proper result. The parties are therefore freed from responsibility for the effects of their own zeal and self-interest, even if excessive. To act in that fashion is accordingly good, not bad.

- The moral calculus is zero-sum. If the patient is right, the physician was wrong. For the physician to be right, the claims of the patient must be wrong. It is a good thing, as well as a necessary thing, to seek to discover which of them is right.

- Right and wrong exist and are opposed. Though the facts may not lead with perfect clarity to one outcome or the other, the physician either satisfied or did not satisfy the standard of professional care.

- No aspect of the humanity of either party needs to be accounted for, except insofar as the rules of law may make individual characteristics relevant to the issues of fault or damages. "Truth" matters more than caring, more than learning, and more than restoration.

- Negligence is morally blameworthy when it causes harm to another. Justice may therefore be retributive as well as corrective and distributive.

This, I want to suggest, is a very comfortable system. It has crisp edges and clear borders. It validates self-interested behaviors and reactive instincts that would be questionable at best in most other arenas of moral life. It does not require much interpersonal engagement, and it characterizes the opposing party (physician and patient equally) as a person whose actions are wrongful and dangerous, justifying whatever consequences and penalties the law and the litigation process might yield. For the patient in particular, in a simpler way, it allows a sublimated satisfaction of the evolutionary need for revenge—made sweeter, perhaps, by the social and contextual inequality of patients and doctors.

The Ethics of Mediation

Mediation is by comparison less comfortable, even considering only those attributes that compare point-by-point with the articulated features of tort litigation. Recall that I am speaking now not of the settlement conference mode, which is itself a reflection of the adversarial nature of litigation, but rather of the interest-based mode. Its principal attributes include these:

- The parties—the patient and the physician and much less so their counsel—are responsible for the outcome of their encounter and therefore responsible for the actions they take within it.

- The process is in fact a personal encounter. The mediator's objective is to provide or to restore communication between the disputants. Each party is encouraged and positioned to communicate with as well as speak to the other. Each is explicitly asked to care about the consequences the event has had on the other, and to examine the event as candidly as possible.

- Individual interests and needs on both sides are equally fair game for discussion and, when possible and appropriate, for recognition and accommodation.

- Right and wrong matter less. It is not necessary in order for the patient's hurt to be validated that the physician's competence be impugned, nor vice versa.

I believe it fair to say that these are ethical propositions. They assign the wrongfulness (or not) of prior acts, and they propose a way of dealing with the person in the aftermath. The "ethics" of mediation, taken in this sense, has not been given much explicit attention in the literature. I believe, however, that interest-based mediation has been well-described by Bender and others who have labeled litigation as remote, non-integrative, and competitive (Bender 1988). The notion of responsibility that means "obligation for" in the litigation system means "responsive to" in mediation. The money into which the tort system converts nearly every other value insulates people from the need to grapple with the affective dimensions of other people. Mediation attempts self-consciously to reverse that translation. The self-interested advocacy accepted in litigation is, in interest-based mediation, supplemented if not replaced by intro-spective candor and respect for a concrete other.

There is, again, a wide diversity, even among mediators, about what media-tion is and what it seeks to accomplish. At one end, it is simply facilitated nego-tiation, reflecting in the parties' conversations not much beyond the language of rights and money that characterizes the more formal litigation process. At the other end, it has been described as nothing short of transformational. The style of post-accident early-intervention mediation I have been referring to in this discussion is closer to—but not nearly at—the latter end of the continuum. It is nevertheless not very far from one experienced mediator's summary view of it: "In mediation, people can recognize and face up to their human responsibilities, not because someone has ordered them to, but because they [are brought] to understand and comprehend someone else's reality and limitations" (Menkel-Meadow 2001, 1087).

It is interesting to note the reflection this texture of mediation has in the cur-rent debate about "care" versus "justice" in medical ethics more generally. Although that literature scarcely mentions mediation, it offers a clear view of what mediation itself can often be (Sharpe 1992; Veatch 1998). On the one hand is the "justice" model, Kantian in tradition, postulating other people as independent, abstract bearers of rights deserving of public (for us, juridical) respect. On the other hand is the "care" model, concerned with the moral qual-ities of relationships among particular people. Justice, to the philosophers of "care," is incomplete without the presence of these other virtues. It is no sur-prise that medical care in particular has attracted the attention of this philos-ophy—for "care" recognizes that, contrary to rights-based ethics, the reality of ordinary life often lies in relationships not of independence and autonomy but of dependence and inequality. Medicine is exactly such a reality. In this setting, some have argued, an ethic based on the postulation of independence and moral impartiality is simply incomplete (A. Baier 1987; Carse 1998; Carse and Nelson 1996). Rights, premised on independence and elevated over care, make up an incomplete ethical vocabulary.

A more comprehensive integration of mediation practice with these devel-oping moral theories has yet to be undertaken. Nor do I mean to suggest that mediation, to be effective, must always or even often be framed by a philosophy that subordinates what is right to what is good (Tong 1998). Nevertheless, when one watches what good mediators actually do, it is tempting to say that, if one wanted a trope for the difference, the ethics of litigation are like those of neo-Kantian liberalism (or social utilitarianism, depending on who is speaking). The ethics of interest-based mediation are closer to those of ethics-of-care feminism (Baier 1994; Clement 1996; Cates and Lauritzen 2001). If this is so, then it is not hard to understand how the difference between them can be jarring. There may simply be an ethical misfit between mediation on the one hand and the conventional legal process on the other.

Implications of the Hypothesis

To summarize the hypothesis, the operatives of the tort system—insurance claims agents, defense lawyers, and to a lesser extent plaintiffs' lawyers—live in and therefore may tend to resonate with an ethical field they find comfortable. Mediation portends a different field, a less certain one, one with rather different values about people and injury and right and wrong. It seems plausible, then, to suppose that some part of the resistance to mediation not otherwise accounted for may be explained by the discomfort some people would feel in moving from the one environment to the other.

It is of course quite a different matter to test this hypothesis; but that is for another day. Assessing its plausibility alone, however, may have been worth the candle. At a practical level, for those of us who believe that using appropriate forms of mediation in appropriate cases offers significant advantages to the world of medical malpractice, including contributions to patient safety, it is good to know what the sources of resistance are. To know them is to have a leg up in meeting them. In addition, it may be useful, in assessing how we shape (or leave unshaped) malpractice litigation itself, to understand something more about its ethical tenor, an enhancement offered by examining the hypothesis even in this preliminary way. Most important, however, if the ideas can be borne out, is our obligation to determine how much law we want to inject into the processes of assuring medical quality. Given the ethical fabric of what we have now, how much of it should there be? Should we offer, as Liang (this volume) and others have suggested, additional room to the practice of medicine to heal itself, apart from the dubious balm of the law? Ethically speaking, maybe so.

Notes

1. Information on file with the author, relating to an early-intervention program now in its third year. As of this date, the organization conducting the program wishes that the data and the company's identity not be published.

2. In *Political Liberalism*, Rawls (1993) identified reciprocity as fundamental to justice and cooperation. Although he emphasizes fair distribution of benefits, the principle can be extended to risks as well.

CHAPTER 12

On Selling "No-Fault"

DAVID M. STUDDERT

Introduction

As an alternative to medical malpractice law for compensating patients who sustain injuries from health care, "no-fault" has a tragic public relations problem. Despite three decades of research painting a cautiously optimistic view of its merits, reasonably positive experiences with no-fault schemes in health care systems abroad, and attitudes among policymakers about the existing malpractice system that fluctuate between tolerance and panic, no-fault continues to live in the policy doghouse. It remains the darling of a small group of medico-legal researchers and is without champions among the most powerful stakeholders in American health care.[1]

Is no-fault's pariah status deserved? Should it remain "championless"? This chapter addresses these questions in the context of recent developments in the field of patient safety and concludes that the answer to both questions is a resounding no. The primary failure of no-fault, and those who support it, has been translating its significant promise to the most important constituency of all—patients. Clear, careful, and broad-based articulation of the potential gains and the likely tradeoffs involved should lead health care consumers to demand, not merely tolerate, experimentation with this alternative approach to compensation.

No-Fault Compensation: Principle and Precedent

The current mechanism used to compensate patients who sustain injuries arising from medical care—the medical malpractice system—is a fault-based model of compensation. To obtain monetary payments for damages, patients must allege and prove that they suffered harm and losses due to a provider's failure to meet the standard expected in their practice community, i.e., negligence (Keeton et al. 1984). By contrast, compensation programs that do not predicate compensation on proof of provider fault are popularly called "no-fault" systems (Bovbjerg and Sloan 1998). To qualify for compensation in these schemes, claimants must still prove that they suffered an injury, and that it was caused by an accident in a specific domain, such as the workplace, road, or hospital, but it is not necessary to demonstrate that the party who caused the accident acted negligently.

Several no-fault compensation systems for medical injury exist abroad. Patients in New Zealand and several Scandinavian countries who believe they have been injured as a result of medical treatment may pursue remedies through no-fault systems in lieu of initiating medical malpractice litigation (Danzon 1994; Brahams 1988; Miller 1993). To be sure, the structures of health care financing and delivery in those countries differ from those in the United States; they have a considerably stronger public bent, and medical no-fault joins other relatively generous layers of social insurance. Nonetheless, I have previously argued that aspects of medical no-fault systems abroad could still provide useful insights for the design of models that would fit within the U.S. health care system (Studdert and Brennan 2001b).

But no-fault systems are not completely foreign to American medicine. In response to soaring malpractice liability premiums in the mid-1980s and fears about the availability of obstetrical services, the legislatures in Florida and Virginia introduced administrative no-fault schemes for compensating the families of infants who sustained severe birth-related neurological injuries (Bovbjerg, Sloan, and Rankin 1997). These "carve out" schemes were supposed to displace tort litigation for this specific class of injuries. There is growing evidence to suggest they have been only moderately successful at achieving such jurisdictional hegemony (Studdert, Fritz, and Brennan 2000; Sloan et al. 1998). Nonetheless, most evaluations of the obstetrical no-fault schemes have reached quite favorable conclusions about their overall performance, especially with respect to their administrative efficiency and the accumulation of case management expertise by the compensation authority (Bovbjerg and Sloan 1998).

For the most significant examples of no-fault compensation in operation in the U.S., however, one must look outside health care. A number of states have embedded no-fault structures into their schemes for compensating automobile injury.[2] In addition, to avoid the onset of costly and complex mass tort litigation, the federal government has utilized a no-fault framework for several specific types of harm—most notably, the Federal Black Lung Program and the National Vaccine Injury Compensation Program. But the most far-reaching and visible examples of administrative no-fault compensation today are the workers' compensation systems in operation in all states. Establishment of workers' compensation regimes throughout the United States in the 1910s and 1920s was arguably the most significant tort reform activity of the last century. It is instructive to reflect on how these regimes came to replace tort law and what their introduction meant for workers, the putative beneficiaries of the reforms.

The Workers' (Non-Faustian) Bargain

Labor historians typically portray the shift from common law remedies to workers' compensation systems as a bargain between employees and employers (Weinstein 1967; Fishback and Kantor 1998). Workers essentially forfeited their rights to pursue common law negligence claims against their employers for workplace accidents in return for remedies that were touted as speedy, cheap, and relatively simple to obtain. Employers, on the other hand, in return for being immunized against this class of lawsuits, were effectively required to pay the costs of medical care, replace a portion of lost earnings, and, in most states, provide limited benefits to the permanently impaired. Thus, the legislation established a kind of "ex ante contract" between workers and employers (Fishback and Kantor 1998).

Each side's motivations for striking this bargain, and precisely what gains they anticipated, have been subjects of extensive historical investigation (and speculation). What seems clear is that for most injured workers early last century, the road to monetary damages through litigation was long and difficult (Epstein 1982). In particular, employers invoked three common law defenses—assumption of risk, the fellow servant rule, and contributory negligence—with considerable success, barring many recoveries. Organized labor was attracted to reforms that would simplify this process and increase payment levels. Employers, for their part, sought peace with organized labor and increased certainty about future liabilities for accidents (Fishback and Kantor 1998). The latter had become quite unpredictable in a number of jurisdictions as courts began to chip away at the defenses that had previously made it so difficult for workers to win lawsuits (Weinstein 1967; Epstein 1982).

Were the anticipated benefits to workers realized? Empirical research on this question suggests a cautiously positive response, with benefits accruing in two key areas.[3] First, statistical modeling of "expected post-accident payments"—calculations that take into account both the average amount of pre-reform damages and the average probability that an injured worker would obtain them—shows that the introduction of workers' compensation regimes was associated with significant increases in the average monetary compensation to injured workers (Fishback and Kantor 1995). There is some evidence, however, that employers passed some of the costs of these higher payments back to workers, particularly nonunion workers, in the form of lower wages (Fishback and Kantor 1995; Hirsch, Macpherson, and DuMond 1997).

Second, there is some evidence of gains in worker safety. Although economic theory suggests that the removal of fault-based liability would decrease incentives to take care and increase the probability of accidents, the leading empirical work on the impact of the workers' compensation systems on injury rates in fact suggests a "powerful safety effect" (Moore and Viscusi 1989; American Law Institute 1991, 31–32). At least part of this seemingly paradoxical finding is explained by the way in which the cost of accident insurance for many large firms was able to be linked to the firms' safety records through "experience rating." The implication here is that the deterrent effect from financial risk was more potent than the one that the threat of litigation had previously generated.

There is certainly no straightforward analogy to be made between the gains enjoyed by workers in the early 1900s and the prospect of gains for patients through tort alternatives in the twenty-first century. However, reflections on the social circumstances that prevailed at the birth of workers' compensation do highlight the contingent nature of public perceptions of alternative compensation models. Today, a shift to no-fault for medical injuries is frequently portrayed as a concession to providers at the expense of patients. Proponents tend to organize their case around rebuttals of this mantra. Yet, as the workers' compensation experience teaches us, assessments of the attractiveness of any alternative compensation model must be anchored in a realistic appraisal of the status quo.

The Status Quo in Health Care

Unlike many other areas of law, a good deal of the data needed for realistic appraisal of the performance of the medical malpractice system is available. Medical malpractice is well-studied. It has been the focus of three of the largest empirical studies of injury and legal process ever conducted (Studdert, Brennan, and Thomas 2000). Unfortunately, what this and other social science research portrays is quite a bleak picture. Malpractice litigation continues to receive failing grades for progress in achieving both of its central goals: compensation and deterrence.

As a system for compensating negligently injured patients, malpractice law falls short on three fronts. First, it is a haphazard compensation mechanism. Most patients who suffer negligent injury never even gain entry into the system; for those who do, the system has shown some success in identifying and compensating worthy litigants (Vidmar 1995; Sloan and Hsieh 1990), although concerns persist about the impact of extraneous considerations on the outcomes of adjudication processes (Brennan, Sox, and Burstin 1996; Edbril and Lagasse 1999; Cheney et al. 1989). In particular, there is evidence to suggest that severity of injury predicts plaintiffs' success in obtaining compensation much more powerfully than negligence (Brennan, Sox, and Burstin 1996). Paul Weiler has likened the situation to a traffic policeman ticketing drivers who do not exceed the speed limit, while allowing many speeders to pass (Weiler, Hiatt, and Newhouse 1993, 75).

Second, the malpractice system delivers compensation inefficiently. Administrative costs consume more than 50 percent of total system costs (Kakalik and Pace 1986), compared to 20 to 30 percent in workers' compensation regimes

(Bovbjerg and Sloan 1998). Third, and most immediate to the current debate around medical injury, the negligence standard is awkwardly out of step with a patient safety movement that "treasures" *all* errors and injuries (Blumenthal 1994)—not just the subset that happen to be associated with negligent care— for the opportunity they present to learn about medical error and improve quality.

With respect to performance of its deterrence function, malpractice law appears to fare little better. Although notions of deterrence have attracted much theoretical interest among legal scholars, available evidence suggests that the deterrent effects of tort law are moderate at best (Schwartz 1994; Sloan et al. 1997). Moreover, where deterrence signals have been detected in the domain of medical malpractice, it is not obvious that their effect is to stimulate high-quality care (Dubay, Kaestner, and Waidmann 1999; Kessler and McClellan 1996).[4]

From a patient safety perspective, perhaps the most damaging feature of malpractice litigation is the adversarial foundation on which it is built. To access compensation, patients must prove liability through allegations of negligence. Through their professional culture and training, physicians tend to conflate negligence with moral turpitude, which cleaves malpractice litigation from the professional drive to provide better quality care. Moreover, because of the sensitive issue of negligence at the core of all claims, the entire process is shrouded in confidentiality, with strict legal rules governing disclosure and protection of information. Institutions are complicit in the cloak of silence, typically forgoing opportunities to learn from the problems that lawsuits can sometimes help to illuminate. These behavioral responses to malpractice law are so ingrained in medical practice that efforts to retrain physicians to better understand the opportunities that a negligence-based system provides for quality improvement are unlikely to provide the necessary breakthrough. Although some commentators continue to hold out hopes that the existing system may adapt, it is increasingly clear that alternative approaches to patient compensation must at least be considered.

No-Fault as an Instrument of Social Justice

The Compensation Objective

Whatever criteria one uses to define eligibility for compensation, a system's capacity to deliver compensation to those individuals who are eligible for it has important implications for distributive justice (Calabresi 1970). As noted above, the malpractice system breaks down badly in this regard. Defenders of the tort system have tended to focus on the adjudication process and argue that the courts (in particular) and the litigation system (in general) do reasonably well at channeling compensation to meritorious litigants who bring claims. But this frame of reference is too narrow. A wider, epidemiological perspective is critical to an evaluation of how adequately and equitably compensation is delivered. This perspective incorporates consideration not just of litigants but also of would-be litigants—individuals who suffer harm and are ostensibly eligible for compensation, but do not or cannot access remedies.

In some instances, not seeking compensation may represent a perfectly rational choice. For example, when an injured patient receives an explanation or apology from his or her provider, accepts this as reasonable redress, and then elects not to sue, this choice cannot legitimately be classified as a failure to litigate. Alternatively, some decisions not to litigate may be the result of the tort system operating efficiently; for example, in cases involving minor or temporary injury, the transaction costs associated with bringing litigation may simply render this course of action cost-ineffective for all parties involved.

However, epidemiological data strongly suggest that this rational patient decision-making explanation cannot come close to realigning the problematic relationship between medical injury and malpractice-claiming behavior (Studdert et al. 2000). Many serious injuries due to negligence never materialize as claims. Especially damning is the evidence that the burden of the compensation-access problem is not borne equally among patients. Nonclaimants are much more likely to be older and poorer (Studdert et al. 2000; Burstin et al. 1993). In other words, the sociodemographic profile of those who fail to access compensation tracks common markers of vulnerability in patient populations. Simply put, medical malpractice litigation has a classic access problem.

Can we expect a no-fault system to do any better in this regard? There are several causes for optimism. First, by definition, no-fault compensation criteria extend eligibility for compensation to a wider population (Studdert et al. 1997). This is an axiomatic result of eliminating the need to prove negligence. Critics of no-fault have argued that expanding the pool of compensable injuries in this way would result in unacceptable increases in system costs. However, there are now reasonable simulations of cost data to suggest that careful formulation of compensation criteria (requiring, for example, that the injuries be due to preventable or avoidable harms, as opposed to negligent ones) and parsimonious design of award packages (for example, replacing lost wages at a portion of pre-injury levels, as most workers' compensation systems currently do) could hold no-fault budgets to levels close to those of existing tort systems (Studdert et al. 1997; Thomas et al. 1999).

Second, the administrative nature of no-fault systems would lessen reliance on attorneys in initiating claims. This aspect of the proposed reform undoubtedly represents one if its biggest political hurdles, but it also promises, contrary to conventional wisdom, certain access gains. One explanation for the access problems faced by non- or low-income earners implicates attorneys. The theory links several well-known features of litigation dynamics: a prospective litigant's ability to claim typically hinges on an attorney's willingness to take on his or her case; the financial return accruing to plaintiffs' attorneys in tort cases is generally tethered to the size of the award through contingency fees; and lost income typically forms a significant component of malpractice awards. Hence, plaintiffs' lawyers tend to maximize their own income by choosing to act for clients with active sources of income. Because the elderly and the poor seldom fit this profile, the economic incentives that attorneys face offer one plausible explanation for the patterns of access problems observed.

Third, injured patients will not seek compensation if they do not know they have been injured. Disentangling iatrogenesis from underlying illness can be extremely difficult, particularly for patients with multiple co-morbidities. There is currently a strong push in the patient safety movement toward more active disclosure of injuries. The Joint Commission on Accreditation of Healthcare Organizations (JCAHO) recently took up this challenge by adopting a standard that promotes disclosure of medical harms as the appropriate and ethical course of action (JCAHO 2001c). However, fear of malpractice repercussions among both practitioners and institutions appears to be a major roadblock to practical progress in this area (Liang 2000e; Lamb et al. 2003). A shift to no-fault should therefore reduce barriers to disclosure that, in turn, would help injured patients better understand when opportunities for accessing compensation exist.

Fourth, and perhaps most importantly from an ethical perspective, an administrative, no-fault compensation system promises to expose the decisions and trade-offs made in determining who does and does not get compensated. No compensation model can avoid the central challenge of distributive justice—how to allocate scarce resources. No-fault merely offers a fresh way to deal with this question. Stakeholders could agree on eligible injuries and reasonable remedies in advance. For example, in order to make compensation available to a broad pool of patients, it may be necessary to impose limits on noneconomic losses and punitive damages, or to make minor injuries, say those lasting less than eight weeks, ineligible for remedies. My colleagues and I have argued previously that this approach would advance equity, predictability, and efficiency in the distribution process (Studdert, Brennan, and Thomas 2000). Some will object that it constitutes an ethically distasteful form of overt rationing. However, the tort system does not avoid such decision making; it merely obscures it. An approach that lays bare the trade-offs involved is surely preferable to the kind of implicit rationing that occurs when patients who suffer medical injury are precluded from compensation because they are unable to navigate their way to, and then through, the tort system.

The Quality Improvement Objective

Besides cost, the primary objection to no-fault compensation models has been the deleterious effect they would have on incentives for physicians to take care. Notwithstanding the questionable role of deterrence in malpractice law, it is appropriate to ask whether implementation of a no-fault model necessarily involves a retreat from deterrence objectives, as critics have traditionally charged. However weak the deterrence signals from malpractice are, runs the critics' argument, surely the relatively less punitive environment of no-fault would weaken them even further, resulting in an increase in the dangerousness of health care.

No-fault advocates have long struggled to make convincing responses to this argument (Bovbjerg and Sloan 1998). Some have turned to the possibility of improved professional oversight, better institutional efforts to monitor and maintain physician quality, and even use of the no-fault adjudication process itself to facilitate disciplinary measures in egregious cases (Abraham and Weiler 1994a). However, concerns about an unchecked medical workforce have generally not been mollified by such arguments.

The new science of patient safety, it turns out, provides the missing piece. Patient safety considerations turn old deterrence arguments on their head. Recall that the objective of deterrence is to reduce the incidence of risky or injurious behavior. By seeking to reduce the incidence of medical error, patient safety initiatives strive to achieve this goal through systematic prevention. Hospital and physician groups, as well as major payers, including large employers, appear eager to support programs that will prevent errors and the injuries they can cause. But as Brennan and I have argued elsewhere, their capacity to do so effectively is inhibited by friction with fundamental tenets of the malpractice system (Studdert and Brennan 2001a).

Thus, the relevant question for advocates of deterrence is: "By which route is the underlying goal of injury reduction best achieved?" The status quo relies on the litigation system, with its limited capacity to leverage quality improvement efforts, together with whatever patient safety advances are achievable in this relatively hostile environment. The alternative I advocate would involve replacing the litigation system with a scheme specifically tailored to achieve compensation goals, and to do so in a manner that is conducive to private and public efforts to reduce error.

Realizing the Gains: Why Can't This Work?

However strong a case empirical research and theoretical analysis may make for no-fault, tangible proof requires operational success. In U.S. health care markets, expressions of consumer preference for a no-fault model that is both workable and affordable will speak far louder than scholarship to legislators, providers, and health insurers. But several significant logistical and political obstacles continue to block states' willingness to test no-fault programs, and must be addressed before any experimentation will be possible.

First, nametags matter. Why should physicians or hospitals that negligently harm patients get special treatment in the civil litigation system, and be allowed to slip away from the accountability that legal liability imposes? In fact, the name "no-fault" is quite misleading. Sophisticated no-fault proposals recognize the need to incorporate incentives to take care, and to penalize financially institutions with poor safety records (Abraham and Weiler 1994a; Sage, Hastings, and Berenson 1994). The most compelling method for doing so involves experience rating of institutions. In much the same way as the calculus of a firm's premium in workers' compensation regimes considers trends in its accident experience, health care institutions with higher injury rates would pay more for indemnity insurance. Hence, the term "no-fault" is unhelpful and should probably be abandoned.[5]

Second, there must be ways of dealing with providers who are dangerous, incompetent, or malevolent (Gawande 2000). There is, of course, ample cause for concern about the performance of professional discipline and self-regulation today.[6] But reforms that jettison options for individual accountability through liability will draw special attention to these weaknesses. To assuage public concerns, a no-fault program will need to exhibit stronger, more active, and better-enforced disciplinary mechanisms than those that are the norm in medicine today.

Third, the fit of no-fault programs with existing health care delivery structures requires more comprehensive consideration than it has received to date. Experience rating mechanisms will not fit easily with every physician's practice. For example, for the solo practitioner who admits patients to several hospitals, the choice of a suitable enterprise to provide coverage may not be straightforward. More fundamentally, the workers' compensation experience indicates that it is not feasible for smaller firms to bear the full costs of injuries through self-insurance (Spieler 1994). Year-to-year fluctuations in injury levels at small firms lead most of them to partially or fully pool their risks. The inability of some organizations to tolerate experience-rated premiums reignites concerns about reduced safety incentives in a shift from tort to no-fault (Ruser 1991). It also raises an important question about the levelness of commercial playing fields; if, as I predict, no-fault allows institutions to outstrip their competitors in terms of their attractiveness to patients and their ability to bring about safety interventions, are physicians or organizations that are not organizationally positioned to take on no-fault unfairly disadvantaged? These are difficult operational issues that will require comprehensive analysis in the context of the markets in which they arise.

Finally, as my experience working with Brennan and Thomas in Utah and Colorado has demonstrated, any radical attempts to reform the tort system will inevitably face formidable opposition from players with strong vested interests in the status quo (Studdert, Brennan, and Thomas 2000). The future role of attorneys, courts, and malpractice insurers in a no-fault program must be carefully considered, with attention to what options will be politically dead at the outset.

Most importantly, patient engagement and input will be critical to breaking the kind of policy deadlocks that so often arise in malpractice reform debates. There are no strong unions to represent patients' interests, educate objectively, weigh alternatives, and bargain, as there were in the workers' compensation reforms of nearly a century ago. But ways must be found to accomplish some of these difficult tasks. It is, after all, an ongoing debate in which combatants with diametrically opposing positions regularly claim to be representing consumer interests above all else. The need to discover who is right and who is mistaken is more urgent than ever.

Acknowledgment

This chapter was supported in part by grant no. KO2HS11285 from the Agency for Healthcare Research and Quality.

Notes

1. Ironically, even the American Medical Association opposed no-fault when it emerged (albeit briefly) as a candidate reform during debates on the Clinton administration's health reform package (Jost 1994, 46).

2. These schemes typically assert jurisdiction over automobile injuries up to a given severity or cost threshold, beyond which injured parties are "freed" to pursue tort remedies.

3. The opportunity costs of not litigating are obviously extremely difficult to estimate, as potential gains to accident victims in the tort system have changed so much over the last eighty years. Hence, this discussion pertains primarily to gains realized in the several decades following introduction of workers' compensation.

4. The story of quality improvements in anesthesia is the most striking exception (Eichhorn et al. 1986).

5. In this sense, it is not unlike a variety of other unfortunate terms in the area of tort reform. "Tort reform," itself, is an ominous phrase. It has grown to be synonymous with a bevy of pro-defendant legislative changes enacted in response to tort crises in the 1970s and 1980s to stem the tide of litigation. "Tort crisis" is another marked term. Is the defendants' tort crisis not the plaintiffs' and the plaintiffs' attorneys' Mardi Gras?

6. Note, however, that this may be a problem with the National Practitioner Data Bank rather than with reporting per se (Baldwin et al. 1999).

CHAPTER 13

Medical Errors: Pinning the Blame versus Blaming the System

E. HAAVI MORREIM

Introduction

In the wake of several prominent national stories and organizational reports about the pervasiveness and seriousness of errors in the nation's health care system, providers are increasingly turning their attention to patient safety. Recently one major medical journal initiated a series of Quality Grand Rounds (QGR) that explores real clinical errors in considerable detail (Chassin and Becher 2002). The inaugural QGR featured a case in which two patients had similar names. Through a series of errors, the person who should have been sent for cerebral angiography was mistakenly sent for the invasive cardiac electrophysiology study that the other patient should have received. The error was discovered approximately one hour into the procedure, which was then aborted.

Two authors were invited to review the numerous individual mistakes that together created the problem; their discussion emphasizes the systemic problems that made this mix-up possible and the kinds of system-oriented improvements that could make this kind of error less likely in the future. For instance, the authors point out how people who work in health care centers are accustomed to poor communication and a lack of teamwork. Hence, when the patient said she hadn't been told she was to receive the electrophysiology study, the nurse did not consider this to be a reason to stop transporting her for the test, since it is not unusual for patients to know rather little about their care. Similarly, when a resident was surprised to see that his patient had been taken for this procedure, he assumed that the attending physician had simply ordered the test and failed to inform him about it—again highlighting the "culture of low expectations" and poor communication endemic in many medical centers. The authors then offer proposals for avoiding similar errors in the future, such as to institute standardized protocols for verifying patient identity. And they discourage punishment. "No single error caused this adverse event; there is no reason to expect that punishing individuals would reduce the likelihood of recurrence" (Chassin and Becher 2002, 831).

In this and other discussions about reducing errors and maximizing patient safety, a certain line of reasoning has become prominent—call it the "common view" or the "standard analysis." Errors are caused by systems, it is said, and rarely if ever by individual people.[1] Accordingly, if we want to prevent errors we must focus on systems rather than individuals, to discover the structures and procedures that make problems likely. That sort of investigation involves finding out how, when, and why errors occur—which requires abundant and specific information from the people actually involved in those errors. However, people are unlikely to report freely about adverse incidents and their personal roles in them unless the information and those who provide it are protected. And that protection, in turn, requires shielding those who report from those who might wish to punish them.

At this point a dilemma is alleged to arise. On the one hand, moral justice traditionally requires blame and sometimes also punishment for those who carelessly or culpably harm someone. Injured individuals are therefore entitled to receive information about the errors that befell them, and to expect compensation for errors that wrongly befell them at providers' hands, whether individual or institutional providers. On this view, if error reports could be used to promote accountability for those who are blameworthy, then injured individuals should have access to this information.

On the other hand, the greater good may require minimizing the impetus toward blame, even where someone has been careless, in order to promote reporting, improve systems, enhance health care safety and thereby harm fewer people overall. If free reporting of errors requires a blame-free atmosphere, then perhaps reports about errors should not be shared with the very patients and families who were harmed. In sum, justice for those who are injured appears to be traded off for the greater good of future patients.

The dilemma is familiar from the peer review setting where, on the one hand, plaintiffs' attorneys have complained that hospitals' peer review reports should not be concealed from injured patients who may be entitled to compensation, whereas, on the other hand, hospitals insist that quality improvement requires confidentiality in at least this setting. Many state legislatures have agreed with hospitals, providing explicit privacy protection for peer review.

In this chapter, I propose, first, that the tension between protecting those who report error and promoting justice for those who are harmed may not be nearly as sharp as it is portrayed to be. There are many ways in which safety can be promoted, and systems improved, that do not involve even potentially depriving injured patients of either information or compensation. Second, I argue that certain kinds of blame should nevertheless play a role in the management of error, and that the legal system can have a legitimate, if circumscribed, role in assigning culpability. That role should not be to punish, per se, but to ensure that those who have caused an injury through culpable careless-ness bear appropriate responsibility for compensating those they have injured. To note a caveat, I focus here on disclosures to patients and other individual persons who may be harmed, plus disclosures within institutions, as those errors are examined. A related but distinct level of disclosure, in which institu-tions such as hospitals are asked to report errors to larger organizations such as government or the Joint Commission on Accreditation of Healthcare Organiza-tions (JCAHO), will not be explored.

Chinks in the Common View of Systems Improvement

The common view holds that only with confidential, blame-free reporting can errors be explored with the detail necessary to improve systems and, in turn, make patient care safer. However, as the study of patient safety becomes increas-ingly sophisticated, it has become evident that safety improvement does not inevitably entail withholding information from injured patients and families (Kraman and Hamm 1999). Further, while exploration of actual errors undoubtedly should play a major role in enhancing safety, it may be a mistake to suppose that it is the only or even invariably the primary tool.

For instance, consider a recently reported case in which an anesthesiologist, during surgery, reached into a drawer containing two vials, sitting side by side. Both had yellow labels and yellow caps. One was a paralytic agent and the other was a reversal agent to be used later, when the paralysis was no longer needed. At the beginning of the procedure, the doctor correctly administered the para-lyzing agent, but then toward the end of the surgery he grabbed the wrong vial and, instead of using the reversal agent, administered additional paralytic. No harm was done in this instance, but in discussing the episode with colleagues, the anesthesiologist found that many of them had committed precisely the same error (Stolberg 1999). All knew of the hazard, yet no one had spoken up about it. And so the situation inviting the error—identical vials sitting side-by-side in the same drawer—continued.

The standard analysis suggests that the optimal way to learn about this hazard is to ask people to "confess," to tell about specific episodes in which they, personally, have made this error. And yet such personal admissions of mistakes are not always needed. Although catastrophic errors may indeed require just such detailed factual investigation, a viable alternative for more routine situa-tions may be to ask staff to identify error scenarios. In the case I have described, it seems unnecessary to know all the names, dates, and particulars from people who actually administered the wrong medication. Many people who work in that operating room (OR) were aware of the potential for that specific error to occur, whether or not they had personally committed it. If appropriately encouraged with administrative emphasis and suitable rewards, staff members could identify hazards like this one and they could be remedied without the need to disclose names and details from specific events. The need for contrasting colors on caps and labels, and the need for separate drawers or some other appropriate system-solution is obvious enough to all who work in that OR. Similarly, in patient mix-ups like the case described above, it does not take detailed exploration of an actual mix-up to figure out that clear, consistent systems for patient identification can reduce the chances of misidentification.

In another "confession-free" approach, institutional leaders can conduct Executive Patient Safety WalkRounds, making frequent, regular inquiries among staff and asking them to identify recent near-misses, problems that make it difficult for them to do their jobs well, solutions they have devised to make their own work safer, and other potential system-improving ideas.[2] That information can be compiled over time, examined for patterns, and put to good use in improving systems. To the extent that system problems and solutions can be identified in these nonthreatening ways, the supposed dilemma pitting justice for patients against protection for error-reporters does not arise.

In a similar vein, we might question whether the proposed protections for error-reporters will actually yield all the hoped-for information. It may be true that people are unlikely to report errors and their role in them if they fear punishment. However, the reciprocal does not necessarily follow: the absence of punishment does not necessarily mean that people will come forward with information. There are many reasons why people may be reluctant to admit their mistakes, such as ego, embarrassment, peer ostracism, loss of reputation (Sage, this volume), skepticism that their reports will actually lead to useful change, or a desire to avoid the inconvenience of explaining what happened, perhaps multiple times.[3] Hence, establishing a no-blame environment may be a necessary, but perhaps not a sufficient, condition for eliciting the kinds and amounts of information required under the standard analysis.

One can also question the premise that protecting those who report errors requires withholding information from patients and families, e.g., on the ground that they could use the information to sue. The premise actually relies on several empirical assumptions, of which three are examined here: first, that patients and families themselves are not likely to be important sources of information about errors; second, that if providers and institutions don't disclose their errors, patients and families won't know about them; and third, that if patients/families are told about an error they will sue, whereas if they are not told, they probably will not sue.

The first assumption is clearly problematic. If one believes that errors can only be fully understood by gathering detailed information about what happened, it makes little sense to exclude information that can only be provided by the people who may have witnessed the entire episode firsthand. If patients and families are to provide this vital information, they obviously cannot be kept in the dark about the fact that an error occurred.

The second and third assumptions are likewise dubious. Patients and families can learn about or at least suspect providers' errors from a number of sources, ranging from knowledgeable friends and acquaintances to health care providers they encounter in subsequent episodes of care (Hickson et al. 1992; Huycke and Huycke 1994).[4] More importantly, a number of studies suggest that patients do not sue because an error was committed, but rather because of poor relationships and poor communication with providers. Patients may sue because they feel the physician has demeaned them and their views and values, because the physician did not seem to care, or because they have no other way to find out what happened (Gilbert 1997; Beckman et al. 1994; Hickson et al. 1992; Huycke and Huycke 1994; Hickson et al. 1994; Levinson 1994; Gilbert, this volume). Indeed, evidence indicates that very few negligent adverse events lead to the filing of a tort claim, whereas, reciprocally, few claims filed are actually connected with a negligent injury.[5] Keeping patients and families in the dark thus cannot be counted on to ward off evil.

Indeed, recent evidence indicates that "extreme honesty"—telling injured parties forthrightly as soon as a significant error is discovered—may actually help to reduce rather than exacerbate the net cost of claims. In one study, a hospital tracked its claims and costs for seven years after adopting a policy in which the institution not only affirmatively informed patients and families about errors that led to serious adverse outcomes, but helped them to find representation and then offered compensation. During the year before the policy was initiated, the hospital lost more than $1.5 million in just two judgments. During the seven ensuing years, although the actual number of claims rose (per the hospital's disclosures), the hospital paid out a total of a little over $1.3 million for the entire period (Kraman and Hamm 1999). While there is no assurance that the results in this Veterans Affairs hospital will be replicated in other settings, the study at least challenges the assumption that honest disclosure is more likely to raise costs than to lower them.[6]

All this is not to deny, of course, that exploring individual errors in depth can be a crucial avenue for improving safety, or that easing the path for disclosure will play an important role. Nevertheless, as the foregoing considerations show, it would be a mistake to suppose that this is the only or invariably the most effective tool. Other approaches can and should play an important role, and, where they succeed, the alleged tension between improving safety and finding justice for injured individuals may not materialize at all.

Still, these encouraging options do not entirely remove the challenges of justice. Surely some errors are the product of an individual provider's inexcusable incompetence, laziness, or recklessness; surely some injured patients deserve recompense well beyond what an institution might offer. Yet at the same time, surely there are some kinds of information about errors that should not be laid open for eager trial lawyers to peruse with glee. Accordingly, we must still inquire what ought to be the role of civil litigation—society's mechanism for resolving disputes that citizens cannot resolve peaceably among themselves—in reconciling justice for injured individuals with improved safety for all patients.

Justice: Systems versus Persons

To identify the most appropriate role for the legal system, we need to examine three possible roles for tort litigation: (1) using it as a means to promote quality improvement, as proposed in theories of enterprise liability; (2) using the tort system as a means to compensate injured parties while avoiding blame for individuals, as embodied in no-fault approaches; and (3) reserving tort law for those instances in which one person has culpably wronged another in ways that require some sort of personal compensation from tortfeasor to victim.

Promoting Safety, Deterring Poor Quality

The principal theory for using tort litigation to promote quality is enterprise liability. In its initial formulation, enterprise liability advocated consolidating tort liability at the locus where most malpractice incidents happen, identified at that time as the hospital (Abraham and Weiler 1994a; Sage, Hastings, and Berenson 1994; Abraham and Weiler 1994b; Sage 1997; Havighurst 1997, 2000). Hospitals bearing all liability for all providers' errors, not just their own, would use their influence to enhance the quality of care delivered within their walls, while, reciprocally, physicians no longer under threat of litigation could avoid the heavy costs of malpractice insurance and might feel less impelled to resort to costly defensive medicine.

Enterprise liability as a hospital-oriented proposal did not gain much foothold, because changing economic conditions soon meant that managed care organizations (MCOs) rather than hospitals became the more important locus of control over the financing, delivery, and thereby accountability of care. However, the essential concept of "enterprise" can be translated easily enough onto MCOs. Clark Havighurst, for instance, proposes a default rule whereby "a health plan is vicariously, and exclusively, liable for medical malpractice and other torts committed by health care providers whom it procures to treat its enrollees" (Havighurst 2000, 8).[7]

Proponents of this approach note that MCOs as the main agents of cost containment may need the threat of legal liability to keep their cost-cutting from paring down quality. At the same time, MCOs are better positioned than individual physicians to be centers for information technology, disease management, investigation of errors, error-reducing system changes, and other population-oriented health care improvements. Since systemwide factors are often the root causes of adverse outcomes, MCOs should bear responsibility on that system level and, in the process, become prime movers for monitoring and improving quality of care. In addition, it might be hoped that physicians, once relieved of many concerns over individual liability, might participate more readily in quality improvement efforts.[8]

If enterprise liability has its strong points, it also has major flaws.[9] For promoting quality, tort litigation is arguably a poor tool. It requires waiting until something untoward happens, then levying a vague even if large financial slap, and hoping the defendant responds in a useful way. As Jeremy Bentham put it:

> Do you know how they make [the common law]? Just as a man makes laws for his dog. When your dog does anything you want to break him of, you wait till he does it, and then beat him for it. This is the way you make laws for your dog; and this is the way the judges make law for you and me. (Bentham 1962, 235)

In the context of health care, tort liability is hardly assured to succeed as a primary vehicle for inspiring safety and quality of care. As I have noted, the filing of tort claims usually has little connection with quality deficiencies or errors. Moreover, litigation takes years to resolve, thus deferring whatever lessons about quality a health plan might glean. After all, the bare fact that someone has sued does not entail that a bona fide quality problem exists, so plans must wait until after the courts rule to determine whether they had a legally cognizable quality deficiency (Dauer, this volume; Studdert, this volume).

Perhaps more importantly, there is no assurance that health plans would respond to tort pressures with actual improvements in quality, rather than with more perverse responses. Two sources of evidence support this last concern. Physicians exposed to tort liability do not always respond by reducing negligent errors or improving the quality of their care—very likely because lawsuits are so rarely associated with negligent care. Instead, physicians have responded with defensive medicine that multiplies diagnostic and therapeutic interventions beyond any medical justification, costing billions every year.[10] There is little reason to assume that hospitals and MCOs would do any better. Indeed, available evidence seems to indicate that provider institutions sometimes act in ways that may threaten quality. One recent study, for instance, indicates that many hospitals credential physicians who bring in large revenues even when those physicians have high rates of malpractice claims (Steinhauer and Fessenden 2001).

Analogously, MCOs' responses to their increasing economic risk may provide clues about how they might respond to increased legal risk. As MCOs assumed increasing economic risk for the care of their patient populations during the late 1980s and early 1990s, many MCOs tried to control that financial risk by exerting clinical controls that ultimately turned out to be naïve, sometimes even medically counterproductive. Some MCOs, for instance, required physicians to seek approval for every intervention over $200, sometimes requiring them to wait for long periods, only to speak with a utilization clerk lacking the education or medical sophistication to understand the question (McDonald 1996). Other MCOs were said to limit specialist referrals to just one visit, thereby introducing considerable inefficiency and discontinuity of care; or to contract with hospitals far from members' homes, potentially exacerbating an illness or injury while a patient is en route to the distant site (Gold et al. 1995; McDonald 1996; Trauner and Chesnutt 1996; Felsenthal 1996). In other cases, tightly constrained pharmaceutical formularies saved short-term drug costs, but with the longer-term consequence of raising rates of hospitalization and emergency room use, as some patients experienced greater side-effects and adherence problems with older, cheaper drugs that were not fully equivalent to their newer counterparts.[11]

Many of these tactics are fading. Standard utilization review and gatekeeping arrangements turned out to be costly and only marginally effective,[12] and restrictions on specialist referrals sometimes generated multiple visits, extensive testing, and treatment failures (Gerber and Bijlefeld 1996; Kirsner and Federman 1996; Gerbert et al. 1996). But the lesson remains: If health plans greeted increased economic risk with such quality-threatening responses, it is not clear why we should expect excellence of quality improvements in response to increased legal risk.

A further concern about enterprise liability is practical. In many parts of the country, physicians have contracts with a number of MCOs, such that no single health plan comprises a majority of that physician's practice. Individual physicians thereby face widely varying policies and procedures, including policies designed to improve safety and quality. Even if a physician wants to conform to them, it may be logistically difficult if not impossible to keep track of, let alone to comply with, so many different sets of rules. This multiplicity of contracts also means that each individual MCO has only limited influence. A physician who does not like its rules—the rules by which that MCO might try to improve quality—can simply refrain from contracting with that MCO.[13]

In sum, it is not clear why we should expect health plans to respond in prudent, clinically well-founded ways if suddenly they bear all legal liability for everyone's errors. Perhaps they would respond magnificently. But bona fide quality improvement is costly and complex. And since the majority of lawsuits arise not from poor care, but from poor relationships,[14] plans may be far more likely to respond to increased legal pressures by improving their public image and by making patients feel loved and cared for, whether or not they are getting good care.[15]

To promote quality and safety, approaches other than after-the-fact tort liability may be considerably more useful. Though the issue is beyond the scope of the present discussion, it might be noted that the use of large-scale purchasing power, exercised by large employers and purchasing pools, appears promising for targeting quality improvement.[16]

Compensating the Injured, Regardless of Blame

Consistent with the theme of forgoing blame in the best interests of improving systems, the no-fault approach would use tort for financial restoration of injury victims, regardless of whether those who erred are blameworthy. No-fault liability, like enterprise liability, is not new. But also like enterprise liability, the idea is now being reframed. Whereas the current tort system focuses on blaming individuals, a no-fault system would shift the emphasis from figuring out who is to blame to a quest to compensate people who are injured by avoidable errors, whether or not those errors resulted from negligence (Studdert and Brennan 2001a; Sage 2001; Studdert and Brennan 2001b; Studdert, this volume). This approach is compatible with enterprise liability, but differs from it in that a no-fault approach can be applied to individual providers, and need not apply exclusively to an institution.

Studdert and Brennan point to two nations that have adopted no-fault approaches with apparent success, New Zealand and Sweden (Studdert and Brennan 2001a, 2001b). Neither nation compensates literally every bad outcome of medical care, as that would be prohibitively costly. Rather, "adjustors ask whether (1) an injury resulted from treatment, (2) the treatment in question was medically justified, and (3) the outcome was unavoidable. If the answer to the first query is 'yes,' and the answer to either the second or third queries is 'no,' the claimant receives compensation" (Studdert and Brennan 2001a, 220). Additionally, only serious injuries are compensated: "New Zealand's Accident Compensation Commission scheme demands fourteen days in a hospital or twenty-eight days of significant disability. Sweden's Patient Insurance Compensation Fund demands ten days in a hospital or thirty sick days" (Studdert and Brennan 2001b, 232). Physicians, rather than being patients' adversaries, often help them to file claims. Successful claims are then paid from a preestablished benefit schedule.

Though attractive in many respects—especially for the fact that it could compensate many more of the people who are injured by their health care than the present system does—a no-fault approach has major drawbacks. In the first place, it does not remove controversy, but rather displaces it to other questions.

Instead of asking about physicians' fault, we can now quarrel about whether the outcome was genuinely an injury, as opposed to an unfortunate outcome emanating from the patient's condition; we can dispute whether the treatment was medically justified; and we can litigate about whether the outcome was genuinely avoidable.[17] Thus, it is not clear that no-fault would reduce litigation or its attendant costs.

Second, we must recognize that a no-fault system in the United States would function very differently from one virtually anywhere else in the industrialized world. In countries with universal access to health care, unlike the United States, such a compensation system typically needs only to encompass some of the nonmedical consequences of injuries, such as lost wages, since future health care costs are already covered. But in the United States, the costs of compensation include future medical care, which can be considerable. In this sense, a no-fault system would represent, not so much a response to injury, as a somewhat disjointed attempt to expand basic access to health care.

Third, the costs of compensating injured people could be far greater than the authors anticipate. If physicians are helping patients to gain compensation, we might expect to see the same kind of "gaming the system" that has become commonplace throughout U.S. medicine in the managed care era (Morreim 1991; Novack et al. 1989; Freeman et al. 1999). Thus, if the compensation system requires that the patient be in the hospital ten or fourteen days, an obliging physician can "find" reasons to keep him there; if a worker must be disabled from working for twenty-eight or thirty days in order to receive compensation, a physician can describe his condition accordingly.

Fourth, once this gaming begins to threaten the financial viability of the no-fault compensation fund, the fund's rules are likely to become increasingly narrow and stringent. In this respect, Studdert and Brennan's comparisons with workers' compensation may be more well-placed, yet considerably more negative, than they realize (Studdert and Brennan 2001a, 219, 221; 2001b, 239; Kohn, Corrigan, and Donaldson 2000, 111; Studdert, this volume). In many states, workers' compensation rules restrict patients' freedom much more tightly than even the most despised cost-containment mechanisms of managed care.

In Colorado, for instance, an injured worker is assigned to a single physician who has the power to determine whether she is injured, what treatment she needs, whether she can benefit from further treatment, and what residual disability she has at the end of treatment.[18] Workers can appeal such determinations, but only by paying fees and hiring their own experts—a daunting, costly prospect for many workers. Further, the physicians who wield this great power sometimes have conflicts of interest as they compete with each other for "business" from the employers or insurers who send them injured patients. If they are too generous in providing care or designating residual disability, those employers and insurers may send injured patients to other occupational physicians in the future. The bottom line, in many cases, is a system in which patients have considerably less freedom of choice over providers and treatments than in the most restrictive managed care systems.

By analogy, in a no-fault system if pro-patient gaming gives rise to unexpected cost increases, and if those in turn give rise to the kinds of stringent restrictions seen in some workers' compensation systems, the gains in compensation for injury will have been bought at the sobering price of substantially reduced freedom for patients.

Blaming the Culpable

The dominant remaining tort theory is an old-fashioned return to personal responsibility and to the debt that one person owes another when he has carelessly caused the latter harm. This approach would recognize that some providers are "incompetent, impaired, or corrupt and make errors repeatedly despite multiple attempts at remediation" (Becher and Chassin 2001, 71).[19]

Fault has been a cornerstone of American tort law ever since Massachusetts Chief Justice Lemuel Shaw asked, in 1850, whether Mr. Kendall was at fault when he accidentally struck Mr. Brown while separating two fighting dogs.[20] Implicit here is a concern for fairness: if someone deliberately, recklessly, or otherwise culpably caused harm to someone else, then that person, not the innocent one who is harmed, should bear the costs. Conversely, when harms simply occur as misfortunes, in the absence of any such culpable error, then the misfortune should lie where it falls because it is not fair to conscript innocent others to pay for damage they did not culpably cause.

In this sense, tort is not fundamentally about punishment (notwithstanding its acknowledged role in determining punitive damages).[21] It is about appropriate assignation of the burdens of injury. Nor should tort be confused with, or seen as a replacement for, professional discipline. Licensing boards, peer review bodies, and others that discipline physicians via restricting their privileges or revoking their licenses are primarily geared toward protecting the public at large from providers who are incompetent, impaired, or unethical. These bodies are neither designed nor empowered to make restitution to individual injured patients. While individual patients' cases may trigger such reviews, the focus of these bodies is not and should not be to exact reparations on behalf of particular patients. Rather, their job is to consider whether this provider should continue to provide services to the public and, if so, under what conditions. Such functions are entirely distinct from the need for person-to-person atonement and recompense that arises when negligence or other blameworthy conduct has harmed individual people.[22]

By the same token, tort should not be seen as a tool for continuing medical education. As noted in the discussion of enterprise liability, at best the messages of tort litigation are delayed and imprecise. Education to remedy inadequate knowledge must be far more timely and specific, and is best meted out by those who are delegated to monitor the profession.

Nor should tort be deemed a device for redistributing wealth—here, via allocating costs to whoever is best able to pay for a mishap. This discussion is not the place to address the complex issues surrounding economic theories of tort, traditionally characterized as a financial balancing in which the costs of preventing the adverse outcome are weighed against the costs of incurring it.[23] Suffice it briefly to say that such an approach can prompt significant distortions of conduct, because where providers perceive that they bear legal and financial risk simply because they may be better able to afford the costs of a mishap, they may be far more likely to undertake the kinds of defensive medicine that not only drive up costs, but can introduce iatrogenic injuries from excessive interventionism. It is a response more likely to thwart than to promote the best interests of patient safety.

Instead, the approach proposed here would limit tort liability to those instances in which the provider has not merely made a mistake, but has fallen below a standard of reasonable conduct and thereby caused the harm. It is the classic definition of tort, long accepted by courts even if in contemporary litigation it is too often submerged in alternative agendas.[24]

If fault should be the pivotal concept, culpability is traditionally defined according to reasonableness. Tort law has never demanded perfection, only reasonableness. Citizens, including physicians, are not expected to avoid all risks of harm, only unreasonable or unnecessary risks, as defined by the "reasonable and prudent person" or, in medicine, the reasonable and prudent physician (Coleman 1982, 380). Accordingly, malpractice law as applied to physicians has long accepted that not every poor outcome, not even every avoidable poor outcome or error, amounts to negligence.[25] Rather, the question is whether the physician breached the duty of reasonable care. It is a process-oriented rather than outcome-oriented standard.[26]

The literature on safety should be brought to enrich this classic definition by tempering our understanding of reasonableness. Although sometimes a lone individual truly should and could quite easily have done other than as he did, careful analyses of the kind now being brought to the study of errors will reveal in many instances that a system may have made it virtually impossible for an individual to have done what, theoretically, he should have done. A system of tort litigation that is faithful to its roots in fairness and reasonableness should begin to take these more complex realities into account as it is determined, in each case, whether someone's conduct was truly unreasonable under the circumstances. This is not to say that tortfeasors should be able blithely to blame "the system" at every turn. But it does mean that evidence regarding the broader circumstances of an error should be taken seriously. Where an institution such as a hospital has established procedures that make it very difficult for individual providers to do their jobs well, such information should serve to shift greater responsibility onto that institution and away from individual providers.

As any first-year student of torts knows, even a clear breach of the duty of care should not trigger liability unless that breach actually caused the injury. Here, too, the literature on safety should bring some important lessons. Causal analyses to determine fault after an adverse event has occurred must begin to recognize that individual conduct is often not the primary causal culprit in an adverse outcome. Accordingly, great care should be taken to determine which defendant(s) actually caused the problem—who had sufficient control, personally, to produce the outcome in question. If recent studies on error and patient safety have one important message in this respect, it is that individuals often do not have any such control. Systems often are far more causally implicated than individuals. Where that is the case, liability should lie where the control and the blame do—with the system that made the errors likely.[27] Indeed, it can be argued that tort law needs to be updated, across the board, to accommodate probabilistic and statistical concepts of causality, as distinct from the sine qua non, rather simplistic "billiard ball" concept that currently predominates (Brennan 1988; Sharpe 1999).

In this context, tort law has begun to recognize that multiple parties can share varying levels of culpability and causal responsibility. For many years, a majority of jurisdictions accepted the theory of joint-and-several liability, also known as "deep pockets" liability, in which anyone who is even slightly to blame for an untoward event can be held liable for the full cost of damages. More recently, however, many jurisdictions have cited fairness concerns in shifting to a "comparative fault" doctrine in which a defendant pays only for the portion of injury he culpably caused.[28] It is a move in the right direction, but as noted above, there is much yet to learn.

Although the foregoing description of how tort should function is based on long-standing historical foundations of tort, those philosophical foundations should not be mistaken for current practice.[29] Current practice is often a confused hodgepodge of competing tort theories, as courts zigzag their way among difficult cases and issues. Accordingly, in concluding this discussion it might make sense to sketch briefly a system into which this renovated but old-fashioned view of tort might fit.

Justice and Errors: A Best-Case Scenario

At the outset, probably the most important element in any system for addressing errors would be to ensure universal access to a reasonable level of health care for all citizens. Aside from the many other reasons to universalize access, in this context its absence creates a major distortion in error management here in the United States. As things currently stand, for someone lacking insured access to care, an adverse outcome can mean suddenly gaining access if that outcome is dubbed a compensable error; alternatively, it can mean a lifetime of medical bills and inadequate care if the event is simply deemed an unfortunate turn of events. It is already a complex enough task to determine whether an adverse event was avoidable and how it should be managed. The haunting fact that this designation can have such an enormous financial impact on the injured person casts a major shadow on the overall process of evaluating errors and fair compensation. Indeed, it is likely that this same phenomenon has been responsible for some of the distortion of classic tort principles over the years. When an infant is born with a major birth injury, for instance, parents suddenly facing a lifetime of huge medical bills they cannot pay may feel they have no alternative but to file a lawsuit even if there is no obvious culpability on anyone's part. Thus, though probably unattainable in the foreseeable future, universal access seems essential to a sound system for addressing the errors that occur during the course of care.

With or without universal access, arguably the ideal approach to compensating those injured by error should be voluntary disclosures and offers of compensation by individual and institutional providers who recognize that they have erred and caused harm. It is an approach being tried, with encouraging success, by an increasing number of medical centers (Kraman and Hamm 1999; Bayley, this volume).[30]

Such direct negotiation, perhaps sometimes facilitated by mediation, affords a host of advantages (Dauer, this volume). Providers can learn important safety information from patients and families who have been injured, and they can offer reasonable compensation to make those who are injured as whole as possible. In the process, patients and families can learn what happened—a vital form of understanding that many victims say they deeply need—and can gain some assurance that appropriate measures are being taken to avoid future recurrences of the same problem. Perhaps even more important, direct negotiation or mediation offers at least the possibility of forgiveness and interpersonal reconciliation that can be an important part of healing for both sides (Berlinger, this volume). As noted by Hilfiker (1984), a great human toll is taken on both patients and physicians when there is no opportunity for either side to seek reconciliation.

Tort should be reserved for those instances where adequate voluntary compensation is not offered, or where there is genuine dispute about whether providers erred or whether any such error caused the patient's adverse outcome. Civil litigation is, after all, society's mechanism for helping citizens to resolve disputes they cannot resolve peaceably among themselves. The focus should not be on punishment, but on ensuring that the costs of the mishap are not imposed unfairly. Through careful weighing of evidence—with appropriate recognition of system factors—the judicial process should then determine whether an injured person should be compensated by providers, or whether his unfortunate condition is just that—an unfortunate event. Courts and society should abjure the temptation to use the tort system to extract money for injured people simply because they need it and because providers have more of it. Such wealth transfers are not the business of the courts, but of the legislature. And as I have noted, the first task of legislatures should be the direct one: to create reasonable access to health care for all citizens.

Acknowledgment

The author acknowledges with gratitude the very helpful comments on earlier drafts of this chapter provided by Ed Dauer, Virginia A. Sharpe, and Brian Liang.

Notes

1. As Lucian Leape put it in summarizing the Institute of Medicine's report *To Err Is Human*: "[E]rrors are caused by faulty systems not by faulty people" (Leape 2001, 145). See also Berwick 1989; Studdert and Brennan 2001a, 2001b; Kohn, Corrigan, and Donaldson 2000; Snook 2000; Krizek 2000.

2. Personal communication, Allan Frankel, Partners Health Care System, 21 June 2002.

3. Similarly, while it may be true that institutions such as hospitals are unlikely to report errors to a central organization such as the Joint Commission on the Accreditation of Healthcare Organizations (JCAHO) if they fear such reports will lead to sanctions or lawsuits, the absence of such fears does not entail that institutions will report. As with individual persons, many other factors may deter reporting, including institutional pride, marketplace concerns, time and personnel constraints, and the like.

4. In one case, an anesthesiologist who had a drug abuse problem and had committed a lethal error in administering epidural anesthesia to a pregnant woman recounted, in a letter to a former girlfriend, that he had killed someone while under the influence of drugs. The letter happened to fall into the patient's hands (Mithoff and Jordan 2000, 7, 14).

5. "On an aggregate basis, there was one malpractice tort claim filed by patients for every 7.5 negligently inflicted injuries. Because about one in two patient claims is ultimately paid, this means that the tort litigation/insurance system paid one claim for every 15 tort incidents" (Weiler et al. 1992, 2355).

"Many more incidents of malpractice occur . . . than result in a claim for damages. Records of patients discharged from two hospitals during 1972 revealed a large number of severe injuries resulting from malpractice; of these, only one in every 15 led to malpractice claims" (Schwartz and Komesar 1978, 1286).

In commenting on a new study, Orentlicher notes: "Eighteen years after landmark California data and 8 years after equally important New York data, malpractice occurrence and malpractice claims data from Colorado and Utah in 1992 paint essentially the same picture as the earlier results: a small percentage of injured patients actually sue, and when claims are brought, a high percentage of them do not involve malpractice. In other words, the tort system includes many false-positives (patients who sue in the absence of negligence) and even more false-negatives (patients who do not sue despite having been harmed by negligence). As a result, the law often subjects the wrong physicians to legal process, it generally does not hold physicians accountable for their negligence, and it fails to ensure adequate compensation for injured patients" (Orentlicher 2000, 247, citing Studdert et al. 2000).

See also Localio et al. 1991; Brennan, Sox, and Burstin 1996; Brennan et al. 1991; Leape, Brennan, et al. 1991; Danzon 1985, 23–25; Wu 1999, 970–71.

6. It is also worth noting that at the level of institutions there is usually no necessary connection between maintaining a blame-free environment for employees such as nurses, and that institution's being willing to be responsible to its patients. In litigation, hospitals are generally regarded as being directly responsible to patients to create an environment in which safe care can be delivered. If harried, short-staffed nurses make mistakes, the hospital will be liable to the injured patient under the legal doctrine of *respondeat superior*, with individual nurses far down the list of attractive defendant-targets. Hence, there is no reason why a hospital cannot maintain a blame-free atmosphere for its employees in an effort to diminish errors and thereby ultimately its own vulnerability to liability, while still itself being directly accountable to patients.

7. Havighurst adds that under his approach MCOs would be free, in turn, to negotiate a downstream allocation of liability to providers via contract (Havighurst 2000, 8).

8. Havighurst also argues that the 1990s backlash against managed care could easily give way to heavy-handed government regulation of managed care organizations (MCOs) if tort and contract law are not seen to provide adequate remedy for quality problems. Such regulatory intrusions could squelch a wide array of potentially useful cost-saving and quality-enhancing innovations in health care delivery (Havighurst 1997, 590–91). See also Sage 1997; Havighurst 2000.

9. This discussion is presented in greater detail in Morreim 2001, 59–64.

10. One estimate pegged the cost of defensive medicine at $13.7 billion per year (Reynolds, Rizzo, and Gonzalez 1987, 2778). See also Bovbjerg 1975, 1397; Zuckerman 1984, 128.

The Office of Technology Assessment concluded that up to 8 percent of diagnostic testing is "consciously defensive," while another study proposed that liability reform might save up to $50 billion per year without compromising outcomes (Anderson 1999, 2399, citing Kessler and McClellan 1996). Anderson (1999) also argues that, aside from defensive medicine that goes beyond the standard of care, that standard itself is inflated by defensive medicine.

11. A variety of studies have come to this conclusion. See, e.g., Horn et al. 1996; Streja et al. 1999; Soumerai et al. 1994; Soumerai et al. 1991; Soumerai et al. 1993; Schroeder and Cantor 1991; Horn, Sharkey, and Phillips-Harris 1998.

12. Utilization review and gatekeeping rules tended to be based on the premise that costs overall could be reduced by directly limiting access to the highest-priced services, without first assessing the overall value of those services to health and outcomes. See, e.g., Goldfarb 1995, 546; Shapiro and Wenger 1995; Bree, Kazerooni, and Katz 1996; Feldstein, Wickizer, and Wheeler 1988; Field and Gray 1989; Rosenberg et al. 1995; Kleinman, Boyd, and Heritage 1997; Zalta 1991; Kapur et al. 2000.

13. A further, somewhat complex issue lies beyond the scope of this discussion. If MCOs are to be held fully and exclusively liable for all the health care that occurs under their aegis,

it is not clear how the standard of care should be set, including for physicians' medical services. For further discussion, see Morreim 2001, 59–64.

14. The strongest predictor of whether a physician will be sued is often the extent to which patients feel that they are being treated with honesty, respect, and personal interest. See Beckman et al. 1994, 1368–69; Hickson et al. 1992, 1362; Hickson et al. 1994, 1586; Huycke and Huycke 1994, 797; Levinson 1994, 1620; Anderson 1995, 39, 42; Kam 1995, 42, 44.

15. Aside from the empirical problems listed here, an even deeper problem with enterprise liability concerns the ways in which courts would set the standard of care to which MCOs and providers would be held accountable. See Morreim 2001, chapter 5.

16. The Pacific Business Group on Health (PBGH), for instance, is a coalition of businesses pooling their purchasing power to buy employees' health care. Recently the PBGH required its health plans to meet specified quality standards, and began to publish patient-reported data on the quality of physicians' care. See Schauffler and Rodriguez 1996; Bodenheimer and Sullivan 1998; Schauffler, Brown, and Milstein 1999; Terry 1998.

On a larger scale, the Leapfrog Group was created by executives of about 100 of the nation's largest corporations, spending $53 billion annually for the care of 31 million enrollees, "to mobilize employer purchasing power and initiate breakthrough improvements in the safety and overall value of health care to American consumers." The group includes such firms as General Electric, General Motors, Delta Air Lines, AT&T, IBM, Boeing, and Xerox. At this time, the group is encouraging members to seek care from providers who satisfy three specific criteria: use of computer entry of medical orders, particularly drug prescriptions; evidence-based hospital referral (for complex treatments, referring patients to hospitals that perform large numbers of that procedure); and critical-care–trained physicians staffing intensive care units. See, e.g., www.leapfroggroup.org.

In a similar vein, health insurers can focus on quality as they assemble their rosters of preferred providers—a move undertaken, for instance, by Blue Shield of California. See Freudenheim 2002.

17. In this connection an interesting question arises. Many treatments have a documented incidence of side-effects or complications. However, the rate of complications, e.g., from a certain surgical procedure, is at least partly a product of surgeons who fail to recognize certain anatomical features intraoperatively and thereby damage them, as when a nerve is accidentally cut. On the one hand, we might say that the cutting of such a nerve is not "avoidable," since it falls under the known incidence of that complication. On the other hand, we might say that it is avoidable because if the surgeon had been more observant and careful, it might not have been cut.

18. See, e.g., Colorado Rev. Stat. 8-43-107 ff., 8-43-301 ff., 8-43-501 ff.

19. Even the most ardent supporters of blame-free systems improvement recognize that alternative remedies must be available for the minority of individuals whose conduct is truly culpable. See, e.g., Kohn, Corrigan, and Donaldson 2000, 169: "The committee recognizes, however, that some individuals may be incompetent, impaired, uncaring, or may even have criminal intent. The public needs dependable assurance that such individuals will be dealt with effectively and prevented from harming patients. Although these represent a small proportion of health care workers, they are unlikely to be amenable to the kinds of approaches described in detail in this chapter. Registration boards and licensure discipline is appropriately reserved for those rare individuals identified by organizations as a threat to patient safety, whom organizations are already required by state law to report."

20. *Brown v. Kendall* (1850). For a historical overview of traditional tort concepts, see White 1980, 14–16; Williams 1984, 554–63; Coleman 1982, 373; Harper and James 1961; Keeton and O'Connell 1975; Wasserstrom 1961.

21. Punitive damages are a more recent addition to tort remedies, and, although media stories might lead one to believe otherwise, such damages are mainly reserved for cases that are particularly outrageous, malicious, or willful. See *BMW of North America, Inc. v. Gore* (1996); Mahoney and Littlejohn 1989.

22. In this sense, the Institute of Medicine is off the mark when it proposes that registration boards and licensure discipline are the appropriate response to providers who are "incompetent, impaired, uncaring, or may even have criminal intent" (Kohn, Corrigan, and Donaldson 2000, 169).

23. In 1947, Judge Hand brought economic concerns within the ambit of reasonableness by asking courts to weigh the seriousness and the likelihood of the harm we wish to avoid against the burdens incurred in avoiding that harm (*United States v. Carroll Towing Co.*, 1947). Note that this appeal to Hand's generally economic approach to tort law is not tantamount to embracing the more purely economic theories of tort offered by Posner and Danzon. That is, we need not resolve tort issues simply by asking who can best afford to pay for the damages. See *Gafner v. Down East Community Hosp.* (1999), rejecting the notion that liability should be placed "on the party most able to pay." See also Morreim 1987, 1758–59.

24. For example, the "Missouri Supreme Court articulated several factors that courts should consider in deciding whether to recognize a legal duty based on public policy. These factors include: (1) the social consensus that the interest is worth protecting, (2) the foreseeability of harm and the degree of certainty that the protected person suffered the injury, (3) the moral blame society attaches to the conduct" (*Millard v. Corrado*, 1999, emphasis added). Other factors the court lists are: "(4) the prevention of future harm, (5) the consideration of cost and ability to spread the risk of loss, and (6) the economic burden upon the actor and the community." Similarly, the New Jersey Supreme Court has said that "whether a duty exists is ultimately a question of fairness. The inquiry involves a weighing of the relationship of the parties, the nature of the risk and the public interest in the proposed solution" (*Reed v. Bojarski*, 2001). See also *Petrovich v. Share Health Plan* (1999): "Physicians have professional ethical, moral and legal obligations to provide appropriate medical care to their patients" (772). See also *Wickline v. State of California* (1986): Courts must look for "'foreseeability for harm to the plaintiff, the degree of certainty that the plaintiff suffered injury, the closeness of the connection between the defendant's conduct and the injury suffered, the moral blame attached to the defendant's conduct, the policy of preventing future harm, the extent of the burden to the defendant and consequences to the community of imposing a duty to exercise care with resulting liability for breach, and the availability, cost, and prevalence of insurance for the risk involved'" (emphasis added; citations omitted).

25. "'A doctor is not negligent simply because his or her efforts prove unsuccessful. The fact a doctor may have chosen a method of treatment that later proves to be unsuccessful is not negligence if the treatment chosen was an accepted treatment on the basis of the information available to the doctor at the time a choice had to be made; a doctor must, however, use reasonable care to obtain the information needed to exercise his or her professional judgment, and an unsuccessful method of treatment chosen because of a failure to use such reasonable care would be negligence'" (*Klisch v. Meritcare Medical Group, Inc.*, 1998, citing *Ouelette v. Subak*, 1986).

See also *Morlino v. Medical Center* (1998); *Brannen v. Prince* (1992); *Deyo v. Kinley* (1989); *Jones v. Chidester* (1992); *Parris v. Sands* (1993); *Riggins v. Mauriello* (1992); *Tefft v. Wilcox* (1870); *Aiello v. Muhlenberg R. Med. Ctr.* (1999); and *Nowatske v. Osterloh* (1996).

26. A number of courts have expressly recognized the need to limit duties of care, and findings of fault, on the basis of reasonableness. In *Creason v. Department of Health Services* (1998), for instance, the California Supreme Court refused to fault a state program for screening newborns, even though its chosen methods of gathering and interpreting data happened to miss a particular infant's congenital illness. In his concurring opinion, Justice Kennard pointed out that "to impose civil liability on the Department here and in any similar future case may well threaten the continuation of a generally beneficial statewide program that has screened millions of California babies for disabling congenital disorders. . . . 'Far more persons would suffer if government did not perform these functions at all than would be benefited by permitting recovery in those cases where the government is shown to have performed inadequately.' . . . The facts of this case are heartrending, and the desire to afford the stricken child and her parents some measure of comfort and financial assistance is strong. But these considerations alone cannot dictate the outcome in this case."

Analogously, in the 1995 case *Doe v. Southeastern Penn. Transp. Auth.* (SEPTA), a self-insured public employer happened to learn, in the course of its program for monitoring drug costs, that an employee had AIDS. The Third Circuit held on various grounds that the employee's privacy had not been violated. The court particularly pointed to the employer's need to track its drug costs, to ensure that drugs are provided only to those authorized to receive them, and to contain costs by requiring generic drugs wherever feasible. "Employers have a legitimate need for monitoring the costs and uses of their employee benefit program, especially employers who have fiscal responsibilities, as does SEPTA, to the public. As health care costs rise, as they have in recent years, and employers become obligated to expand employee coverage with greater protection for more illnesses and health conditions, health care costs become a major concern for employers as well as for Congress."

27. One promising development is the Supreme Court's decision, in *Daubert v. Merrell Dow Pharmaceuticals* (1993), that judges must screen empirical testimony more rigorously than previous rules of evidence required. In the case of systems-based errors, defendants should be permitted to introduce evidence of the broad causal etiology of the injury in question.

28. In *Baer v. Regents of University of California* (1998), the New Mexico court cites the Restatement (Third) of Torts (Proposed Final Draft 1998), Section 50(b)(1) and (2), which "addresses the apportionment of liability when damages can be divided by causation":

> (b) Damages can be divided by causation when there is a reasonable basis for the factfinder to determine:
> (1) that any legally culpable conduct of a party or other relevant person to which the factfinder assigns a percentage of responsibility was a legal cause of less than the entire damages for which the plaintiff has recovery and
> (2) the amount of damages separately caused by that conduct.

As noted in that court's earlier decision in *Scott v. Rizzo* (1981), by 1981 some thirty-five states had replaced old doctrines such as an all-or-none contributory negligence with comparative fault. "Regardless of the degrees of comparative fault of the parties, the principle of requiring wrongdoers to share the losses caused, at the ratio of their respective wrongdoing, more fairly distributes the burden of fault" (1241).

See also *McIntyre v. Balentine* (1992); *Harlow v. Chin* (1989); *Smith v. Department of Ins.* (1987); and *Lujan v. HealthSouth Rehabilitation Corp.* (1995).

29. This is not to say that tort as it is actually employed at the present time remains within the confines of this traditional view. As noted by Latham: "Tort law used to unambiguously be about redressing wrongs and compensating victims for harms caused wrongfully. The

development of the theory of tort law as a scheme of social insurance against the harms that flow from social activity, along with the view that the tort system is supposed to prevent harms, have undermined this original common law understanding" (Latham 2001, 177).

30. It is worth noting that the entire Veterans Affairs hospital system has embraced this approach. See Quality Interagency Coordination Task Force 2000. Such "early offers" of compensation were also cited favorably in Department of Health and Human Services 2002a, 20.

CASES CITED

Aiello v. Muhlenberg R. Med. Ctr., 733 A.2d 433, 438 (N.J. 1999)

Arana v. Koerner, 735 S.W.2d 729, 737 (Mo. App. 1987)

Atlantic Coast Line Railroad Co. v. Whitney, 56 So. 937, 938 (Fla. 1911)

Baer v. Regents of University of California, 972 P.2d 9, 13 (N.M. App. 1998)

Berlin v. Nathan, 381 N.E.2d 1367, 1371 (Ill. App. 1978)

BMW of North America, Inc. v. Gore, 116 S.Ct. 1589 (1996)

Brannen v. Prince, 421 S.E.2d 76, 80 (Ga. App. 1992)

Brown v. Foley, 218 Cal. App. 2d 430, 437 (Cal. App. 1963)

Brown v. Kendall, 60 Mass. (6 Cush.) 292 (1850)

Burgos v. Giannakakos, 1998 Conn. Super. LEXIS 3328 (Conn. Super. 1998)

Carruth v. Stoike, 80 Cal. App. 3d 215, 217 (1978)

Clark v. Gibbons, 66 Cal. 2d 399, 417–18 (1967)

Commission on Medical Discipline v. McDonnell, 467 A.2d 1072, 1075, 1079 (Md. App. 1983)

Creason v. Department of Health Services, 957 P.2d 1323 (Cal. 1998)

Daubert v. Merrell Dow Pharmaceuticals, Inc., 113 S.Ct. 2786 (1993)

Deese v. Carroll City County Hospital, 416 S.E.2d 127 (Ga. 1992)

Deyo v. Kinley, 565 A.2d 1286 (Vt. 1989)

Doe v. Southeastern Penn. Transp. Auth. (SEPTA), 72 F.3d 1133 (3rd Cir. 1995)

Elbaor v. Smith, 845 S.W.2d 240, 253 (Tex. 1992)

Foster v. Thornton, 170 So. 459 (Fla. 1936)

Friedman v. Dozorc, 312 N.W.2d 585, 602 (Mich. 1981)

Gafner v. Down East Community Hosp., 735 A.2d 969, 978 (Me. 1999)

Gannett Co. v. Kanaga, 750 A.2d 1174 (Del. 2000)

Harlow v. Chin, 545 N.E. 2d 602, 608 (Mass. 1989)

Hinson v. Clairemont Community Hospital, 218 Cal. App. 1110, 1121–22 (Cal. App. 1990)

Holtman v. Hoy, 8 N.E. 832, 833 (Ill. 1886)

Jones v. Chidester, 610 A.2d 964 (Pa. 1992)

Klisch v. Meritcare Medical Group, Inc., 134 F.3d 1356, 1360 (8th Cir. 1998)

Lujan v. HealthSouth Rehabilitation Corp., 902 P.2d 1025 (N.M. 1995)

McIntyre v. Balentine, 833 S.W. 2d 52 (Tenn. 1992)

Michael O'Neil v. Gerard Bancker, New York Medical and Physical Journal 6: 145–52 (1827)

Millard v. Corrado, 14 S.W.3d 42, 47 (Mo. App. E.D. 1999)

Morlino v. Medical Center, 706 A.2dD 721, 731 (N.J. 1998)

Morrman v. Khan, 2002 Conn. Super. LEXIS 1942 (2002)

Nowatske v. Osterloh, 543 N.W.2d 265 (Wis. 1996)

Ouelette v. Subak, 391 N.W.2d 810, 816 (Minn. 1986)

Parris v. Sands, 25 Cal. Rptr. 2d 800 (Cal. App. 2 Dist. 1993)

Petrovich v. Share Health Plan, 719 N.E.2d 756 (Ill. 1999)

Phinney v. Vinson, 605 A.2d 849 (Vt. 1992)

Potvin v. Metropolitan Life Insurance Co., 22 Cal. 4th 1060 (2000)

Raine v. Drasin, 621 S.W.2d 895, 899 (Ky. 1981)

Reed v. Bojarski, 764 A.2d 433, 443 (N.J. 2001)

Riggins v. Mauriello, 603 A.2d 827 (Del. 1992)

Scott v. Rizzo, 634 P.2d 1234, 1237 (N.M. 1981)

Sedlitsky v. Pareso, 625 A.2d 71, 73 (Pa. Super. 1993)

Senesac v. Associates in Obstetrics and Gynecology, 449 A.2d 900 (Vt. 1982)

Shuster v. South Broward Hospital District Physicians' Professional Liability Insurance Trust, 570 So. 2d 1362 (Fla. App. 1990)

Smith v. Department of Ins., 507 So.2d 1080, 1090–92 (Fla. 1987)

Tefft v. Wilcox, 6 Kan. 46 (1870)

United States v. Carroll Towing Co., 159 F.2d 169 (2d Cir. 1947)

Wickline v. State of California, 228 Cal. Rptr. 661, 670 (Cal. App. 2 Dist. 1986)

Zaretsky v. Jacobson, 126 So. 2d 757, 758 (Fla. App. 1961)

REFERENCES

Abraham, K. S., and P. C. Weiler. 1994a. Enterprise medical liability and the evolution of the American health care system. *Harvard Law Review* 108: 381–486.

———. 1994b. Enterprise medical liability and the choice of the responsible enterprise. *American Journal of Law and Medicine* 20: 29–36.

American Heritage Dictionary of the English Language. 2000. 4th ed. New York: Houghton Mifflin.

American Law Institute. 1991. Reporters' Study: *Enterprise responsibility for personal injury.* Philadelphia: American Law Institute.

American Medical Association (AMA). 1847. *Code of medical ethics.* New York: William Wood and Company.

American Medical Association (AMA), Council on Ethical and Judicial Affairs. 1997. *Code of medical ethics: Current opinions with annotations.* Chicago: AMA.

———. 1999. *Code of medical ethics: Current opinions with annotations.* Chicago: AMA.

Anbar, M. 1984. Penetrating the black box: Physical principles behind health care technology. In *The machine at the bedside,* edited by S. J. Reiser and M. Anbar, 23–45. New York: Cambridge University Press.

Anderson, E. G. 1995. Why some patients sue: Learning from a plaintiffs' lawyer. *Physician's Management* 35, no. 4: 39–45.

Anderson, R. E. 1999. Billions for defense: The pervasive nature of defensive medicine. *Archives of Internal Medicine* 159: 2399–2402.

Andrews, R., M. Biggs, M. Seidel, et al., eds. 1996. *The Columbia world of quotations.* New York: Columbia University Press. www.bartleby.com/66/.

Aristotle. 1999. *Nicomachean ethics.* Translated by Terence Irwin. Indianapolis, Ind.: Hackett Co.

Arrow, K. J. 1963. Uncertainty and the welfare economics of medical care. *American Economic Review* 53, no. 5: 941–73.

———. 1972. Social responsibility and economic efficiency. *Public Policy* 21, no. 3: 303–17.

Ashton, D., ed. 1988. *Picasso on art: A selection of views.* Cambridge, Mass.: Da Capo Press.

Associated Press. 2002a. SAS flight circles airport after traffic controller fails to show up after vacation. 26 August.

———. 2002b. Ohio atomic plant investigated over acid leaks. *New York Times,* 1 September.

Australian Safety and Quality Council. 2000. Sequential list. www.safetyand quality.org/definition/smsequential.htm (accessed 8 October 2003).

Baier, A. C. 1987. The need for more than justice. *Canadian Journal of Philosophy* supp. vol. 13: 41–56.

———. 1994. *Moral prejudices: Essays on ethics.* Cambridge, Mass.: Harvard University Press.

Baier, K. 1987. Moral and legal responsibility. In *Medical innovation and bad outcomes: Legal, social, and ethical responses,* edited by S. Toulmin, F. E. Zimring, and K. F. Schaffner, 101–29. Ann Arbor, Mich.: Health Administration Press.

Baldwin, L. M., L. G. Hart, R. E. Oshel, M. A. Fordyce, R. Cohen, and R. A. Rosenblatt. 1999. Hospital peer review and the National Practitioner Data Bank: Clinical privileges action reports. *Journal of the American Medical Association* 282: 349–55.

Barrett Browning, E. 1900. A curse for a nation. In *The complete works of Elizabeth Barrett Browning.* Volume 3. New York: Thomas Y. Crowell.

Bartholomew, L. 1999. *Medical malpractice mediation.* Physician Insurers Association of America, unpublished (on file with Edward A. Dauer).

Bates, D. W. 1996. Medication errors: How common are they and what can be done to prevent them? *Drug Safety* 15: 303–10.

Bates, D. W., D. J. Cullen, N. Laird, L. A. Peterson, et al. 1995. Incidence of adverse drug events and potential adverse drug events: Implications for prevention. *Journal of the American Medical Association* 274: 29–34.

Beauchamp, T. L., and J. Childress. 1994. *Principles of Biomedical Ethics.* 4th ed. New York: Oxford University Press.

Becher, E. E., and M. R. Chassin. 2001. Improving quality, minimizing error: Making it happen. *Health Affairs* 20, no. 3: 68–81.

Beckman, H. B., K. M. Markakis, A. L. Suchman, and R. M. Frankel. 1994. The doctor-patient relationship and malpractice: Lessons from plaintiff depositions. *Archives of Internal Medicine* 154: 1365–70.

Bedell, S. E., D. C. Deitz, D. Leeman, and T. L. Delbanco. 1991. Incidence and characteristics of preventable iatrogenic cardiac arrests. *Journal of the American Medical Association* 265: 2815–20.

Bender, L. 1988. A lawyer's primer on feminist theory and tort. *Journal of Legal Education* 38: 3–37.

Bentham, J. 1962. Truth versus Ashhurst; Or, law as it is, contrasted with what it is said to be. In *The works of Jeremy Bentham*, vol. 5, edited by J. Bowring, 231–37. New York: Russell and Russell.

Berlinger, Nancy. 2004. Avoiding cheap grace: Medical harm, patient safety, and the culture(s) of forgiveness. *Hastings Center Report* 33, no. 6: 28–36.

Berwick, D. M. 1989. Continuous improvement as an ideal in healthcare. *New England Journal of Medicine* 320: 53–56.

Black, W. C., and H. G. Welch. 1993. Advances in diagnostic imaging and over-estimations of disease prevalence and the benefits of therapy. *New England Journal of Medicine* 173: 1237–43.

Blumenthal, D. 1994. Making medical errors into "medical treasures." *Journal of the American Medical Association* 272: 1867–68.

Bodenheimer, T, and K. Sullivan. 1998. How large employers are shaping the health care marketplace (first of two parts). *New England Journal of Medicine* 338: 1003–7.

Bok, S. 1993. Impaired physicians: What should patients know? *Cambridge Quarterly of Healthcare Ethics* 2: 331–40.

Bonhoeffer, D. [1937] 2001. *Discipleship*. In *Works*, edited by G. Kelly and J. Godsey. Volume 4. Translated by B. Green and R. Krauss. Minneapolis: Fortress Press.

———. [1949] 1995. *Ethics*. Translated by N. H. Smith. New York: Simon and Schuster.

———. [1951] 1997. *Letters and Papers from Prison*. Edited by E. Bethge. Translated by R. Fuller, F. Clark, et al. New York: Simon and Schuster, 1997.

Boodman, S. G. 1996. Diagnosing medical errors: In the wake of widely publicized mistakes, doctors try to make hospitals safer. *Washington Post*, 19 November: A12.

Bosk, C. L. 1979. *Forgive and remember: Managing medical failure*. Chicago: University of Chicago Press.

———. 2000. Understanding harm. *Hastings Center Report* 30, no. 4: 44–45.

———. 2001. Seminar comments. *Promoting Patient Safety Meeting II*, Hastings Center, Garrison, N.Y., 21 and 22 June.

Bovbjerg, R. R. 1975. The medical malpractice standard of care: HMOs and customary practice. *Duke Law Journal* 1975: 1375–1414.

Bovbjerg, R. R., and F. A. Sloan. 1998. No-fault for medical injury: Theory and evidence. *University of Cincinnati Law Review* 67: 53–123.

Bovbjerg, R. R., F. A. Sloan, and P. J. Rankin. 1997. Administrative performance of no-fault compensation for medical injury. *Law and Contemporary Problems* 60, nos. 1–2: 71–113.

Brahams, D. 1988. No fault compensation Finnish style. *Lancet* 2, no. 8613: 733–36.

Brandes, S. 1997. The cremated Catholic: A tale of one dead body in two countries. Unpublished paper presented at the American Anthropological Association, Washington, D.C. (on file with Sandra M. Gilbert).

Brazeau, C. 2000. Disclosing the truth about a medical error. *American Family Physician* 62: 315.

Bree, R. L., E. A. Kazerooni, and S. J. Katz. 1996. Effect of mandatory radiology consultation on inpatient imaging use. *Journal of the American Medical Association* 276: 1595–98.

Brennan, T. A. 1988. Causal chains and statistical links: The role of scientific uncertainty in hazardous-substance litigation. *Cornell Law Review* 73, no. 3: 469–533.

———. 1990. Ethics of confidentiality: The special case of quality assurance research. *Clinical Research* 38, no. 3: 551–57.

———. 1999. Medical malpractice reform—The long view. Editorial. *Journal of Clinical Anesthesiology* 11: 265–66.

———. 2000. The Institute of Medicine Report on medical errors—Could it do harm? *New England Journal of Medicine* 342: 1123–25.

———. 2002. Luxury primary care: Market innovation or threat to access? *New England Journal of Medicine* 346: 1165–68.

Brennan, T. A., L. L. Leape, N. M. Laird, L. Hebert, A. R. Localio, A. G. Lawthers, J. P. Newhouse, P. C. Weiler, and H. H. Hiatt. 1991. Incidence of adverse events and negligence in hospitalized patients: Results of the Harvard Medical Practice Study I. *New England Journal of Medicine* 324: 370–76.

Brennan, T. A., C. M. Sox, and H. R. Burstin. 1996. Relation between negligent adverse events and the outcomes of medical malpractice litigation. *New England Journal of Medicine* 335: 1963–67.

Burke, K. 2002. Doctor says some hospitals too ready to apologise. *British Medical Journal* 324: 256.

Burstin, H. R., W. G. Johnson, S. R. Lipsitz, and T. A. Brennan. 1993. Do the poor sue more? A case-control study of malpractice claims and socioeconomic status. *Journal of the American Medical Association* 270: 1697–1701.

Calabresi, G. 1970. *The cost of accidents: A legal and economic analysis.* New Haven, Conn.: Yale University Press.

California Evidence Code. 2000. Admissibility of expressions of sympathy or benevolence. California Evidence Code §1160. St. Paul: West Publishers.

Callum, J. L., H. S. Kaplan, L. L. Merkley, P. H. Pinkerton, B. Rabin Fastman, R. A. Romans, A. S. Coovadia, and M. D. Reis. 2001. Reporting of near-miss events for transfusion medicine: Improving transfusion safety. *Transfusion* 41: 1204–11.

Campaigne, C., et al. 2000. Evidence; Particular types of evidence; Admissions and Declarations; Person making or affected by statement; Agents and employees. In *American jurisprudence*. 2d ed. Rochester, N.Y.: Lawyers Co-Operative Publishing Co.

Campbell, M. L. 1994. Breaking bad news to patients. *Journal of the American Medical Association* 271: 1052.

Carse, A. L. 1998. Impartial principle and moral context: Securing a place for the particular in ethical theory. *Journal of Medicine and Philosophy* 23, no. 2: 153–69.

Carse, A. L., and H. L. Nelson. 1996. Rehabilitating care. *Kennedy Institute of Ethics Journal* 6, no. 1: 19–35.

Cashdollar, C. D. 1976. European positivism and American unitarianism. *Church History* 45: 119–37.

———. 1978. Social implications of the doctrine of divine providence: A nineteenth century debate in American theology. *Harvard Theological Review* 71: 265–84.

Castiglioni, A. 1941. *A history of medicine*. Translated by E. B. Krumbhaar. New York: Knopf.

Cates, D. F., and P. Lauritzen. 2001. *Medicine and the ethics of care*. Washington, D.C.: Georgetown University Press.

Chamberlain, G., and A. Turnbull. 1989. The continuity of obstetrics. In *Obstetrics*, edited by G. Chamberlain and A. Turnbull. New York: Churchill Livingstone.

Charles, S. C. 1985. Sued and non-sued physicians' self-reported reactions to malpractice litigation. *American Journal of Psychiatry* 142: 437–40.

Chassin, M. R., and E. C. Becher. 2002. The wrong patient. *Annals of Internal Medicine* 136: 826–33.

Chassin, M. R., R. W. Galvin, and the National Roundtable on Health Care Quality. 1998. The urgent need to improve health care quality. *Journal of the American Medical Association* 280, no. 11: 1000–1005.

Cheney, F. W., K. Posner, R. A. Caplan, and R. J. Ward. 1989. Standard of care and anesthesia liability. *Journal of the American Medical Association* 261: 1599–1603.

Christensen, J. F., W. Levinson, and P. M. Dunn. 1992. The heart of darkness: The impact of perceived mistakes on physicians. *Journal of General Internal Medicine* 7: 424–31.

Christian Spectator. 1823. Religious doctrine of Providence vindicated. *Christian Spectator* 5: 169–75.

———. 1836. The doctrine of a particular Providence. *Christian Spectator* 8: 1–12.

Clark, C. E. 1965. Science, reason, and an angry God: The literature of an earthquake. *New England Quarterly* 13: 340–62.

Clement, G. 1996. *Care, autonomy, and justice: Feminism and the ethic of care*. Boulder, Colo.: Westview Press.

Clemments, B. 1992. Claims against primary care physicians rise. *American Medical News*, 14 September.

Code of Federal Regulations. 2000. Security and privacy: Privacy of individually identifiable health information. *Code of Federal Regulations* 45, §164.508 (d).

Cohen, J. R. 2000. Apology and organizations: Exploring an example from medical practice. *Fordham Urban Law Journal* 27: 1447–82.

Coleman, J. L. 1982. Moral theories of torts: Their scope and limits. *Law and Philosophy* 1982: 371–90.

Conrad, D., P. Milgrom, C. Whitney, D. O'Hara, and L. Fiset. 1998. The incentive effects of malpractice liability rules on dental practice behavior. *Medical Care* 36: 706–19.

Cook, R. I, D. D. Woods, and C. Miller. 1998. A tale of two stories: Contrasting views of patient safety. Report from a Workshop on Assembling the Scientific Basis for Progress on Patient Safety. Chicago: National Patient Safety Foundation. www.npsf.org/exec/front.html (accessed 29 September 2002).

Cooper, J. B., R. S. Newbower, and R. J. Kitz. 1984. An analysis of major errors and equipment failures in anesthesia management: Considerations for prevention and detection. *Anesthesiology* 60: 34–42.

Cooper-White, P. 1995. *The cry of Tamar: Violence against women and the church's response*. Minneapolis: Fortress Press.

Corrigan, J., A. Greiner, and S. Erickson, eds. 2002. *Fostering rapid advances in health care: Learning from system demonstrations*. Washington, D.C.: National Academy Press.

Council on Scientific Affairs, American Medical Association. 1993. The use of pulse oximetry during conscious sedation. *Journal of the American Medical Association* 270: 1463–68.

Crawley, L., M. Shultz, and J. Weinberg. 2000. Truth and consequences: Moving patients from the periphery to the center. Unpublished paper (on file with Sandra M. Gilbert).

Cross, F. L., ed. 1997. *The Oxford dictionary of the Christian church*. 3d ed. New York: Oxford University Press.

Cullen, D. J., A. R. Nemeskal, J. B. Cooper, A. Zaslavsky, and M. J. Dwyer. 1992. Effect of pulse oximetry, age, and ASA physical status on the frequency of patients admitted unexpectedly to a postoperative care unit. *Anesthesia and Analgesia* 74: 181–88.

Danzon, P. M. 1985. *Medical malpractice: Theory, evidence, and public policy*. Cambridge, Mass.: Harvard University Press.

———. 1994. The Swedish patient compensation system: Lessons for the United States. *Journal of Legal Medicine* 15: 199–248.

———. 2000. Liability for medical malpractice. In *Handbook of health economics*, 1339–1404. Amsterdam: Elsevier.

Danzon, P. M., M. V. Pauly, and R. S. Kington. 1990. The effects of malpractice litigation on physicians' fees and incomes. *Papers and Proceedings of the American Economics Association* 80, no. 2: 122–27.

Dauer, E. A., and D. W. Becker. 2000. Conflict management in managed care. In *Health care dispute resolution manual: Techniques for avoiding litigation*, edited by E. A. Dauer, K. K. Kovach, B. A. Liang, R. B. Mathews, D. Richardson, and P. S. Walker. Gaithersburg, Md.: Aspen Publishers.

Dauer, E. A., and L. J. Marcus. 1997. Adapting mediation to link resolution of medical malpractice disputes with health care quality improvement. *Law and Contemporary Problems* 60, no. 1: 185–218.

Dauer, E. A., L. J. Marcus, and S. M. C. Payne. 2000. Prometheus and the litigators: A mediation odyssey. *Journal of Legal Medicine* 21: 159–86.

Davidoff, F. 2002. Shame: The elephant in the room; Managing shame is important for improving health care. *British Medical Journal* 324: 623–24.

Davis, D. S. 1999. It ain't necessarily so: Clinicians, bioethics, and religious studies. In *Notes from a narrow ridge: Religion and bioethics*, edited by D. S. Davis and L. Zoloth. Hagerstown, Md.: University Publishing Group.

De Ville, K. A. 1990. *Medical malpractice in nineteenth-century America: Origins and legacy*. New York: New York University Press.

———. 1998. Medical malpractice in twentieth-century United States: The interaction of technology, law, and culture. *International Journal of Technology Assessment in Health Care* 14, no. 2: 197–211.

Deason, E. E. 2002. Predictable mediation confidentiality in the U.S. federal system. *Ohio State Journal of Dispute Resolution* 17: 239–319.

Defoe, D. 1895. *Serious reflections during the life and surprising adventures of Robinson Crusoe*. Edited by George A. Aitken. London: J. M. Dent.

Dembner, A. 2002. Doctor awarded $4M from *Globe*, cancer institute. *Boston Globe*, 13 February, B1.

Deming, W. E. 1986. *Out of the crisis*. Cambridge, Mass.: MIT Center for Applied Engineering Studies.

Demorest, B. H. 2001. When it's okay to say you're sorry. *Survey of Ophthalmology* 46, no. 2: 190–91.

Department of Health and Human Services. 2002a. Confronting the new health care crisis: Improving health care quality and lowering costs by fixing our medical liability system. 24 July. Available at http://aspe.hhs.gov/daltcp /reports/litrefm.pdf (accessed 29 September 2002).

———. 2002b. Standards for privacy of Individual Identifiable Health Information: Final Rule *Federal Register* 67, no. 157 (14 August): 53182–201. Available at www.hhs.gov/ ocr/hipaa/privrulepd.pdf (accessed 17 August 2002).

Donchin, Y., D. Gopher, M. Olin, Y. Badihi, M. Biesky, C. L. Sprung, R. Pizov, and S. Cotev. 1995. A look into the nature and causes of human errors in the intensive care unit. *Critical Care Medicine* 23: 294–300.

Dowling, G. 2001. *Creating corporate reputations: Identity, image and performance.* Oxford: Oxford University Press.

Drayer, J. 1999. The culture of secrecy. Salon.com, 2 December. www.salon .com/health/feature/1999/12/02/meaculpa/print.html (accessed 29 September 2002).

Dubay, L., R. Kaestner, and T. Waidmann. 1999. The impact of malpractice fears on cesarean section rates. *Journal of Health Economics* 18, no. 4: 491–522.

Dujarier, M. 1979. *A history of the catechumenate: The first six centuries.* Translated by E. J. Haasl. New York: Sadlier.

Dwyer, S. 1999. Reconciliation for realists. *Report of the Institute of Philosophy and Public Policy*, spring/summer: 18–23.

Edbril, S. D., and R. S. Lagasse. 1999. The relationship between malpractice litigation and human errors. *Anesthesiology* 91: 848–55.

Editor's Choice. 2002. Informed compliance. *British Medical Journal* 324: 648.

Eichhorn, J. H., J. B. Cooper, D. J. Cullen, W. R. Maier, J. H. Philip, and R. G. Seeman. 1986. Standards for patient monitoring during anesthesia at Harvard Medical School. *Journal of the American Medical Association* 256, no. 8: 1017–20.

Elliott, C. 1999. *A philosophical disease: Bioethics, culture, and identity.* New York and London: Routledge.

Elwell, J. 1860. *A medico-legal treatise on medical malpractice and medical evidence.* New York: John S. Voorhis.

English, P. C. 1980. *Shock, physiological surgery, and George Washington Crile: Medical innovation in the Progressive Era.* Westport, Conn.: Greenwood Press.

Epstein, R. 1982. The historical origins and economic structure of workers' compensation law. *Georgia Law Review* 16: 775.

Fadiman, A. 1997. *The spirit catches you and you fall down: A Hmong child, her American doctors, and the collision of two cultures.* New York: Farrar, Straus and Giroux.

Feldstein, P. J., T. M. Wickizer, and J. R. C. Wheeler. 1988. Private cost containment: The effects of utilization review programs on health care use and expenditures. *New England Journal of Medicine* 318: 1310–14.

Felsenthal, E. 1996. When HMOs say no to health coverage, more patients are taking them to court. *Wall Street Journal*, 5 May: B-1, B-6.

Field, M. J., and B. H. Gray. 1989. Should we regulate "utilization-management"? *Health Affairs* 8, no. 4: 103–12.

Fishback, P. V., and S. E. Kantor. 1995. Did workers pay for the passage of workers' compensation laws? *Quarterly Journal of Economics* 110, no. 3: 713–42.

———. 1998. The adoption of workers' compensation in the United States, 1900–1930. *Journal of Law and Economics* 16; 305–33.

Fombrun, C. J. 1996. *Reputation: Realizing value from the corporate image.* Boston: Harvard Business School Press.

Fonseka, C. 1996. To err was fatal. *British Medical Journal* 313: 1640–42.

Fortune, M. M., and J. Poling. 1995. Calling to accountability: The church's response to abusers. In *Violence against women and children: A Christian theological sourcebook*, edited by C. J. Adams and M. M. Fortune. New York: Continuum.

Fourier, Charles. 1829. *Le nouveau monde industriel et sociétaire, Ou invention du procédé d'industrie attrayante et naturelle distribuée en séries passionnées.* Paris: Bossange père.

Foushee, H. C., and R. L. Helmreich. 1988. Group interaction and flight crew performance. In *Human factors in aviation*, edited by E. L. Wiener and D. C. Nagel. San Diego: Academic Press.

Freedman, D. N., ed. 1992. *The Anchor Bible dictionary.* Volume 6. New York: Doubleday.

Freedman, S. R., and R. D. Enright. 1996. Forgiveness as an intervention goal with incest survivors. *Journal of Consulting and Clinical Psychology* 64, no. 5: 983–92.

Freeman, V. G., S. S. Rathore, K. P. Weinfurt, K. A. Schulman, and D. P. Sulmasy. 1999. Lying for patients: Physician deception of third-party payers. *Archives of Internal Medicine* 159: 2263–70.

Freudenheim, M. 2002. Quality goals in incentives for hospitals. *New York Times*, 26 June. www.nytimes.com/2002/06/26/business/26CARE.html (accessed 26 June 2002).

Fried, C. 1976. The lawyer as friend. *Yale Law Journal* 85: 1060–89.

Frisch, P. R., S. C. Charles, R. D. Gibbons, and D. Hedeker. 1995. Role of previous claims and specialty on the effectiveness of risk-management education for office-based physicians. *Western Journal of Medicine* 163: 346–50.

Gaba, D. M. 1989. Human errors in anesthetic mishaps. *International Anesthesiology Clinics* 27: 137–47.

Gaba, D. M., and A. DeAnda. 1988. A comprehensive anesthesia simulation environment: Recreating the operating room for research and training. *Anesthesiology* 69: 387–94.

Gawande, A. 1999. When doctors make mistakes. *The New Yorker*, 1 February: 40–55.

———. 2000. When good doctors go bad. *The New Yorker*, 7 August 7: 60–69.

Gerber, P. C., and M. Bijlefeld. 1996. Watch out for these malpractice hot spots. *Physician's Management* 36, no. 5: 37–50.

Gerbert, B., T. Maurer, T. Berger, S. Pantilat, S. J. McPhee, M. Wolff, A. Bronstone, and N. Caspers. 1996. Primary care physicians as gatekeepers in managed care: Primary care physicians' and dermatologists' skills at secondary prevention of skin cancer. *Archives of Dermatology* 132: 1030–38.

Gilbert, S. M. [1995a] 1997. *Wrongful death: A medical tragedy.* New York: W. W. Norton.

————. 1995b. *Ghost volcano: Poems.* New York: W. W. Norton.

Gilmore, G. 1974. *The death of contract.* Columbus: Ohio State University Press.

Gilson, R. J., and R. Kraakman. 1984. The mechanisms of market efficiency. *Virginia Law Review* 70: 549–644.

Glaser, J. 1994. *Three realms of ethics.* Kansas City, Mo.: Sheed and Ward.

Gold, M. R., R. Hurley, T. Lake, T. Ensor, and R. Berenson. 1995. A national survey of the arrangements managed-care plans make with physicians. *New England Journal of Medicine* 333: 1678–83.

Goldfarb, S. 1995. Physicians in control of the capitated dollar: Do unto others... *Annals of Internal Medicine* 123: 546–47.

Gorovitz, S., and A. MacIntyre. 1976. Toward a theory of medical fallibility. *Journal of Medicine and Philosophy* 1: 51–71.

Gosfield, A., et al. 1992. Report of the Institutional Transformations Panel. In *Health care delivery and tort: Systems on a collision course?*, edited by E. Rolph. Santa Monica, Calif.: Rand.

Grady, M. F. 1988. Why are people negligent? Technology, nondurable precautions, and the medical malpractice explosion. *Northwestern Law Review* 82: 293–334.

Graveson, R. H. 1941. The movement from status to contract. *Modern Law Review* 4: 261–67.

Gray, J. G., Jr. 1986. *Managing the corporate image: The key to public trust.* Westport, Conn.: Quorum Books.

Gribbin, W. 1972. Divine providence or miasma? The yellow fever epidemic of 1822. *New York History* 53: 283–98.

Grimes, R. L. 1996. Ritual criticism and infelicitous performances. In *Readings in Ritual Studies*, edited by R. L. Grimes. Upper Saddle River, N.J.: Prentice Hall.

Guinther, J. 1978. *The malpractitioners.* New York: Doubleday.

Habeeb, W. R. 1960. Malpractice: Propriety and effect of instruction or argument directing attention to injury to defendant's professional reputation or standing. *American Law Review* 2d ed. 74: 662.

Hall, M. A., Elizabeth Dugan, B. Zheng, and A. K. Mishra. 2001. Trust in physicians and medical institutions: What is it, can it be measured, and does it matter? *Milbank Quarterly* 79, no. 4: 613–33.

Hamilton, F. H. 1886. Suits for malpractice in surgery: Their cause and their remedies. In *Papers read before the Medico-Legal Society of New York.* 3d ser. New York: Medico-Legal Society of New York.

Hampton, J. 1988. Forgiveness, resentment, and hatred. In *Forgiveness and mercy*, edited by J. G. Murphy and J. Hampton. Cambridge: Cambridge University Press.

Hanawalt, B. A. 1998. *Of good and ill repute: Gender and social control in medieval England.* New York: Oxford University Press.

Harper, F. V., and F. James. 1961. Accidents, fault, and social insurance. In *Freedom and responsibility*, edited by H. Morris, 267–73. Stanford: Stanford University Press.

Hatchett, M. J. 1980. *Commentary on the American prayer book.* New York: Seabury Press.

Havighurst, C. C. 1997. Making health plans accountable for the quality of care. *Georgia Law Review* 31, no. 2: 587–647.

———. 2000. Vicarious liability: Relocating responsibility for the quality of medical care. *American Journal of Law and Medicine* 26: 7–29.

Hebert, P. C., A. V. Levin, and G. Robertson. 2001. Bioethics for clinicians: 23. Disclosure of medical error. *Canadian Medical Association Journal* 164, no. 4: 509–13.

Hiatt, H. H., B. A. Barnes, T. A. Brennan, N. M. Laird, A. G. Lawthers, L. L. Leape, A. R. Localio, J. P. Newhouse, L. M. Peterson, and K. E. Thorpe. 1989. Special report: A study of medical injury and medical malpractice. *New England Journal of Medicine* 321: 480–84.

Hiatt, H. H., et al. 1990. *Harvard Medical Practice Study: Patients, doctors, and lawyers: Medical injury, malpractice litigation, and patient compensation in New York.* Cambridge, Mass.: Harvard University Press.

Hickson, G., E. W. Clayton, P. B. Githens, and F. A. Sloan. 1992. Factors that prompted families to file medical malpractice claims following perinatal injuries. *Journal of the American Medical Association* 267: 1359–63.

Hickson, G. B., E. W. Clayton, S. S. Entman, C. S. Miller, P. B. Githens, K. Whetten-Goldstein, and F. A. Sloan. 1994. Obstetricians' prior malpractice experience and patients' satisfaction with care. *Journal of the American Medical Association* 272: 1583–87.

Hickson, G. B., C. F. Federspiel, J. W. Pichert, C. S. Miller, J. Gauld-Jaeger, and P. Bost. 2002. Patient complaints and malpractice risk. *Journal of the American Medical Association* 287, no. 22: 2951–57.

Hilfiker, D. 1984. Facing our mistakes. *New England Journal of Medicine* 310: 118–222.

———. 2001. From the victim's point of view. *Journal of Medical Humanities* 22, no. 4: 255–63.

Hingorani, M., T. Wong, and G. Vafidis. 1999. Patients' and doctors' attitudes to amount of information given after unintended injury during treatment: Cross sectional, questionnaire survey. *British Medical Journal* 318: 640–41.

Hippocrates. 1923–1988. Epidemics I. In *Hippocrates*, translated by W. H. S. Jones. Loeb Classical Library. Cambridge, Mass.: Harvard University Press.

Hirsch, B. T., D. A. Macpherson, and J. M. DuMond. 1997. Workers' compensation recipiency in union and nonunion workplaces. *Industrial and Labor Relations Review* 50, no. 2: 213–36.

Hofer, T. P., and R. A. Hayward. 2002. Are bad outcomes from questionable clinical decisions preventable medical errors? A case of cascade iatrogenesis. *Annals of Internal Medicine* 137: 227–333.

Hofer, T. P., E. A. Kerr, and R. A. Hayward. 2000. What is an error? *Effective Clinical Practice* 6: 261–69.

Hooker, W. 1849. *Physician and patient; Or a practical view of the mutual duties, relations, and interests of the medical profession and the community*. New York: Baker and Scribner.

Horn, S. D., P. D. Sharkey, and C. Phillips-Harris. 1998. Formulary limitations and the elderly: Results from the managed care outcomes project. *American Journal of Managed Care* 4: 1105–13.

Horn, S. D., P. D. Sharkey, D. M. Tracy, C. E. Horn, B. James, and F. Goodwin. 1996. Intended and unintended consequences of HMO cost-containment strategies: Results from the managed care outcomes project. *American Journal of Managed Care* 2: 253–64.

Howell, J. D. 1995. *Technology in the hospital: Transforming patient care in the early twentieth century*. Baltimore: Johns Hopkins University Press.

Hunter, V. J. 1994. *Policing Athens: Social control in the Attic lawsuits, 420–320 B.C.* Princeton, N.J.: Princeton University Press.

Hupert, N., A. G. Lawthers, T. A. Brennan, and L. M. Peterson. 1996. Processing the tort deterrent signal: A qualitative study. *Social Science and Medicine* 43, no. 1: 1–11.

Huycke, L., and M. Huycke. 1994. Characteristics of potential plaintiffs in malpractice litigation. *Annals of Internal Medicine* 120: 792–98.

Hyman, D. M. 1998. Lies, damned lies, and narrative. *Indiana Law Journal* 73: 797–865.

iHealthBeat. 2002. Policy: Kennedy, House dems seek to amend HIPPA privacy rule. 14 August. Available at www.ihealthbeat.org/members/basecontent.asp?oldcoll=&program=1&contentid=23619&collectionid=100 (accessed 4 November 2002).

Johns Hopkins Medical Institutions. 2001. *Johns Hopkins Hospital interdisciplinary clinical practice manual*. Baltimore, Md.: Johns Hopkins Medical Institutions.

Joint Commission on Accreditation of Healthcare Organizations (JCAHO). 2001a. *Revisions to Joint Commission standards in support of patient safety and medical/health care error reduction*. Available at www.dcha.org/JCAHO Revision.htm (accessed 20 January 2004).

————. 2001b. *Facts about the sentinel event policy.* Available at www.jcaho.org/sentinel/se_pp.htm (accessed 1 September 2001).

————. 2001c. Standard RI 1.2.2. Available at www.jcaho.org/standards_frm.html (accessed 14 September 2001).

————. 2002. *2002 Comprehensive accreditation manual for hospitals: The official handbook.* Oakbrook Terrace, Ill.: JCAHO.

Jones, K., and P. H. Rubin. 2001. Effects of harmful environmental events on the reputations of firms. *Advances in Financial Economics* 6: 161–82.

Jones, L. G. 1994. The cost of forgiveness: Grace, Christian community, and the politics of worldly discipleship. In *Theology and the practice of responsibility: Essays on Dietrich Bonhoeffer*, edited by W. W. Floyd and C. Marsh. Valley Forge, Pa.: Trinity Press International.

Jost, K. 1994. Fault-free malpractice. *American Bar Association Journal* 80: 46–49.

Juran, J. M., and F. M. Gryna, eds. 1988. *Juran's quality control handbook.* 4th ed. New York: McGraw-Hill.

Kahan, D. M. 1996. What do alternative sanctions mean? *University of Chicago Law Review* 63: 591–653.

Kakalik, J. S., and N. M. Pace. 1986. *Costs and compensation paid in tort litigation.* Santa Monica, Calif.: Rand (R-3391-ICJ).

Kam, K. 1995. Why doctors get sued. *Hippocrates* 9, no. 10: 42–53.

Kaminer, D. A., D. J. Stein, I. Mbanga, and N. Zungu-Dirwayi. 2001. The Truth and Reconciliation Commission in South Africa: Relation to psychiatric status and forgiveness among survivors of human rights abuses. *British Journal of Psychology* 178: 373–77.

Kapur, K., G. F. Joyce, K. A. van Vorst, and J. J. Escarce. 2000. Expenditures for physician services under alternative models of managed care. *Medical Care Research and Review* 57: 161–81.

Keeton, R. E., and J. O'Connell. 1975. Why shift loss? In *Philosophy of law*, edited by J. Feinberg and H. Gross, 389–92. Encino, Calif.: Dickenson Publishing Company, Inc.

Keeton, W. P., D. B. Dobbs, R. E. Keeton, and D. G. Owens. 1984. *Prosser and Keeton on the law of torts.* 5th ed. St. Paul, Minn: West Publishing Co.

Kern, K. A. 1992. Risk management goals involving injury to the common bile ducts during laparoscopic cholecystectomy. *American Journal of Surgery* 163: 551–52.

————. 1994. A medicolegal analysis of the bile duct injury during open cholecystectomy and abdominal surgery. *American Journal of Surgery* 168: 17–20.

Kessler, D., and M. McClellan. 1996. Do doctors practice defensive medicine? *American Journal of Economics* 111, no. 2: 353–90.

————. 1997. The effects of malpractice pressure and liability reforms on physicians' perceptions of medical care. *Law and Contemporary Problems* 60, no. 1: 81–106.

————. 2002. Malpractice law and health care reform: Optimal liability in an era of managed care. *Journal of Public Economics* 84: 175–97.

Kett, J. F. 1977. *Rites of passage: Adolescence in America, 1790 to the present*. New York: Basic Books.

Kirsner, R. S., and D. B. Federman. 1996. Lack of correlation between internists' ability in dermatology and their patterns of treating patients with skin disease. *Archives of Dermatology* 132: 1043–46.

Kleinman, A. 1995. *Writing at the margin: Discourse between anthropology and medicine*. Berkeley: University of California Press.

Kleinman, L. C., E. A. Boyd, and J. C. Heritage. 1997. Adherence to prescribed explicit criteria during utilization review: An analysis of communications between attending and reviewing physicians. *Journal of the American Medical Association* 278: 497–501.

Kohn, L. T., J. M. Corrigan, and M. S. Donaldson, eds. 2000. *To err is human: Building a safer health system*. Washington, D.C.: National Academy Press.

Kolata, G. 2000. Web research transforms visit to the doctor. *New York Times*, 6 March: A1.

Korn, P. 2000. When doctors make mistakes. *Ladies Home Journal*, March: 100–105, 236.

Kraman, S. S., and G. Hamm. 1999. Risk management: Extreme honesty may be the best policy. *Annals of Internal Medicine* 131: 963–67.

Krizek, T. J. 2000. Surgical error: Ethical issues of adverse events. *Archives of Surgery* 135: 1359–66.

Lamb, R. M., D. M. Studdert, R. M. J. Bohmer, D. M. Berwick, and T. A. Brennan. 2003. Hospital disclosure practices: Results of a national survey. *Health Affairs* 2: 73–83.

Latham, S. R. 2001. System and responsibility: Three readings of the IOM report on medical error. *American Journal of Law and Medicine* 27: 163–79.

Lauber, J. K., and P. J. Kayten. 1990. Sleepiness, circadian dysrhythmia, and fatigue in transportation system accidents. *Sleep* 11: 503–12.

Leape, L. L. 1993. Preventing medical injury. *Quality Review Bulletin* 81: 144–49.

————. 1994. Error in medicine. *Journal of the American Medical Association* 272: 1851–57.

————. 1999. Why should we report adverse events? *Journal of the Evaluation of Clinical Practice* 5: 1–4.

————. 2001. Forward: Preventing medical accidents: Is "systems analysis" the answer? *American Journal of Law and Medicine* 27: 145–48.

Leape, L. L., D. W. Bates, D. J. Cullen, J. Cooper, H. J. Demonaco, T. Gallivan, R. Hallisey, J. Ives, N. Laird, G. Laffel, et al. for the ADE Prevention Study

Group. 1995. Systems analysis of adverse drug events. *Journal of the American Medical Association* 274: 35–43.

Leape, L. L., T. A. Brennan, N. Laird, A. G. Lawthers, A. R. Localio, B. A. Barnes, L. Hebert, J. P. Newhouse, P. C. Weiler, and H. Hiatt. 1991. The nature of adverse events in hospitalized patients: Results of the Harvard Medical Practice Study II. *New England Journal of Medicine* 324: 377–84.

Leape, L. L., D. S. Swankin, and M. R. Yessian. 1999. A conversation on medical injury. *Public Health Reports* 114: 302–17.

Leape, L. L., D. D. Woods, M. J. Hatlie, K. W. Kizer, S. A. Schroeder, and G. D. Lundberg. 1998. Promoting patient safety by preventing medical error. *Journal of the American Medical Association* 280: 1444–47.

Leary, F., Jr., and R. S. Hudson. 1985. Unfair credit reporting and wrongful dishonor: Two wrongs made from the same right. *Delaware Journal of Corporate Law* 10: 1–43.

Legorreta, A. P., J. H. Silber, G. N. Constantino, R. W. Kobylinski, and S. L. Zatz. 1993. Increased cholecystectomy rate after the introduction of laparoscopic cholecystectomy. *Journal of the American Medical Association* 270: 1429–32.

Lester, G. W., and S. G. Smith. 1993. Listening and talking to patients: A remedy for malpractice suits? *Western Journal of Medicine* 158: 268–72.

Levinson, W. 1994. Physician-patient communication: A key to malpractice prevention. *Journal of the American Medical Association* 272: 1619–20.

Levinson, W., D. L. Roter, J. P. Mullooly, V. T. Dull, and R. M. Frankel. 1997. Physician-patient communication: The relationship with malpractice claims among primary care physicians and surgeons. *Journal of the American Medical Association* 277: 553–59.

Levmore, S. 1993. *Foundations of tort law.* New York: Oxford University Press.

Liang, B. A. 1997a. An overview and analysis of challenges to medical exclusive contracts. *Journal of Legal Medicine* 18: 1–45.

———. 1997b. Deselection under *Harper v. Healthsource*: A blow for maintaining patient-physician relationships in the era of managed care? *Notre Dame Law Review* 72: 799–861.

———. 1997c. Assessing medical malpractice jury verdicts: A case study of an anesthesiology department. *Cornell Journal of Law and Public Policy* 7: 121–64.

———. 1998. Patient injury incentives in law. *Yale Law and Policy Review* 17: 1–93.

———. 1999. Error in medicine: Legal impediments to U.S. reform. *Journal of Health Politics, Policy, and Law* 24: 28–57.

———. 2000a. ADR in health care: An overview of the ADR landscape. In *Health care dispute resolution manual: Techniques for avoiding litigation*, edited by E. A. Dauer, K. K. Kovach, B. A. Liang, R. B. Mathews, D. Richardson, and P. S. Walker. Gaithersburg, Md.: Aspen Publishers.

————. 2000b. Comment: Other people's money: A reply to the Joint Commission. *Journal of Health Law* 33: 657–64.

————. 2000c. Concepts of law. In B. A. Liang, *Health law and policy*. Boston: Butterworth-Heinemann.

————. 2000d. Promoting patient safety through reducing medical error: A paradigm of cooperation between patient, physician, and attorney. *SIU Law Journal* 24: 541–68.

————. 2000e. Risks of reporting sentinel events. *Health Affairs* 19, no. 5: 112–20.

————. 2000f. The effectiveness of physician risk management: Potential problems for patient safety. *Risk Decision Policy* 5: 183–202.

————. 2001a. The adverse event of unaddressed medical error: Identifying and filling the holes in the health-care and legal systems. *Journal of Law, Medicine, and Ethics* 29, nos. 3 and 4: 346–68.

————. 2001b. The perils of law and medicine: Avoiding litigation to promote patient safety. *Preventive Law Reporter* 19, no. 4: 10–12.

————. 2002a. A system of medical error disclosure. *Quality and Safety in Health Care* 11, no. 1: 64–68.

————. 2002b. Lies on the lips: Dying declarations, Western legal bias, and unreliability as reported speech. *Law/Text/Culture* 5, no. 2: 113–56.

Liang, B. A., and S. D. Small. 2003. Communicating about care: Addressing federal-state issues in peer review and mediation to promote patient safety. *Houston Journal of Health Law and Policy* 3: 219–64.

Liang, B. A., and K. Storti. 2000. Creating problems as part of the "solution": The JCAHO sentinel event policy, legal issues, and patient safety. *Journal of Health Law* 33: 263–85.

Localio, A. R., A. G. Lawthers, T. A. Brennan, N. M. Laird, L. E. Hebert, L. M. Peterson, J. P. Newhouse, P. C. Weiler, and H. H. Hiatt. 1991. Relation between malpractice claims and adverse events due to negligence. Results of the Harvard Medical Practice Study III. *New England Journal of Medicine* 325, no. 4: 245–51.

Lovern, B. 2001. JCAHO's new tell-all; Standards require that patients know about below-par care. *Modern Healthcare* 1 January: 2.

Mahoney, R. J., and S. E. Littlejohn. 1989. Innovation on trial: Punitive damages versus new products. *Science* 246: 1395–99.

Maine, H. 1884. *Ancient law*. New York: Henry Holt.

Mann, R. J. 1999. Verification institutions in financing transactions. *Georgetown Law Journal* 87: 2225–72.

Many, C. 2000. How to be a smarter patient. *Ladies Home Journal*, March: 101.

Marconi, J. 2001. *Reputation marketing: Building and sustaining your organization's greatest asset*. Chicago: McGraw-Hill.

Marty, M. E. 1970. From providence to progress. In *Righteous empire: The Protestant experience in America*. New York: Dial Press, 188–98.

Massachusetts General Laws. 2000. Admissibility of benevolent statements, writings, or gestures relating to accident victims. Massachusetts General Laws, ch. 233, §23D. St. Paul: West Publishers.

Maurino, D., J. Reason, and R. Lee. 1995. *Beyond aviation human factors*. Aldershot, U.K.: Avery Press.

May, H. F. 1983. The decline of providence? In *Ideas, faiths, and feelings: Essays on American intellectual and religious history*, edited by H. F. May. New York: Oxford University Press.

May, L., and S. Hoffman. 1991. *Collective responsibility: Five decades of debate in theoretical and applied ethics*. Savage, Md.: Rowman and Littlefield.

May, M., and D. Stengel. 1990. Who sues their doctors? How patients handle medical grievances. *Law and Society Review* 24: 105–20.

McAdams, R. H. 1997. The origin, development, and regulation of norms. *Michigan Law Review* 96: 343–433.

McCormick, B. 1996. Liability rates: Mixed signals. *American Medical News*, 30 January.

McDonald, C. J., M. Weiner, and S. L. Hui. 2000. Deaths due to medical errors are exaggerated in Institute of Medicine report. *Journal of the American Medical Association* 284: 93–95.

McDonald, R. K. 1996. My practice almost destroyed me. *Medical Economics* 73, no. 5: 181–87.

McKinlay, J. B. 1981. From "promising report" to standard procedure: Seven stages in the career of a medical innovation. *Milbank Memorial Fund Quarterly* 59: 374–411.

Meadows, K. K. 1999. Resolving medical malpractice disputes in Massachusetts: Statutory and judicial alternatives in alternative dispute resolution. *Suffolk Journal of Trial and Appellate Advocacy* 4: 165–85.

Menkel-Meadow, C. 2001. And now, a word about secular humanism, spirituality, and the practice of justice and conflict resolution. *Fordham Urban Law Journal* 28: 1073–87.

Merry, A., and A. M. Smith. 2001. *Errors, medicine, and the law*. Cambridge: Cambridge University Press.

Metzloff, T. B. 1991. Resolving medical malpractice disputes: Imaging the jury's shadow. *Law and Contemporary Problems* 54: 43–115.

———. 1992. Alternative dispute resolution strategies in medical malpractice. *Alaska Law Review* 9: 429–55.

Michael O'Neil v. Gerard Bancker. 1827. *New York Medical and Physical Journal* 6: 145–52.

Milgrom, P., and J. Roberts. 1992. *Economics, organization, and management*. Englewood Cliffs, N.J.: Prentice-Hall.

Miller, P. 1939. *The New England mind: The seventeenth century*. Cambridge, Mass.: Harvard University Press.

————. 1953. *The New England mind: From colony to providence.* Cambridge Mass.: Harvard University Press.

Miller, R. S. 1993. An analysis and critique of the 1992 changes to New Zealand's accident compensation scheme. *Maryland Law Review* 52: 1070–92.

Mithoff, R. W., and J. L. Jordan. 2000. Proving the impossible: Patient safety and the peer review process. *Health Law News* (University of Houston) 13, no. 3 (March): 7, 14.

Mohr, J. C. 1993. *Doctors and the law: Medical jurisprudence in nineteenth-century America.* New York: Oxford University Press.

Moore, D. 1998. JCAHO urges "do tell" in sentinel event fight: Aviation's lesson—Learn from experience. *Modern Healthcare* (2 March): 60.

Moore, M. J., and W. K. Viscusi. 1989. Promoting safety through workers' compensation: The efficacy and net wage costs of injury insurance. *Rand Journal of Economics* 20, no. 4: 499–515.

Morantz-Sanchez, R. 1999. *Conduct unbecoming a woman: Medicine on trial in turn-of-the-century Brooklyn.* New York: Oxford University Press.

Morreim, E. H. 1987. Cost containment and the standard of medical care. *California Law Review* 75, no. 5: 1719–63.

————. 1991. Gaming the system: Dodging the rules, ruling the dodgers. *Archives of Internal Medicine* 151, no. 3: 443–47.

————. 2001. *Holding health care accountable: Law and the new medical marketplace.* New York: Oxford University Press.

Ness, G., and C. Cordess. 2002. Promoting patient safety in primary care: Honesty and openness may not be the best policy [letter]. *British Medical Journal* 324: 109.

Nock, S. L. 1993. *The costs of privacy: Surveillance and reputation in America.* New York: Aldine de Gruyter.

Nolan, R. E. 2001. Analysis of HHS Cost Estimates for the Final HIPAA Privacy Regulation. March 2001. Available at http://bcbshealthissues.com /relatives/17340.pdf (accessed 4 November 2002).

Novack, D. H., B. J. Detering, R. Arnold, L. Forrow, M. Ladinsky, and J. C. Pezzullo. 1989. Physicians' attitudes toward using deception to resolve difficult ethical problems. *Journal of the American Medical Association* 261: 2980–85.

Nuland, S. B. 1994. *How we die: Reflections on life's final chapter.* New York: Knopf.

Nutting, P. A. 1986. Health promotion in primary medical care: Problems and potential. *Preventive Medicine* 15: 537–48.

Office of Management and Budget. 2002. Draft report to Congress on the costs and benefits of federal regulations; Notice. *Federal Register* 67: 15014–45.

Ohio Medical Society. 1856. Report on difficulties growing out of alleged mal-practice in the treatment of fractures. *Transactions of the Ohio Medical Society* 11: 53–66.

Ordronaux, J. 1869. *The jurisprudence of medicine.* Philadelphia: T. and J. W. Johnson; reprint, New York: Arno Press, 1973.

Orentlicher, D. 2000. Medical malpractice: Treating the causes instead of the symptoms. *Medical Care* 38: 247–49.

Osterweil, N. 1999. Truth or consequences: Does disclosure reduce risk exposure? Admitting errors makes process less adversarial, MDs, lawyers agree. *WebMD Medical News*, 20 December. http://my.webmd.com/content /article/1728.53548 (accessed 9 September 2002).

Owen, D. G. 1995. *Philosophical foundations of tort law.* Oxford: Clarendon Press.

Paget, M. 1993. *A complex sorrow: Reflections on cancer and an abbreviated life.* Philadelphia: Temple University Press.

Passineau, T. 1998. Why burned-out doctors get sued more often. *Medical Economics* 75 (May): 210–18.

———. 2000. *Physician litigation stress.* Unpublished (on file with Edward A. Dauer).

Pellegrino, E. D. 1977. The expansion and contraction of "discretionary space." *Priorities for the use of resources in medicine*, 99–112. National Institutes of Health, DHEW Publication No. (NIH) 77-1288. Washington, D.C.: U.S. Government Printing Office.

———. 1979. Toward a reconstruction of medical morality: The primacy of the act of profession and the fact of illness. *Journal of Medicine and Philosophy* 4: 32–55.

———. 1982. Editorial: The ethics of collective judgments in medicine and health care. *Journal of Medicine and Philosophy* 7, no. 1: 3–10.

———. 1983. The healing relationship: Architectonics of clinical medicine. In *The clinical encounter*, edited by E. Shelp, 153–72. Dordrecht: D. Reidel.

———. 2000. Bioethics at century's turn: Can normative ethics be retrieved? *Journal of Medicine and Philosophy* 25: 655–75.

———. 2001. The internal morality of clinical medicine: A paradigm for the ethics of the helping and healing professions. *Journal of Medicine and Philosophy* 26, no. 6: 559–79.

Pellegrino, E. D., and D. C. Thomasma. 1988. *For the patient's good: The restoration of beneficence in health care.* New York: Oxford.

Percival, T. 1803. *Medical ethics, or A code of institutes and precepts adapted to the professional conduct of physicians and surgeons.* Manchester: S. Russell.

Perrow, C. 1999. *Normal accidents: Living with high-risk technologies.* 2d ed. Princeton, N.J.: Princeton University Press.

Peters, G. 1999. *Waltzing with the raptors: A practical roadmap to protecting your company's reputation*. New York: John Wiley and Sons.

Pinker, S. 2002. *The blank slate: The modern denial of human nature*. New York: Viking Press.

Plato. 1983. *The collected dialogues*. Edited by E. Hamilton and H. Cairns. Princeton, N.J.: Princeton University Press.

Postema, G. J. 2001. *Philosophy and the law of torts*. New York: Cambridge University Press.

Pound, R. 1953. *The lawyer from antiquity to modern times: With particular reference to the development of bar associations in the United States*. St. Paul, Minn.: West Publishing.

Powers, J. F. 2000. *Wheat that springeth green*. New York: New York Review Books.

Quality Interagency Coordination Task Force (QuIC). 2000. *Doing what counts for patient safety: Federal actions to reduce medical errors and their impact*. February 2000. www.quic.gov/report/toc.htm (accessed 29 September 2002).

Quill, T. E., R. M. Arnold, and F. Platt. 2001. I wish things were different: Expressing wishes in response to loss, futility, and unrealistic hopes. *Annals of Internal Medicine* 135, no. 7: 551–55.

Rabin, R. L. 1995. *Perspectives on tort law*. Boston: Little, Brown.

Rawls, J. 1993. *Political liberalism*. New York: Columbia University Press.

Reason, J. 1990. *Human error*. New York: Cambridge University Press.

———. 1998. *Managing the risks of organizational accidents*. Aldershot, U.K.: Ashgate.

———. 2000. Human error: Models and management. *British Medical Journal* 320: 768–70.

Reiser, S. J. 1994. Criteria for standard versus experimental therapy. *Health Affairs* 13, no. 3: 127–36.

Reynolds, R. A., J. A. Rizzo, and M. L. Gonzalez. 1987. The cost of medical professional liability. *Journal of the American Medical Association* 257: 2776–81.

Richards, E. P., and C. W. Walter. 1991. How effective safety devices lead to secondary litigation. *IEEE: Engineering in Medicine and Biology* 10: 66–68.

Rosenberg, C. 1962. *The cholera years: The United States in 1832, 1849, and 1866*. Chicago: University of Chicago Press.

Rosenberg, S., D. R. Allen, J. S. Handte, T. C. Jackson, L. Leto, B. M. Rodstein, S. C. Stratton, G. Westfall, and R. Yasser. 1995. Effect of utilization review in a fee-for-service health insurance plan. *New England Journal of Medicine* 333: 1326–30.

Rostow, V., M. Osterweis, and R. J. Bulger. 1989. Medical professional liability and the delivery of obstetrical care. *New England Journal of Medicine* 291: 1057–60.

Rothstein, W. G. 1972. *American physicians in the nineteenth century: From sects to science*. Baltimore: Johns Hopkins University Press.

Ruser, J. W. 1991. Workers' compensation and occupational injuries and ill-nesses. *Journal of Labor Economics* 9, no. 4: 325–50.

Sage, W. M. 1997. Enterprise liability and the emerging managed health care system. *Law and Contemporary Problems* 60, no. 2: 159–210.

———. 1999. Regulating through information: Disclosure laws and American health care. *Columbia Law Review* 99, no. 7: 1701–1829.

———. 2001. Principles, pragmatism, and medical injury. *Journal of the American Medical Association* 286: 226–28.

———. 2002. Putting the patient in patient safety. *Journal of the American Medical Association* 287, no. 22: 3003–5.

Sage, W. M., K. E. Hastings, and R. A. Berenson. 1994. Enterprise liability for medical malpractice and health care quality improvement. *American Journal of Law and Medicine* 10, nos. 1 and 2: 1–28.

Sandor, A. A. 1957. The history of professional liability suits in the United States. *Journal of the American Medical Association* 163: 459–66.

Saum, L. O. 1976. Providence in the popular mind of pre–Civil War America. *Indiana Magazine of History* 72: 341–42.

Schauffler, H. H., C. Brown, and A. Milstein. 1999. Raising the bar: The use of performance guarantees by the Pacific Business Group on Health. *Health Affairs* 18, no. 2: 134–42.

Schauffler, H. H., and T. Rodriguez. 1996. Exercising purchasing power for preventive care. *Health Affairs* 15, no. 1: 73–85.

Schroeder, S. A., and J. C. Cantor. 1991. On squeezing balloons: Cost control fails again. *New England Journal of Medicine* 325: 1099–1100.

Schultz, M, M. J. Hatch, and M. H. Larsen. 2000. *The expressive organization: Linking identity, reputation, and the corporate brand.* Oxford: Oxford University Press.

Schwartz, G. T. 1994. Reality in the economic analysis of tort law: Does tort law really deter? *UCLA Law Review* 42: 377–444.

Schwartz, W. B., and N. K. Komesar. 1978. Doctors, damages, and deterrence. *New England Journal of Medicine* 298: 1282–89.

Shakespeare, W. 1993. *Henry IV Part I. Norton Anthology of English Literature*, 6th ed., volume I. New York: W. W. Norton.

Shapiro, A. 1997. The doctor. In *The vigil.* Chicago: University of Chicago Press.

Shapiro, M. F., and N. S. Wenger. 1995. Rethinking utilization review. *New England Journal of Medicine* 333: 1353–54.

Shapiro, R. S., D. E. Simpson, S. L. Lawrence, A. M. Talsky, K. A. Sobocinski, and D. L. Schiedermayer. 1989. A survey of sued and nonsued physicians and suing patients. *Archives of Internal Medicine* 149: 2190–96.

Sharpe, V. A. 1992. Justice and care: The implications of the Kohlberg-Gilligan debate for medical ethics. *Theoretical Medicine* 13: 295–318.

————. 1999. "No tribunal other than his own conscience": Historical reflections on error and responsibility in medicine. In *Proceedings of the National Patient Safety Foundation conference on enhancing patient safety and reducing errors in health care*. Chicago: NPSF.

————. 2000a. "Behind closed doors": Accountability and responsibility in patient care. *Journal of Medicine and Philosophy* 25: 28–47.

————. 2000b. Taking responsibility for medical mistakes. In *Margin of error: The ethics of mistakes in the practice of medicine*, edited by S. B. Rubin and L. Zoloth, 183–92. Hagerstown, Md.: University Publishing Group.

————. 2003. Promoting patient safety: An ethical basis for policy deliberation. *Hastings Center Report* 33 (supplement): S1–S20.

————. 2004. Patient safety and the role of hospital boards. In *The ethics of hospital trustees*, edited by B. Jennings, V. A. Sharpe, B. H. Gray, and A. R. Fleischman. Washington, D.C.: Georgetown University Press.

Sharpe, V. A., and A. Faden. 1998. *Medical harm: Historical, conceptual, and ethical dimensions of iatrogenic illness*. Cambridge: Cambridge University Press.

Shekelle, P. G. 2002. Why don't physicians enthusiastically support quality improvement programs? *Quality and Safety in Health Care* 11: 6.

Shimmel, E. M. 1964. The hazards of hospitalization. *Annals of Internal Medicine* 60: 100–110.

Shriver, D. W. 1995. *An ethic for enemies: Forgiveness in politics*. New York and Oxford: Oxford University Press.

Simanowitz, A. 1993. Accountability. In *Medical accidents*, edited by C. Vincent et al. Oxford: Oxford University Press.

Simon, Y. 1986. *The definition of moral virtue*. New York: Fordham University Press.

Simpson, J. B., comp. 1988. *Simpson's contemporary quotations*. Boston: Houghton Mifflin. www.bartleby.com/63/ (accessed 29 September 2002).

Sloan, F. A., S. S. Entman, B. A. Reilly, C. A. Glass, G. B. Hickson, and H. H. Zhang. 1997. Tort liability and obstetricians' care levels. *International Review of Law and Economics* 17, no. 2: 245–60.

Sloan, F. A., P. B. Githens, E. W. Clayton, G. B. Hickson, D. A. Gentile, and D. F. Partlett. 1993. *Suing for medical malpractice*. Chicago: University of Chicago Press.

Sloan, F. A., and C. R. Hsieh. 1990. Variability in medical malpractice payments: Is the compensation fair? *Law and Society Review* 24, no. 4: 997–1039.

Sloan, F. A., K. Whetten-Goldstein, E. M. Stout, S. S. Entman, and G. B. Hickson. 1998. No-fault system of compensation for obstetric injury: Winners and losers. *Obstetrics and Gynecology* 60, nos. 1–2: 35–70.

Smith, R. 2002. The discomfort of patient power: Medical authorities will have to learn to live with "irrational" decisions by the public. *British Medical Journal* 324: 497–98.

Snook, S. A. 2000. *Friendly fire: The accidental shootdown of U.S. Black Hawks over northern Iraq.* Princeton: Princeton University Press.

Sokol, D. J. 1985. The current status of medical malpractice countersuits. *American Journal of Law and Medicine* 10: 439–57.

Soloski, J., and R. P. Bezanson. 1992. *Reforming libel law.* New York: The Guilford Press.

Soper, N. J., P. T. Stockmann, D. L. Dunnegan, and W. E. Ashley. 1992. Laparoscopic cholecystectomy: The new "gold" standard. *Archives of Surgery* 127: 917–23.

Soumerai, S. B., T. J. McLaughlin, D. Ross-Degnan, C. S. Caswteris, and P. Bollini. 1994. Effects of limiting Medicaid drug-reimbursement benefits on the use of psychotropic agents and acute mental health services by patients with schizophrenia. *New England Journal of Medicine* 331: 650–55.

Soumerai, S. B., D. Ross-Degnan, J. Avorn, T. J. McLaughlin, and I. Choodnovskiy. 1991. Effects of Medicaid drug-payment limits on admission to hospitals and nursing homes. *New England Journal of Medicine* 325: 1072–77.

Soumerai, S. B., D. Ross-Degnan, E. E. Fortess, and J. Abelson. 1993. A critical analysis of studies of state drug reimbursement policies: Research in need of discipline. *Milbank Quarterly* 7, no. 2: 217–52.

Spieler, E. 1994. Perpetuating risk? Workers' compensation and the persistence of occupational injuries. *Houston Law Review* 31: 119–264.

Starr, P. 1982. *The social transformation of American medicine.* New York: Basic Books.

State of Pennsylvania. 2002. Pennsylvania Medical Care Availability and Reduction of Error Act (MCARE Act), March 2002. www.legis.state.pa.us /WU01/LI/BI/BT/2001/0/HB1802P3420.HTM (accessed 29 September 2002).

Steiner, C. A., E. B. Bass, M. A. Talmini, H. A. Pitt, and E. P. Steinberg. 1994. Surgical rates and operative mortality for open and laparoscopic cholecystectomy in Maryland. *New England Journal of Medicine* 330: 403–8.

Steinhauer, J., and F. Fessenden. 2001. Medical retreads: Punished by state but prized at the hospitals. *New York Times,* 27 March: A1.

Stolberg, S. G. 1999. Breaking down "culture of silence" in medicine. *Memphis Commercial Appeal,* 12 December: B-1, B-6.

Streja, D. A., R. L. Hui, E. Streja, and J. S. McCombs. 1999. Selective contracting and patient outcomes: A case study of formulary restrictions for selective serotonin reuptake inhibitor antidepressants. *American Journal of Managed Care* 5: 1133–42.

Studdert, D. M., and T. A. Brennan. 2000. The problem of punitive damages in lawsuits against managed-care organizations. *New England Journal of Medicine* 342: 280–84.

———. 2001a. No-fault compensation for medical injuries: The prospect for error-prevention. *Journal of the American Medical Association* 286: 217–23.

———. 2001b. Toward a workable model of "no-fault" compensation for medical injury in the United States. *American Journal of Law and Medicine* 27: 225–52.

Studdert, D. M., T. A. Brennan, and E. J. Thomas. 2000. Beyond dead reckoning: Measures of medical injury burden, malpractice litigation, and alternative compensation models from Utah and Colorado. *Indiana Law Review* 33: 1643–86.

Studdert, D. M., L. Fritz, and T. A. Brennan. 2000. The jury is still in: Florida's Birth-Related Neurological Injury Compensation Association after a decade. *Journal of Health Politics, Policy, and Law* 25, no. 3: 499–526.

Studdert, D. M., E. J. Thomas, H. R. Burstin, B. I. Zbar, E. J. Orav, and T. A. Brennan. 2000. Negligent care and malpractice claiming behavior in Utah and Colorado. *Medical Care* 38, no. 3: 250–60.

Studdert, D. M., E. J. Thomas, B. I. Zbar, J. P. Newhouse, P. C. Weiler, and T. A. Brennan. 1997. Can the United States afford a no-fault system of compensation for medical injury? *Law and Contemporary Problems* 60: 1–34.

Sulmasy, D. P. 1993. What's so special about medicine? *Theoretical Medicine* 14, no. 1: 27–42.

Sunnybrook and Women's College Health Sciences Centre. 2001. Policy statement on disclosure of adverse medical events and unanticipated outcomes of care. In *Sunnybrook and Women's College Health Sciences Centre administrative manual.* www.utoronto.ca/jcb/sunnybrook.html (accessed 16 January 2004).

Sweet, M. P., and J. L. Bernat. 1997. A study of the ethical duty of physicians to disclose errors. *Journal of Clinical Ethics*, no. 4 (winter): 341–48.

Syverud, K. D. 1990. The duty to settle. *Virginia Law Review* 76: 1113–1209.

Tadelis, S. 2002. The market for reputations as an incentive mechanism. *Journal of Political Economy* 110: 854–82.

Terry, K. 1998. Look who's rating doctors on clinical quality—patients. *Medical Economics* 75, no. 7: 50–51.

Texas Civil Practice and Remedies Code. 2000. Communication of sympathy. Texas Civil Practice and Remedies Code, §18.061. St. Paul: West Publishing.

Thacker, S. B. 1989. The impact of technology assessment and medical malpractice on the diffusion of medical technologies: The case of electronic fetal monitoring. In *Medical professional liability and the delivery of obstetric care*, vol. 2., edited by V. P. Roston and R. J. Bulger, 9–26. Washington D.C.: National Academy Press.

Thomas, E. J., D. M. Studdert, and T. A. Brennan. 2002. The reliability of medical record review for estimating adverse event rates. *Annals of Internal Medicine* 136: 812–15.

Thomas, E. J., D. M. Studdert, J. P. Newhouse, B. I. Zbar, K. M. Howard, E. J. Williams, and T. A. Brennan. 1999. Costs of medical injuries in Colorado and Utah in 1992. *Inquiry* 36: 255–64.

Thomas, K. 1971. *Religion and the decline of magic: Studies in popular beliefs in the sixteenth and seventeenth centuries in England.* London: Wiedenfeld.

Tilton, E. M. 1940. Lightning rods and the earthquake of 1775. *New England Quarterly* 13: 85–97.

Tong, R. 1998. The ethics of care: A feminist virtue ethics of care for healthcare practitioners. *Journal of Medicine and Philosophy* 23, no. 2: 131–52.

Trauner, J. B., and J. S. Chesnutt. 1996. Medical groups in California: Managing care under capitation. *Health Affairs* 15, no. 1: 159–70.

U.S. Department of Health, Education, and Welfare. 1973. *Report of the Secretary's Commission on Medical Malpractice.* Washington, D.C.: U.S. Government Printing Office.

Veatch, R. M. 1998. The place of care in ethical theory. *Journal of Medicine and Philosophy* 23, no. 2: 210–24.

Vidmar, N. 1995. *Medical malpractice and the American jury: Confronting the myths about jury incompetence, deep pockets, and outrageous damage awards.* Ann Arbor: University of Michigan Press.

Vincent, C., S. Taylor-Adams, E. J. Chapman, D. Hewett, S. Prior, P. Strange, and A. Tizzard. 2000. How to investigate and analyse clinical incidents: Clinical risk unit and association of litigation and risk management protocol. *British Medical Journal* 320: 777–81.

Vincent, C., M. Young, and A. Phillips. 1994. Why do people sue doctors? A study of patients and relatives taking legal action. *Lancet* 343: 1609–13.

Voelker, R. 1996. "Treat systems, not errors," experts say. *Journal of the American Medical Association* 276: 1537–38.

Waddams, S. M. 2000. *Sexual slander in nineteenth-century England: Defamation in the ecclesiastical courts, 1815–1855.* Toronto: University of Toronto Press.

Walker, W. J. 1848. On the treatment of compound and complicated fractures. *Medical Communications of the Massachusetts Medical Society* 7: 171–215.

Walsh, K., and M. Dineen. 1998. *Clinical risk management in the NHS: Making a difference?* Birmingham, U.K.: NHS Confederation.

Walters, R. G. 1978. *American reformers, 1815–1860.* New York: Hill and Wang.

Wasserstrom, R. A. 1961. Strict liability in the criminal law. In *Freedom and responsibility*, edited by H. Morris, 273–81. Stanford: Stanford University Press.

Weiler, P. 1991. *Medical malpractice on trial.* Cambridge, Mass.: Harvard University Press.

Weiler, P. C., H. H. Hiatt, and J. P. Newhouse. 1993. *A measure of malpractice: Medical injury, malpractice litigation, and patient compensation.* Cambridge, Mass.: Harvard University Press.

Weiler, P. C., J. P. Newhouse, and H. H. Hiatt. 1992. Proposal for medical liability reform. *Journal of the American Medical Association* 267: 2355–58.

Weinstein, J. 1967. Big business and the origins of workmen's compensation. *Labor History* 8: 156–74.

Weinstein, M. M. 1998. Checking medicine's vital signs. *New York Times Magazine,* 19 April: 36.

Wennberg, J. E. 1999. Understanding geographic variations in health care delivery. *New England Journal of Medicine* 340, no. 1: 52–53.

Werblowsky, R. J. Z., and G. Wigoder, eds. 1997. *The Oxford dictionary of the Jewish religion.* New York and Oxford: Oxford University Press.

Wexler, D., and B. Winick. 1996. *Law in a therapeutic key.* Durham, N.C.: Carolina Academic Press.

White, C., and L. Boucke. 2001. *The undutchables: An observation of the Netherlands, its culture, and its inhabitants.* Lafayette, Colo.: White-Boucke Publishing.

White, G. 1980. *Tort law in America.* New York: Oxford University Press.

Whitman, J. Q. 1998. What is wrong with inflicting shame sanctions? *Yale Law Journal* 107: 1055–92.

Williams, P. C. 1984. Abandoning medical malpractice. *The Journal of Legal Medicine* 5: 549–94.

Winthrop, J. 1908. *Winthrop's journal: History of New England, 1630–1649,* 2 vols., edited by J. K. Hosmer. New York: Charles Scribner's Sons.

Witman, A. B., D. M. Park, and S. B. Hardin. 1996. How do patients want physicians to handle mistakes? A survey of internal medicine patients in an academic setting. *Archives of Internal Medicine* 156, no. 22: 2565–69.

Wu, A. W. 1999. Handling hospital errors: Is disclosure the best defense? *Annals of Internal Medicine* 131, no. 12: 970–72.

———. 2001. A major medical error [commentary]. *American Family Physician* 63: 985–88.

Wu, A. W., T. A. Cavanaugh, S. J. McPhee, B. Lo, G. P. Micco. 1997. To tell the truth: Ethical and practical issues in disclosing medical mistakes to patients. *Journal of General Internal Medicine* 12, no. 12: 770–75.

Wu, A. W., S. Folkman, S. J. McPhee, and B. Lo. 1991. Do house officers learn from their mistakes? *Journal of the American Medical Association* 265: 2089–94.

———. 1993. How house officers cope with their mistakes. *Western Journal of Medicine* 159: 565–69.

Wu, A. W., P. Pronovost, and L. Morlock. 2002. ICU incident reporting systems. *Journal of Critical Care* 17: 86–94.

Yardley, M. J. 1984. Malicious prosecution: A physician's need for reassessment. *Chicago-Kent Law Review* 60: 317–48.

Zalta, E. 1991. Utilization review works—most of the time. *Medical Economics* 68, no. 13: 23–27.

Zuckerman, S. 1984. Medical malpractice: Claims, legal costs, and the practice of defensive medicine. *Health Affairs* 3: 128–33.

CONTRIBUTORS

CAROL BAYLEY, Ph.D. Vice President for Ethics and Justice Education, Catholic Healthcare West, San Francisco, California.

NANCY BERLINGER, Ph.D., M.Div. Deputy Director, The Hastings Center, Garrison, New York.

EDWARD A. DAUER, LL.B., M.P.H. Dean Emeritus and Professor of Law, University of Denver College of Law, Denver, Colorado.

KENNETH DE VILLE, Ph.D., J.D. Administrative Director, University and Medical Center Institutional Review Board, and Professor, Department of Medical Humanities, Brody School of Medicine, East Carolina University, Greenville, North Carolina.

SANDRA M. GILBERT, Ph.D. Distinguished Professor of English, University of California, Davis.

ROXANNE GOELTZ is an air traffic controller and a patient safety advocate in Minneapolis, Minnesota. She is cochair of the Partnership for Patient Safety (p4ps) advisory board and consumer spokesperson for the National Patient Safety Foundation's (NPSF) Stand Up for Patient Safety Campaign.

CAROL LEVINE, Director, Families and Health Care Project, United Hospital Fund of New York.

BRYAN A. LIANG, M.D., Ph.D., J.D. Professor and Director, Institute of Health Law Studies, California Western School of Law, San Diego, California.

E. HAAVI MORREIM, Ph.D. Professor, College of Medicine, University of Tennessee, Memphis, Tennessee.

EDMUND D. PELLEGRINO, M.D. Professor Emeritus of Medicine and Medical Ethics, Center for Clinical Bioethics, Georgetown University Medical Center, Washington, D.C.

WILLIAM M. SAGE, M.D., J.D. Professor, Columbia Law School, New York.

VIRGINIA A. SHARPE, Ph.D. Visiting Scholar, Center for Clinical Bioethics, Georgetown University Medical Center, Washington, D.C.

DAVID M. STUDDERT, LL.B, Sc.D., M.P.H. Associate Professor for Law and Public Health, Department of Health Policy and Management, Harvard School of Public Health, Boston, Massachusetts.

ALBERT W. WU, M.D., M.P.H. Associate Professor, Health Policy and Management, Bloomberg School of Public Health, Johns Hopkins University, Baltimore, Maryland.

INDEX